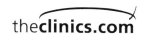

INFECTIOUS DISEASE CLINICS OF NORTH AMERICA

Fungal Infections

GUEST EDITOR
Thomas F. Patterson, MD

CONSULTING EDITOR
Robert C. Moellering, Jr, MD

September 2006 • Volume 20 • Number 3

SAUNDERS

An Imprint of Elsevier, Inc.
PHILADELPHIA   LONDON   TORONTO   MONTREAL   SYDNEY   TOKYO

W.B. SAUNDERS COMPANY
A Division of Elsevier Inc.

Elsevier, Inc., 1600 John F. Kennedy Blvd., Suite 1800, Philadelphia, PA 19103-2899.

http://www.theclinics.com

**INFECTIOUS DISEASE CLINICS
OF NORTH AMERICA**
September 2006
Editor: Karen Sorensen

Volume 20, Number 3
ISSN 0891–5520
ISBN 1-4160-3866-3

The ideas and opinions expressed in *Infectious Disease Clinics of North America* do not necessarily reflect those of the Publisher. The Publisher does not assume any responsibility for any injury and/or damage to persons or property arising out of or related to any use of the material contained in this periodical. The reader is advised to check the appropriate medical literature and the product information currently provided by the manufacturer of each drug to be administered to verify the dosage, the method and duration of administration, or contraindications. It is the responsibility of the treating physician or other health care professional, relying on independent experience and knowledge of the patient, to determine drug dosages and the best treatment for the patient. Mention of any product in this issue should not be construed as endorsement by the contributors, editors, or the Publisher of the product or manufacturers' claims.

Infectious Disease Clinics of North America (ISSN 0891–5520) is published in March, June, September, and December (For Post Office use only: volume 20 issue 3 of 4) by Elsevier Inc., 360 Park Avenue South, New York, NY 10010-1710. Business and Editorial Offices: 1600 John F. Kennedy Blvd., Suite 1800, Philadelphia, PA 19103-2899. Customer Service Office: 6277 Sea Harbor Drive, Orlando, FL 32887-4800. Periodicals postage paid at New York, NY and additional mailing offices. Subscription prices are $170.00 per year for US individuals, $285.00 per year for US institutions, $85.00 per year for US students, $200.00 per year for Canadian individuals, $345.00 per year for Canadian institutions, $225.00 per year for international individuals, $345.00 per year for international institutions, and $110.00 per year for Canadian and foreign students. To receive student rate, orders must be accompanied by name of affiliated institution, date of term, and the *signature* of program/residency coordinator on institution letterhead. Orders will be billed at individual rate until proof of status is received. Foreign air speed delivery is included in all *Clinics* subscription prices. All prices are subject to change without notice. **POSTMASTER**: Send address changes to *Infectious Disease Clinics of North America*, Elsevier Periodicals Customer Service, 6277 Sea Harbor Drive, Orlando, FL 32887-4800. **Customer Service: 1-800-654-2452 (US). From outside of the US, call 1-407-345-4000. E-mail: hhspcs@wbsaunders.com**.

Infectious Disease Clinics of North America is also published in Spanish by Editorial Inter-Médica, Junin 917, 1er A 1113, Buenos Aires, Argentina.

Reprints. For copies of 100 or more, of articles in this publication, please contact the Commercial Reprints Department, Elsevier Inc., 360 Park Avenue South, New York, New York 10010-1710. Tel. (212) 633-3813, Fax: (212) 462-1935, email: reprints@elsevier.com.

Infectious Disease Clinics of North America is covered in *Index Medicus, Current Contents/Clinical Medicine, Science Citation Alert, SCISEARCH,* and *Research Alert.*

Printed in the United States of America.

CONSULTING EDITOR

ROBERT C. MOELLERING, Jr, MD, Shields Warren-Mallinckrodt Professor of Medical Research, Harvard Medical School; Department of Medicine, Beth Israel Deaconess Medical Center, Boston, Massachusetts

GUEST EDITOR

THOMAS F. PATTERSON, MD, FACP, The University of Texas Health Science Center at San Antonio; Professor of Medicine and Director, San Antonio Center for Medical Mycology, San Antonio, Texas

CONTRIBUTORS

ELIAS ANAISSIE, MD, Professor of Medicine and Director of Clinical Affairs, Division of Supportive Care, Myeloma Institute for Research and Therapy, University of Arkansas for Medical Sciences, Little Rock, Arkansas

DAVID ANDES, MD, Department of Medicine, Infectious Diseases Section; Department of Medical Microbiology and Immunology, University of Wisconsin, Madison, Wisconsin

GREGORY M. ANSTEAD, MD, PhD, Assistant Professor, Department of Medicine, Division of Infectious Diseases, The University of Texas Health Science Center at San Antonio; Staff Physician, Research Service, South Texas Veterans Healthcare System, San Antonio, Texas

PENELOPE D. BARNES, MBBS, PhD, Research Associate, Program in Infectious Diseases, Fred Hutchinson Cancer Research Center; Acting Instructor, University of Washington, Seattle, Washington

METHEE CHAYAKULKEEREE, MD, Assistant Professor, Department of Medicine, Division of Infectious Diseases and International Health, Duke University Medical Center, Durham, North Carolina; Division of Infectious Diseases and Tropical Medicine, Department of Medicine, Faculty of Medicine, Siriraj Hospital, Mahidol University, Bangkok, Thailand

ANNETTE W. FOTHERGILL, MA, MBA, MT(ASCP), CLS(NCA), Assistant Professor, Department of Pathology, The University of Texas Health Science Center at San Antonio; Technical Director, Fungus Testing Laboratory, San Antonio, Texas

JOHN R. GRAYBILL, MD, Professor, Department of Medicine, Division of Infectious Diseases, The University of Texas Health Science Center at San Antonio, San Antonio, Texas

CAROL A. KAUFFMAN, MD, Professor of Internal Medicine, University of Michigan Medical School; Chief, Infectious Diseases Section, Veterans Affairs Ann Arbor Healthcare System, Ann Arbor, Michigan

DIMITRIOS P. KONTOYIANNIS, MD, ScD, FIDSA, Department of Infectious Diseases, Infection Control and Employee Health, The University of Texas M. D. Anderson Cancer Center, Houston, Texas

RUSSELL E. LEWIS, PharmD, FCCP, Department of Clinical Sciences and Administration, University of Houston College of Pharmacy, Houston, Texas

KIEREN A. MARR, MD, Associate Member, Program in Infectious Diseases, Fred Hutchinson Cancer Research Center; Associate Professor of Medicine, University of Washington, Seattle, Washington

MONIQUE A.S.H. MENNINK-KERSTEN, PhD, Department of Medical Microbiology, Radboud University Nijmegen Medical Center; Nijmegen University Center for Infectious Diseases, Nijmegen, The Netherlands

MARCIO NUCCI, MD, Associate Professor, Hematology Service, Department of Internal Medicine, University Hospital, Universidade Federal do Rio de Janeiro, Rio de Janeiro, Brazil

PETER G. PAPPAS, MD, Professor, Division of Infectious Diseases, Department of Medicine, University of Alabama at Birmingham, Birmingham, Alabama

JOHN R. PERFECT, MD, Professor, Departments of Medicine and Microbiology and Molecular Genetics, Division of Infectious Diseases and International Health, Duke University Medical Center, Durham, North Carolina

SANJAY G. REVANKAR, MD, Associate Professor of Medicine, Division of Infectious Diseases, Harper University Hospital, Wayne State University, Detroit, Michigan

MICHAEL G. RINALDI, PhD, Director, Fungus Testing Laboratory; Professor of Pathology, Microbiology, and Medicine, The University of Texas Health Science Center at San Antonio; Director of Clinical Microbiology, Audie L. Murphy Veterans Administration Health System; Director, Veterans Administration Mycology Reference Laboratory, San Antonio, Texas

WILLIAM J. STEINBACH, MD, Assistant Professor of Pediatrics, Molecular Genetics, and Microbiology; Department of Pediatrics, Division of Pediatric Infectious Diseases; Department of Molecular Genetics and Microbiology, Duke University Medical Center, Durham, North Carolina

DEANNA A. SUTTON, PhD, MT, SM(ASCP), SM, RM(NRM), Assistant Professor, Department of Pathology, The University of Texas Health Science Center at San Antonio; Administrative Director, Fungus Testing Laboratory, San Antonio, Texas

PAUL E. VERWEIJ, MD, PhD, Department of Medical Microbiology, Radboud University Nijmegen Medical Center; Nijmegen University Center for Infectious Diseases, Nijmegen, The Netherlands

THOMAS J. WALSH, MD, Senior Investigator, Immunocompromised Host Section, Pediatric Oncology Branch, National Cancer Institute, Bethesda, Maryland

CONTENTS

Invasive candidiasis (IC) remains an important nosocomial infection. Changes in its epidemiology have occurred for many reasons, including the extensive use of prophylactic antifungal agents, broad-spectrum antibacterial agents, and medical devices. The diagnosis of IC remains elusive in many patients, and there is a critical need for improved diagnostics that will provide clinicians the opportunity to intervene earlier in the course of disease. Newer antifungal agents offer promise in the treatment of candidemia and other forms of IC. Despite an overwhelming amount of data concerning risk factors and excess mortality associated with the development of IC, there is no consistent approach to treatment and primary prevention among individuals who are deemed to be at the highest risk for this complication.

In the past 2 decades, *Cryptococcus* has emerged in its clinical significance and as a model yeast for understanding molecular pathogenesis. *C neoformans* and *C gattii* are currently considered major primary and secondary pathogens in a wide array of hosts that are known to be immunocompromised or apparently immunocompetent. A recent outbreak of *C gattii* infections further underscores the clinical importance of the yeast through its epidemiology and pathogenicity features. With an enlarging immunosuppressed population caused by HIV infection, solid organ transplantation, and clinical use of potent immunosuppressives, such as cancer chemotherapy, monoclonal antibodies, and corticosteroids, this fungus has become a well-established infectious complication of modern medicine. This article examines current issues in cryptococcal infections, including new classification, epidemiology, pathogenesis, and specific clinical aspects.

Aspergillosis: Spectrum of Disease, Diagnosis, and Treatment

Penelope D. Barnes and Kieren A. Marr

Infections by *Aspergillus* species present a particular challenge. The organism, which is ubiquitous in the environment, causes allergic disease in otherwise healthy individuals and devastating disease in the immunosuppressed. This article examines the range of infections caused by *Aspergillus* species, the challenges of diagnosis, and current treatment options.

Emerging Fungi

Marcio Nucci and Elias Anaissie

The epidemiology of invasive fungal infections is evolving. Molds other than *Aspergillus* have emerged as significant pathogens in severely immunosuppressed patients. In most cases, the emergence of these infections seems to be a consequence of changes in the host accompanying more severe immunosuppression. The hyalohyphomycetes (molds that present in tissue as hyaline septate fungi) are a group of such emerging fungi. This article reviews the clinical spectrum, diagnosis, and management of infection caused by these pathogens, with a special emphasis on infection caused by *Fusarium* species.

Invasive Zygomycosis: Update on Pathogenesis, Clinical Manifestations, and Management

Dimitrios P. Kontoyiannis and Russell E. Lewis

Zygomycosis is an increasingly common infection in immunocompromised patients. Advances in the understanding of Zygomycetes pathobiology and the introduction of new drugs with improved activity and tolerability for treatment of zygomycosis have improved the prospects of effectively controlling this devastating infection. Further reductions in mortality will require improved diagnostic and novel therapeutic approaches for this group of aggressive opportunistic molds.

Phaeohyphomycosis

Sanjay G. Revankar

Phaeohyphomycosis is a term for infections caused by dematiaceous fungi that encompasses many clinical syndromes, from local infections caused by trauma to widely disseminated infection in immunocompromised patients. These fungi are unique owing to the presence of melanin in their cell walls, which imparts the characteristic dark color to their spores and hyphae. Melanin may also be a virulence factor in these fungi. Therapy depends on the clinical syndrome. Local infection may be cured with excision alone, whereas systemic disease is often refractory to therapy. Azoles such as itraconazole and voriconazole have the most consistent in vitro activity, although there is more clinical experience with itraconazole. Further studies are needed to better understand the pathogenesis and treatment of these uncommon infections.

Coccidioidomycosis is an infection caused by dimorphic fungi of the genus *Coccidioides*, soil-dwelling fungi endemic in semiarid to arid life zones in the southwestern United States, northern Mexico, and scattered areas of Latin America. This article discusses populations at particular risk, diagnosis, clinical presentation, outcomes, and treatment of this potentially horrific disease.

The endemic mycoses are a diverse group of fungi that share several characteristics. They are able to cause disease in healthy hosts, they each occupy a specific ecologic niche in the environment, and they exhibit temperature dimorphism, existing as molds in the environment at temperatures of 25°C to 30°C, and as yeasts, or spherules in the case of coccidioidomycosis, at body temperatures. This article discusses histoplasmosis and blastomycosis. Sporotrichosis, which differs in that it is usually a localized lymphocutaneous infection, is included because it shares the characteristics of endemic mycoses.

This article provides a brief overview of some of the unique differences in invasive fungal infections in children compared with those of adults and then focuses on the key differences in antifungal pharmacology and use in children. The specific pathogens are covered in greater detail elsewhere in this issue.

Application of pharmacodynamic principles to antifungal drug therapy of *Candida* and *Aspergillus* infections has provided an understanding of the relationship between drug dosing and treatment efficacy. Observations of the pharmacodynamics of triazoles and amphotericin B have correlated with the results of clinical trials and have proven useful for validation of in vitro susceptibility breakpoints. Although there remain many unanswered questions regarding antifungal pharmacodynamics, available data suggest usefulness in the application of pharmacodynamics to antifungal clinical development. Future application of these principles should aid in the design of optimal combination antifungal therapies.

Antifungal susceptibility testing has been a recognized tool for more than 15 years. Despite this tenure, interpretation of the results and determining how best to use these results continues to be controversial. Although initially laboratories hesitated to initiate antifungal susceptibility testing into their workflow, advances by industry have made this testing more attractive to even smaller institutions. As a result, much information has been generated regarding susceptibility patterns between specific species and specific antifungal agents. By understanding the available testing methods and by using the susceptibility patterns, physicians are better equipped to use the results provided by the laboratory to make treatment decisions.

The value of the diagnostic markers galactomannan and 1,3-β-D-glucan for the diagnosis of opportunistic fungal infections is reviewed in this article. Both markers have undergone clinical evaluation, and increasing insight is emerging with respect to the causes of false-negative or false-positive reactivity. These data will help design protocols in which single or multiple markers are used to identify patients who require antifungal therapy.

FORTHCOMING ISSUES

RECENT ISSUES

ELSEVIER
SAUNDERS

Infect Dis Clin N Am
20 (2006) xi–xii

INFECTIOUS
DISEASE CLINICS
OF NORTH AMERICA

Preface

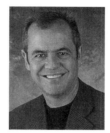

Thomas F. Patterson, MD
Guest Editor

Since the last comprehensive issues of the *Infectious Disease Clinics of North America* dedicated to medical mycology, edited by Drs. Walsh and Rex in 2002, this field has continued to see major advances in new therapies, diagnostic tools, and strategies for treatment and prevention. Despite these encouraging developments, large numbers of patients are at risk for infectious diseases, and the epidemiology of invasive mycoses continues to emerge. The diagnosis of these infections remains difficult, and treatment outcomes in highly immunosuppressed patients remain poor. Thus, this issue is devoted to state-of-the-art updates on fungal infections by internationally recognized authorities in this field.

The initial articles, by Drs. Pappas and Chayakulkeeree and by Dr. Perfect, address recent advances in invasive candidiasis and in cryptococcosis, respectively. Invasive candidiasis is the most common nosocomial infection worldwide and has been the focus of outstanding clinical and basic research efforts to improve outcomes in this ubiquitous pathogen. Cryptococcosis remains an important cause of meningitis worldwide.

Infections due to molds, including aspergillosis, reviewed by Drs. Barnes and Marr, have emerged as major causes of morbidity and mortality in immunosuppressed patients. Other previously rare molds, like *Fusarium*, with distinct epidemiological features and management strategies, are discussed by Drs. Nucci and Anaissie. Drs. Kontoyiannis and Lewis review the importance of Zygomycetes, which have been particularly recognized as emerging pathogens in recent years, and infections due to darkly pigmented fungi—the phaeohyphomycoses—are addressed by Dr. Revankar.

0891-5520/06/$ - see front matter © 2006 Elsevier Inc. All rights reserved.
doi:10.1016/j.idc.2006.07.003   *id.theclinics.com*

Infections due to endemic fungi, coccidioidomycosis, and other endemic organisms, remain important pathogens in specific geographic regions and can now be managed with a variety of treatment options, which are discussed by Drs. Anstead and Graybill and by Dr. Kauffman, respectively.

The epidemiology, presentation, and management of mycoses in pediatric populations can be distinct, as outlined by Drs. Steinbach and Walsh. Dr. Andes reviews important pharmacokinetic and pharmacodynamic properties of the growing antifungal armamentarium. Finally, the role of the laboratory is discussed, in terms of susceptibility testing by Ms. Fothergill and Drs. Rinaldi and Sutton and the use of non-culture-based assays by Drs. Mennink-Kersten and Verweij.

We hope this volume will provide a timely, comprehensive, and practical guide for the diagnosis and management of invasive mycoses.

Thomas F. Patterson, MD
The University of Texas Health Science Center
7703 Floyd Curl Drive—MSC 7881
San Antonio, TX 78229-3900, USA

E-mail address: patterson@uthscsa.edu

ELSEVIER
SAUNDERS

Infect Dis Clin N Am
20 (2006) 485–506

INFECTIOUS
DISEASE CLINICS
OF NORTH AMERICA

Invasive Candidiasis

Peter G. Pappas, MD

*Division of Infectious Diseases, Department of Medicine, University of Alabama
at Birmingham, 1530 3rd Avenue South, THT 229, Birmingham, AL 35294-0006, USA*

The term "invasive candidiasis" (IC) encompasses a wide variety of severe and invasive disorders that include candidemia, disseminated candidiasis, endocarditis, meningitis, endophthalmitis, and other deep organ involvement; it excludes more superficial and less severe diseases, such as oropharyngeal and esophageal candidiasis. IC is a problem of increasing relevance in the modern health care setting, and is particularly prevalent in ICUs [1–12]. A direct result of the tremendous advances in health care technology over the last several decades, IC is largely a disease of medical progress. Among the most important of these advances include the use of broad-spectrum antimicrobials; the use of chronic, indwelling, and central venous catheters; the use of acute hemodialysis in the intensive care setting; the extensive use of chronic immunosuppressive agents, including glucocorticosteroids and other immunomodulators; the use of other internal prosthetic devices; and aggressive chemotherapy for a variety of neoplastic conditions [1–19]. Not surprisingly, IC generally is more common in tertiary medical centers with highly specialized clinical care and access to many of these interventions.

As the fourth most common cause of nosocomial bloodstream infection in the United States, IC is the most common invasive mycosis in the developed world [1–12,20–28]. As such, IC has a significant impact on patient outcomes and on the health care economy. It has been estimated that the attributable mortality of IC is as high as 47% [29–31], although most authorities estimate the attributable mortality to be between 15% and 25% for adults and approximately 10% to 15% for neonates and children [5,7,11,32,33]. Economically, the costs of IC are staggering; it has been estimated that each episode of IC in adults costs approximately $40,000 [5,11,18,34].

E-mail address: pappas@uab.edu

doi:10.1016/j.idc.2006.07.004

The pathogen

Candida exists predominantly as unicellular yeasts with small (4–6 μm), thin-walled ovoid cells that reproduce by budding. Fresh preparations often show budding yeast, hyphae, and pseudohyphae. These organisms grow well on most artificial media and generally do not require special conditions for growth. On artificial media, *Candida* are identifiable as smooth, creamy white colonies. There are more than 150 species of *Candida*, but only about 15 are recognized as frequent human pathogens, including *C albicans*, *C glabrata*, *C tropicalis*, *C parapsilosis*, *C krusei*, *C guilliermondii*, *C lusitaniae*, *C dubliniensis*, *C pelliculosa*, *C kefyr*, *C lipolytica*, *C famata*, *C inconspicua*, *C rugosa*, and *C norvegenis* [35–40]. Among these, *C albicans* is by far the most common species isolated from humans, and is a frequent denizen of the oropharynx, the skin, and mucous membranes, and the lower respiratory, gastrointestinal, and genitourinary tracts. Identification of these organisms to the species level is critically important, not only because of issues related to antifungal susceptibility, but also because of differences in virulence potential among the different species of *Candida* [7,10,41–45].

Pathogenesis

There are three major components to the pathogenesis of IC including, (1) increased fungal burden or colonization, typically resulting from the use of broad spectrum antimicrobial agents; (2) breakdown of normal mucosal and skin barriers as a result of the use of chronic indwelling intravascular devices, recent surgery or trauma, and severe mucositis associated with cytotoxic chemotherapy and radiation; and (3) immune dysfunction (eg, neutropenia) that leads to dissemination and proliferation in deep tissues [46–49].

Candida adheres to vaginal, gastrointestinal, and oral epithelial cells, fibronectin, platelet fibrin clots, acrylic material, endothelium, lymphocytes, and plastic material. The importance of biofilm in the development and propagation of IC is an area of intense investigation. When compared with planktonic (free-living) organisms, *Candida* spp that live within the biofilm matrix of an intravascular catheter or other prosthetic device develop several unique phenotypic and genotypic characteristics, including resistance to a variety of antifungal agents [50,51].

All arms of the immune system are involved in the control of candidal infections. Lymphocytes are crucial in the development of cell-mediated immunity to *Candida* spp and in the prevention of mucosal candidiasis. Patients who have a global T-cell deficient-state (eg, advanced HIV disease) or a more specific T-cell defect (eg, as seen among patients who have chronic mucocutaneous candidiasis) have a strong propensity to develop recurrent/persistent mucocutaneous candidiasis, but rarely invasive disease [52,53].

Monocytes and polymorphonuclear cells damage and kill pseudohyphae and blastospores [54]. In contrast to patients who have cell-mediated immune dysfunction, patients who have conditions that are associated with neutropenia or significant neutrophil dysfunction have a strong propensity toward the development of IC and candidemia. Complement and immunoglobulins are necessary for efficient opsonization and intracellular killing of the organism, and deficiency of either of these components can be associated with more complicated or refractory disease [55]. Despite these important considerations of host immune function, iatrogenic factors are, by far, the most influential in the pathogenesis of IC.

Epidemiology

Recent surveys indicate that *Candida* spp are the fourth most common nosocomial bloodstream isolates in the United States; there are similar trends in other parts of the developed world [1–12,20–28]. A little more than half of all cases occur in the context of ICU care, and virtually all patients who have IC have one or more identifiable risk factors. The most common of these risk factors are demonstrated in Box 1. Perhaps the most important risk factor is the length of stay in the ICU, with most studies indicating that the peak

---

Box 1. Risk factors for invasive candidiasis

Adults
Prolonged length of stay in an ICU
High Acute Physiology and Chronic Health Evaluation
   II score (eg, >20)
Renal failure
Hemodialysis
Broad-spectrum antibiotics
Central venous catheter
Parenteral nutrition
Immunosuppressive drugs
Cancer and chemotherapy
Severe acute pancreatitis
Candida colonization at multiple sites
Surgery
Transplantation

Neonates and children
In addition to the adult risk factors:
   Prematurity
   Low Apgar score
   Congenital malformations

incidence of IC is at around day 10 of the ICU stay [56,57]. This generally corresponds with observations that suggest that *Candida* colonization increases dramatically after day 8. Other important risk factors among adults include the use of central venous catheters, broad-spectrum antimicrobial agents, or parenteral nutrition; the development of acute renal insufficiency; hemodialysis (acute or chronic); severe pancreatitis; neutropenia; diabetes mellitus; immunosuppressive therapy; any surgery that requires general anesthesia, but especially upper gastrointestinal tract surgery, and solid organ or stem cell transplantation; and *Candida* colonization [31,46].

Infants in the neonatal ICU also are at high risk for developing IC [7,11,49]. This is especially true for infants with low gestational age, low Apgar scores, and congenital malformations. A unique characteristic of IC in the neonatal ICU is the overrepresentation of *C parapsilosis* compared with adult populations. In the neonatal population, *C parapsilosis* accounts for more than 30% of all *Candida* bloodstream isolates compared with only 10% to 15% of *Candida* bloodstream isolates in adults [7,10,42,49]. With the exception of prematurity and congenital abnormalities, risk factors for the development of IC in infants and children are similar to those in adults.

The significance of *Candida* colonization as a predictor of invasive disease has been an issue of debate over the last 2 decades. *Candida* "colonization intensity" has been examined in several single-center studies, with results suggesting that certain levels of colonization predict invasive disease [58–60]. In the largest multicenter study performed to date, however, there was no correlation between the number of sites colonized and the likelihood of developing IC [46,48]. Rather, the presence or absence of colonization was the most important risk factor. Thus, it is most appropriate to view *Candida* colonization at any clinically important site as a risk factor and not as a disease. Conversely, the absence of *Candida* colonization in patients who are at risk strongly suggests that IC is not present.

The last 2 decades also have witnessed an important shift in the species of *Candida* that cause invasive disease. There has been a proportional decrease of *C albicans* and a corresponding proportional increase in non-albicans *Candida* isolates from patients who have IC [7,11,36]. Table 1 provides a list of the most common isolates that cause IC and the reported range of frequency for each of these species. Driving this change are multiple factors, but the most important ones include the widespread use of prophylactic antifungal therapy and the increased use of chronic indwelling multipurpose intravascular catheters [61–64]. Each of the more common non-albicans *Candida* spp has been associated with a specific patient population and associated risk factors based on published reports. For example, *C glabrata* is reported more commonly isolated from older patients and those who have underlying neoplastic disease [44,64,65]; *C tropicalis* is recognized more commonly among patients who have leukemia and neutropenia [41,43]; *C parapsilosis* is seen more commonly among neonates and patients with chronic indwelling intravenous catheters [7,11,12]; and *C*

Table 1
Most common *Candida* bloodstream isolates and range of distribution

Organism	Range of distribution	
	Adults (%)	Children (%)
C albicans	44%–71	49%–63
C glabrata	9%–24	0%–7
C parapsilosis	8%–13	19%–45
C tropicalis	7%–19	0%–8
C krusei	0%–2	0%–1
Other Candida spp	<1	<1

krusei is seen most commonly among stem cell transplant recipients and patients who have leukemia who receive fluconazole prophylaxis [63].

Diagnostic assays and antifungal susceptibility testing

Blood cultures are an insensitive means of identifying patients who have IC. As many as 50% of patients with autopsy-proven disease have negative blood cultures antemortem. Newer blood culture techniques probably have increased overall sensitivity to around 70%, but there remain significant numbers of patients who have IC in whom all routine blood cultures are negative [66]. Because of the difficulty in establishing a firm diagnosis of IC clinically and the limited usefulness of blood cultures, nonculture diagnostic techniques have great potential value. Among the diagnostic assays that are approved by the U.S. Food and Drug Administration (FDA), the 1,3 β-glucan assay probably is the most reliable, with a sensitivity and specificity of 70% and 87%, respectively, among patients who have proven IC [67]. The assay is approved as an adjunct for the diagnosis of IC. Its role in the early diagnosis of IC is being determined; however, this assay represents an important step forward toward reliance on nonculture methodologies in the diagnosis of this disorder.

The Platellia Aspergillus ELISA (PA-ELISA) is an FDA-approved test for invasive aspergillosis that is based on its ability to identify galactomannan, a cell wall component of many fungi. The assay is not approved for use as a diagnostic adjunct for IC. Thus, its role in IC is uncertain; however, the PA-ELISA has been evaluated in a select population of patients that has IC with promising preliminary results. Other newer diagnostic assays include polymerase chain reaction–based assays, but none of these promising diagnostic tests have been approved.

The identification of clinically relevant *Candida* isolates to the species level is critically important. The germ tube test is a reliable and inexpensive means of identifying *C albicans*. This test is performed by placing the organism in serum and observing for germ tube formation, which usually is apparent within 2 hours. The newly developed peptide nucleic acid fluorescent in situ hybridization (PNA-FISH) can distinguish *C albicans* from non-albi-cans *Candida* spp [68]. This assay is more rapid than the germ tube but is considerably more expensive and provides only a modest improvement in sensitivity. CHROMagar, a specialized media for *Candida* isolation and identification, readily distinguishes *C albicans*, *C tropicalis*, and *C krusei* based on distinctive pigments observed for each of these individual species. Despite these new innovations, most laboratories still rely upon a battery of biochemical tests offered in the API-20C strip to identify *Candida* to the species level.

Antifungal susceptibility testing is not performed routinely at most small-to modest-sized laboratories. The need for antifungal susceptibility testing for all clinically significant *Candida* isolates is debatable, because there are ample data to suggest that the determination of *Candida* spp allows an accurate prediction of antifungal susceptibility. As such, in hospitals where *Candida* identification to the species level is performed routinely, antifungal susceptibility testing generally is not necessary, except on a selected basis among patients with disease that is refractory to conventional therapy and among patients with unusual isolates. Currently available Clinical Labora-tory Standards Institute-approved antifungal susceptibility testing techniques include microtiter dilution methodology, E-Test, and disc diffusion method-ology [69–73]. The susceptibility patterns of the more common species of *Candida* are shown in Table 2.

Clinical manifestations of invasive candidiasis

Invasive candidiasis can involve virtually any organ, and, as such, has a variety of clinical manifestations. With few exceptions, there are no dis-tinctive and unique clinical features that are sufficiently predictive of IC

Table 2
Common susceptibility patterns of *Candida* species

Species	Common susceptibility patterns				
	Amphotericin B	5-FC	Fluconazole and itraconazole	Voriconazole and posaconazole[a]	Echinocandin[b]
C albicans	S	S	S	S	S
C glabrata	S to I	S	S-DD to R	S to S-DD?	S
C krusei	S to I	I to R	R	S to S-DD?	S
C lusitaniae	S to R	S	S	S	S
C parapsilosis	S	S	S	S	S to I?
C tropicalis	S	S	S	S	S

Abbreviations: 5-FC, 5-fluorocytosine; I, intermediate; R, resistant; S, susceptible; S-DD, susceptible dose-dependent (dose needs to be increased to achieve therapeutic efficacy).
  [a] Posaconazole is approved in Europe, awaiting approval in the United States.
  [b] Caspofungin, micafungin, anidulafungin.

to guide specific antifungal therapy. A review of the more common clinical syndromes that are associated with IC follows.

Candidemia

Candidemia, the isolation of *Candida* spp in one or more blood cultures, is the most commonly recognized manifestation of IC, and occurs in 50% to 70% of patients with this disorder. The demonstration of candidemia always should be taken seriously; a positive blood culture for *Candida* spp never should be regarded as merely a contaminant, and should trigger immediate intervention with effective antifungal therapy and other appropriate interventions (eg, intravascular catheter removal). Based on recently published studies, the all-cause mortality for adults who have candidemia (complicated and uncomplicated) approximates 40% [7,11,12,33]. For neonates and children, the all-cause mortality approximates 20% [7,11,12,33]. It is important to recognize that candidemia is the "tip of the iceberg" with regard to all patients who have IC, and that candidemic patients provide a broad spectrum of clinical illness that ranges from "transient" or self-limited candidemia secondary to a contaminated central venous catheter, to sepsis, multiorgan failure, and rapid demise. Clinically, it is difficult to determine disease severity and the propensity for development of complicated disease; therefore, most authorities recommend antifungal therapy for any episode of candidemia [74,75].

Acute disseminated candidiasis

This form of candidiasis is seen most commonly among patients who are neutropenic as a result of cytotoxic chemotherapy for an underlying hematologic malignancy. Most of these patients have documented candidemia, most are acutely ill, and many have multiple organ involvement or failure [76]. Among patients who are neutropenic, many have a discrete erythematous or hemorrhagic palpable rash, which is consistent with small vessel vasculitis, as a major manifestation of this form of IC (Fig. 1).

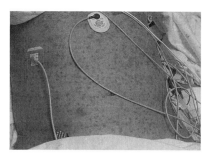

Fig. 1. The rash of acute disseminated candidiasis in a patient who had recently diagnosed acute myelogenous leukemia, profound neutropenia, and *C krusei* fungemia.

Infective endocarditis

Infective endocarditis that is due to *Candida* spp is uncommon and is seen mostly among individuals who have chronic indwelling intravenous catheters (eg, Hickman, Broviac) or large-caliber hemodialysis catheters. Other important risk factors for *Candida* endocarditis include an abnormal native valve, a prosthetic valve, congenital cardiac abnormalities (eg, ventriculo-septal defect), and a history of injection of illicit drugs, especially heroin. Any cardiac valve may be involved and most patients are fungemic. Valvular vegetations may be large and may be associated with more frequent systemic embolic events. Although a rare disorder, *Candida* is by far the most common cause of fungal endocarditis and accounts for more than two thirds of cases [77].

Vertebral osteomyelitis and diskitis

Vertebral osteomyelitis, with or without diskitis, has become an increasingly common disorder that is associated with unrecognized or untreated candidemia [78]. This disorder may be caused by any of the pathogenic *Candida* spp, and symptoms usually are manifest several weeks to several months after an episode of candidemia. The lumbosacral vertebral disks and vertebral bodies are preferred sites of involvement, and patients typically present with chronic progressively severe local back pain, usually without concomitant fever, weight loss, or other constitutional symptoms [79]. As with other forms of vertebral osteomyelitis and diskitis, nerve root compression syndromes, including complete loss of function, are associated with advanced disease.

Endophthalmitis

Untreated candidemia has been associated with retinal lesions in up to 37% of patients [80]; however, *Candida* endophthalmitis is uncommon in its full-blown clinical form. In an era of effective azole antifungal therapy, fewer than 1% of patients that have proven candidemia and are treated with a full 2-week course of systemic antifungal therapy develops retinitis or endophthalmitis. *Candida* endophthalmitis begins as a choroidal lesion that progresses to an area of retinal necrosis followed by full-blown vitreitis and endophthalmitis [81]. Untreated, this condition leads to blindness. Unilateral involvement is the rule, although bilateral endophthalmitis leading to total blindness has been reported. A disproportionate number of cases (~90%) of *Candida* endophthalmitis is due to *C albicans*, which confirms the significant invasive potential for this organism through its ability to attach to and invade endothelial cells [81].

Chronic disseminated candidiasis (hepatosplenic candidiasis)

Chronic disseminated candidiasis is seen almost exclusively among patients who have undergone myeloablative chemotherapy and have developed IC during the period of neutropenia [82]. Upon recovery from neutropenia, patients with this disorder develop low-grade fever and right upper quadrant pain, often associated with a palpable and tender liver, splenomegaly, and an elevated serum alkaline phosphatase. Imaging studies (CT or ultrasound) may reveal multiple focal lesions in the liver, spleen, kidneys, or rarely, the lungs (Fig. 2). The development of parenchymal lesions after neutrophil recovery suggests that an adequate host inflammatory response is a prerequisite to the development of radiographically visible lesions. In a patient with a history of documented candidemia, the diagnosis can be inferred on the basis of the clinical laboratory and radiographic findings. In the absence of documented candidemia, however, a CT-directed liver biopsy for histopathology and culture generally is recommended to rule out other infectious and noninfectious processes [82].

Other forms of visceral candidiasis

Candida spp may cause meningitis, septic arthritis, tenosynovitis, isolated involvement of the kidney, and pneumonia, which are less common manifestations of IC and are not discussed in detail. The diagnosis of septic arthritis and tenosynovitis involves the isolation of the organism from synovial fluid [83]. Similarly, the diagnosis of *Candida* meningitis is confirmed by isolation of *Candida* spp from cerebrospinal fluid or histopathologic evidence in tissue or cerebrospinal fluid [84]. *Candida* pneumonia is a rare disorder that is seen almost exclusively among severely immunocompromised patients; the

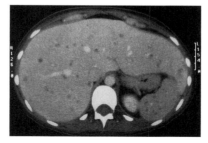

Fig. 2. CT scan of the abdomen demonstrating findings consistent with chronic disseminated candidiasis in a 21-year-old woman who had acute lymphocytic leukemia. She had experienced an episode of *C tropicalis* fungemia during a recent course of myeloablative chemotherapy, and had received 10 days of amphotericin B before discharge. She returned 7 days later with right upper quadrant pain, low-grade fever, and an elevated serum alkaline phosphatase.

diagnosis of this disorder requires isolation of the organism from a respiratory sample and histopathologic evidence of deep tissue invasion that is due to *Candida* spp [85].

Treatment

The treatment of IC is based largely on data from randomized controlled clinical trials among patients who had proven candidemia, with a much smaller proportion of the data coming from patients who had proven IC, but who did not have candidemia. There are only anecdotal reports of antifungal therapy for the less common forms of IC, including endocarditis, endophthalmitis, osteomyelitis, septic arthritis, and meningitis.

General principles of therapy

The Infectious Diseases Society of America treatment guidelines that were published in 2004 are being updated, but remain a useful guide for the general approach to treatment of the common forms of IC [74]. These general recommendations, demonstrated in Table 3, are based on recently published data and include primary therapy and suggested alternatives. Since guidelines were published, four new compounds have been approved for treatment of candidemia in the United States and Europe, or are in late development and supported by clinical trials and favorable anecdotal results. These compounds include micafungin, anidulafungin, voriconazole, and posaconazole; the role for each of these compounds in the treatment of IC is being examined.

Several important considerations dictate the choice of initial antifungal therapy in a patient who has proven or suspected IC. What is the recent history of azole exposure? What are the susceptibility patterns of *Candida* spp in this health care setting? What are the dominant *Candida* spp in this particular unit/location and in this particular situation? What are the comorbidities and underlying disorders? How acutely ill is this patient? Is there clinical evidence to suggest involvement of the central nervous system, cardiac valves, liver, spleen, or kidneys? Is there a patient history of intolerance to an antifungal agent? Each of these questions must be addressed specifically to make an informed choice relative to the most suitable antifungal agent.

Fluconazole and itraconazole

Fluconazole remains a standard of primary therapy for selected patients who have proven and probable IC. There is little role for itraconazole in the treatment of IC given the similar antifungal spectrum, ease of administration, superior pharmacokinetics, and better tolerability of fluconazole. Fluconazole should be considered for first-line therapy among patients who do not have previous azole exposure, with mild to moderate illness, and who are not at high risk for *C glabrata* (elderly patients, patients who have neoplasia, diabetics) [74,75]. It also is the drug of choice for patients who have suspected genitourinary candidiasis because of its excellent urinary concentration. Selected patients who probably should not receive fluconazole as primary therapy for proven or suspected IC include patients with the following characteristics: neutropenia, severe illness (eg, Acute Physiology and Chronic Health Evaluation [APACHE] > 20), suspected involvement of cardiac valves or myocardium, and suspected central nervous system (CNS) involvement. Fluconazole is a reasonable "step-down therapy" for patients who are improving on more aggressive initial antifungal therapy (eg, echinocandin or amphotericin B), who are infected with a susceptible organism, and who are ready for transition to oral therapy [74,75].

Voriconazole and posaconazole

A recently published trial demonstrated that voriconazole is an effective alternative to amphotericin B induction therapy for 4 to 7 days, followed by fluconazole, 400 mg daily—both regimens administered for at least 2 weeks—for candidemia and other forms of invasive candidiasis [86]. Voriconazole has broad activity against most *Candida* spp, including *C krusei*, and most *C glabrata*. There are several disadvantages to voriconazole, however, including more frequent administration (twice a day), unpredictable pharmacokinetics, more drug interactions, and poor tolerance of the drug when compared with other systemic antifungals [87]. Because of these disadvantages, parenteral or oral voriconazole has not been a popular selection for primary therapy of IC by most clinicians. The agent, does, however, fill a niche among patients with potentially fluconazole-resistant isolates, such as *C. krusei* or *C. glabrata*, who are clinically stable and ready for transition to oral therapy [35]. Among those select patients, voriconazole is an excellent oral alternative to intravenous amphotericin B or an echinocandin. Patients who have underlying liver disease should not be given voriconazole [87].

Like voriconazole, posaconazole has excellent in vitro activity against most *Candida* spp, although there is a paucity of clinical data to support its use among patients who have IC [88]. Posaconazole recently was approved in Europe for prophylaxis of invasive fungal infections among recipients of stem cell transplants, and it is awaiting FDA approval in the United States. Based on available data, it is difficult to envision a major role for posaconazole in the treatment of IC other than in select patients for whom transition therapy to an expanded-spectrum triazole is warranted.

Echinocandins

Currently, there are three FDA-approved echinocandins that have been elevated for the treatment of candidemia and IC: caspofungin, micafungin,

Table 3
Treatment for candidemia and other forms of invasive candidiasis

Condition	Therapy		Duration	Comments
	Primary	Alternative		
Candidemia				
Non-neutropenic adults	AmB, 0.6–1.0 mg/kg/d IV; or Flu, 400–800 mg/d IV or by mouth; or Caspo, 50 mg/d; Mica, 100 mg/d; or Anid, 100 mg/d	AmB, 0.7 mg/kg/d + Flu, 800 mg/d for 4–7 d, then Flu, 800 mg/d	14 days after last positive blood culture and resolution of signs and symptoms	Remove all intravascular catheters, if possible
Children	AmB, 0.6–1.0 mg/kg/d IV; or Flu, 6 mg/kg every 12 h IV or by mouth	Caspo, Mica	14–21 days after resolution of signs and symptoms and negative repeat blood cultures	
Neonates	AmB, 0.6–1.0 mg/kg/d IV; or Flu, 5–12 mg/kg/d IV	Caspo, Mica	14–21 days after resolution of signs and symptoms and negative repeat blood cultures	
Neutropenia	AmB, 0.7–1.0 mg/kg/d IV; or LFAmB, 3.0–6.0 mg/kg/d; or Caspo, 50 mg/d; Mica, 100 mg/d; or Anid, 100 mg/d	Flu, 6–12 mg/kg/d IV or by mouth	14 days after last positive blood culture and resolution of signs and symptoms and resolved neutropenia	Removal of all intravascular catheters is controversial in neutropenic patients; gastrointestinal source is common.
Chronic disseminated candidiasis	AmB, 0.6–0.7 mg/kg/d; or LFAmB, 3–5 mg/kg/d; Caspo, 50 mg/d; Mica, 100 mg/d; or Anid, 100 mg/d	Flu, 6 mg/kg/d	3–6 mo and resolution or calcification of radiologic lesions	Flu may be given after 1–2 wk of AmB or echinocandin therapy if clinically stable or improved

Endocarditis	AmB, 0.6–1.0 mg/kg/d IV; or LFAmB, 3–6 mg/kg/d ± 5-FC, 25–37.5 mg/kg by mouth qid; Caspo, 50 mg/d; Mica, 100 mg/d; Anid, 100 mg/d	Flu, 6–12 mg/kg/d IV or by mouth; Caspo, 50 mg/d; Mica, 100 mg/d; Anid, 100 mg/d	At least 6 wk after valve replacement	Valve replacement is almost always necessary; long-term suppression with Flu has been successful among selected patients who cannot undergo valve replacement
Endophthalmitis	AmB, 0.7–1.0 mg/kg/d IV; or Flu, 6–12 mg/kg/d IV or by mouth	Caspo, 50 mg/d; Mica, 100 mg/d; Anid, 100 mg/d	6–12 wk after surgery	Vitrectomy usually is performed when vitreitis is present
Urinary/renal	Flu, 6–12 mg/kg/d IV or by mouth; AmB, 0.7–1.0 mg/kg/d	Unclear role for echinocandins	2 wk	

Abbreviations: 5-FC, 5-fluoroctosine; AmB, amphotericin B; Anid, anidulafungin; Caspo, caspofungin; Flu, fluconazole; IV, intravenously; LFAmB, lipid formulation of amphotericin B; Mica, micafungin; qid, four times a day.

and anidulafungin [89]. Each must be administered intravenously once daily and each has a favorable safety profile and few drug interactions. Three large, controlled, randomized phase III studies that examined the safety, tolerability, and efficacy of these compounds in the treatment of candidemia and other forms of IC demonstrated remarkably consistent efficacy, with successful outcomes in approximately 75% of patients in each of these trials (Reboli et al, submitted from publication, 2006) [90,91]. Consequently, the echinocandins have become extraordinarily popular agents as primary therapy for patients who have proven or suspected IC because of their ease of administration, safety, few drug interactions, and broad fungicidal activity against all *Candida* spp. The compounds have similar pharmacokinetics and excellent in vitro activity against all *Candida* spp [89,92]. Each agent demonstrates diminished activity and higher minimum inhibitory concentrations versus *C parapsilosis*, and there is a suggestion in clinical trials that these compounds may be less effective than fluconazole or amphotericin B deoxycholate against this organism. When all of the clinical data are examined carefully, they suggest that the echinocandins are sufficiently similar that they probably are interchangeable in most clinical circumstances pertaining to IC. Few reports of echinocandin resistance are documented [93,94].

Clinical circumstances in which an echinocandin should be considered as first-line therapy include, but are not limited to, patients who have any of the following characteristics: recent exposure to an azole as therapy or prophylaxis for invasive fungal infection, ongoing neutropenia, a history of allergy to azoles or intolerance to amphotericin B, high risk for infection with *C krusei* or *C glabrata* (neutropenic patients, patients who have leukemia, and elderly patients), and moderate to severe disease (eg, APACHE > 20) [74,75]. A strategy of initial echinocandin therapy followed by transition to oral fluconazole or voriconazole (depending on the *Candida* isolate or susceptibility data) is a reasonable approach to the treatment of candidemia and other forms of IC. Patients in whom echinocandins should be avoided include those who have suspected CNS involvement (echinocandins penetrate the CNS poorly and there are several reports of relapsing or persistent CNS candidiasis with echinocandin therapy) and the rare patients who are unable to tolerate any one of the echinocandins.

Amphotericin B formulations

Among the amphotericin B formulations, amphotericin B deoxycholate has been the most studied antifungal agent in the treatment of candidemia and other forms of IC. It has been the standard agent in at least four large, randomized and controlled trials [95–97]. In three of these studies, amphotericin B demonstrated numerical, but not statistical, superiority when compared with fluconazole, 400 mg/d or 800 mg/d [95–97]. In the first trial that compared amphotericin B deoxycholate with an echinocandin, caspofungin was numerically, but not statistically, superior to amphotericin B but was significantly less toxic [90]. Finally, recent data suggest a potential role for continuous infusion of amphotericin B deoxycholate as a therapeutic option for IC [98], but most authors generally discourage this approach to therapy because of limited clinical information, the pharmacodynamic information against this approach, and the availability of many other therapeutic alternatives.

Among the lipid formulations of amphotericin B, only liposomal amphotericin B (LAmB) and amphotericin B lipid complex (ABLC) have been studied in large prospective, randomized trials for the treatment of candidemia. In the most recent of these studies, micafungin, 100 mg/d, was compared with LAmB for candidemia [91]. Micafungin was noninferior to LAmB in this trial, but it demonstrated an improved safety profile. There are no published data from large randomized controlled trials that compared ABLC or amphotericin B colloidal dispersion with another agent for the treatment of IC. Thus, all of the recent experience with these two formulations of amphotericin B is anecdotal or based on information from treatment registries and salvage protocols.

Prevention

Prevention of IC has been an important priority, particularly among intensivists and those caring for high-risk patients in ICUs. Single-center studies that were performed in surgical ICUs demonstrated a benefit to fluconazole when administered to patients in ICUs with certain characteristics that were defined as "high risk" [47,56,57,99]. These studies have not been multicenter, and may not be generalizable to ICU patients at large, although most analyses of the data suggest a potential benefit for a subset of these high-risk patients (Ostrosky-Zeichner and colleagues, unpublished manuscript) [100–106]. Consequently, most clinicians in the ICU setting establish their own set of "risks" and implement antifungal prophylaxis in a manner that seems most appropriate to their unique situation. This nonstandardized approach to antifungal prophylaxis has led to tremendous overuse of all antifungal agents, especially fluconazole, in the ICU setting despite the lack of compelling clinical data to demonstrate a survival benefit among the recipients of intervention.

To address the important problem, the Bacteriology and Mycoses Study Group recently designed and implemented a study among patients in the ICU who are determined to be at high risk for candidemia and other forms of IC by using a "rule" to determine individual risk for development of IC (Ostrosky-Zeichner and colleagues, unpublished manuscript) (Box 2). In this double-blinded study, patients who met eligibility requirements based on this rule and who agreed to participate in the study were randomized to one of the two arms: one group received caspofungin, 50 mg/d, and the other group received placebo. Unfortunately, the study accrual was poor

---

Box 2. A predictive rule for invasive candidiasis among patients in the ICU for Bacteriology and Mycoses Study Group study 2-01

<u>All</u> patients must be in the ICU for at least 4 days

> *plus either*

Any antibiotic use

> *or*

A central venous catheter D 1–3

> *in addition to the above criteria*

At least two of the following:
- Any surgery, D 7 to 0
- Immunosuppressive use, D 7 to 0
- Pancreatitis, D 7 to 0
- Total parenteral nutrition, D 1 to 3
- Any dialysis, D 1 to 3
- Steroid use, D 7 to 3

Abbreviation: D, day relative to ICU admission.

Adapted from Ostrosky-Zeichner L, Sable C, Sobel JD, et al. Multicenter retrospective development and validation of a clinical predictive rule for nosocomial invasive candidiasis in the intensive care setting; unpublished manuscript.

---

and the study was terminated prematurely. A modified version of the study, with a more inclusive rule, is being designed with plans to implement it in the near future. If successful, this trial would help to define the role of antifungal prophylaxis in the ICU setting, and it could create a new paradigm approach to these patients.

Summary

Invasive candidiasis remains an important nosocomial infection that continues to present major diagnostic and therapeutic challenges to the clinician. Changes in the epidemiology of this disorder have occurred for many reasons, and include especially the extensive use of prophylactic antifungal agents, broad-spectrum antibacterial agents, and medical devices (eg, chronic indwelling intravascular catheters). The diagnosis of IC remains elusive in many patients, and there is a critical need for improved diagnostics that will provide clinicians the opportunity to intervene earlier in the course of disease. Newer antifungal agents offer promise in the treatment of candidemia and other forms of IC, but the optimal use of these agents, particularly in the approach to non-albicans *Candida* infections, needs to be explored in more detail. Furthermore, despite an overwhelming amount of data concerning risk factors and excess mortality associated with the development of IC, there is no consistent approach to treatment and primary prevention among individuals who are deemed to be at highest risk for this complication. Research that focuses on these important clinical areas could provide valuable insights into the diagnosis and management of this common and evolving infection.

References

[1] Fridkin SK. The changing face of fungal infections in health care settings. Clin Infect Dis 2005;41:1455–60.

[2] Kao AS, Brandt ME, Pruitt WR, et al. The epidemiology of candidemia in two United States cities: results of a population-based active surveillance. Clin Infect Dis 1999;29: 1164–70.

[3] Diekema DJ, Messer SA, Brueggemann AB, et al. Epidemiology of candidemia: 3-year results from the Emerging Infections and the Epidemiology of Iowa Organisms study. J Clin Microbiol 2002;40:1298–302.

[4] Abi-Said D, Anaissie E, Uzan O, et al. The epidemiology of hematogenous candidiasis caused by different *Candida* species. Clin Infect Dis 1997;24:1122–8.

[5] Morgan J, Meltzer MI, Plikaytis BD, et al. Excess mortality, hospital stay, and cost due to candidemia: a case-control study using data from population-based candidemia surveillance. Infect Control Hosp Epidemiol 2005;26:540–7.

[6] Asmundsdottir LR, Erlendsdottir H, Gottfredsson M. Increasing incidence of candidemia: results of 20 year nationwide study in Iceland. J Clin Micro 2002;40:3489–92.

[7] Pappas PG, Rex JH, Lee J, et al. A prospective observational study of candidemia: epidemiology, therapy, and influences on mortality in hospitalized adult and pediatric patients. Clin Infect Dis 2003;37:634–43.

[8] Tortorano AM, Peman J, Bernhardt H, et al. Epidemiology of candidemia in Europe: results of 28-month European Confederation of Medical Mycology (ECMM) hospital-based surveillance study. Eur J Clin Microbiol Infect Dis 2004;23:317–22.

[9] Trick WE, Fridkin SK, Edwards JR, et al. Secular trend of hospital-acquired candidemia among intensive care unit patients in the United States during 1989–1999. Clin Infect Dis 2002;35:622–30.

[10] Wisplinghoff H, Bischoff T, Tallent SM, et al. Nosocomial bloodstream infections in US hospitals: analysis of 24,179 cases from a prospective nationwide surveillance study. Clin Infect Dis 2004;39:309–17.

[11] Zaoutis TE, Argon J, Chu J, et al. The epidemiology and attributable outcomes of candidemia in adults and children hospitalized in the United States: a propensity analysis. Clin Infect Dis 2005;41:1232–9.

[12] Edmond MB, Wallace SE, McClish DK, et al. Nosocomial bloodstream infections in United States hospitals: a three-year analysis. Clin Infect Dis 1999;29:239–44.

[13] Harbarth S, Ferriere K, Hugonette S, et al. Epidemiology and prognostic determinants of bloodstream infections in surgical intensive care. Arch Surg 2002;137:1353–9.

[14] Malani A, Bradley SF, Little RS, et al. Trends in species causing fungemia in a tertiary care medical centre over 12 years. Mycoses 2002;44:446–9.

[15] Martin GS, Mannino DM, Eaton S, et al. The epidemiology of sepsis in the United States from 1979 through 2000. N Engl J Med 2003;348:1546–54.

[16] Marr KA, Seidel K, White TC, et al. Candidemia in allogeneic blood and marrow transplant recipients: evolution of risk factors after the adoption of prophylactic fluconazole. J Infect Dis 2000;181:309–16.

[17] Viscoli C, Girmenia C, Marinus A, et al. Candidemia in cancer patients: a prospective, multicenter surveillance study by the Invasive Fungal Infection Group (IFIG) of the European

Organizaiton for Research and Treatment of Cancer (EORTC). Clin Infect Dis 1999;28: 1071–9.

[18] Wenzel RP, Edmonds MB. The impact of hospital-acquired bloodstream infections. Emerg Infect Dis 2001;7:174–7.

[19] Antoniadou A, Torres HA, Lewis RE, et al. Candidemia in a tertiary care center: in vitro susceptibility and its association with outcome of initial antifungal therapy. Medicine 2003; 82:309–21.

[20] Arendrup MC, Fuursted K, Gahrn-Hansen B, et al. Seminational surveillance of fungemia in Denmark: notably high rates of fungemia and number of isolates with reduced azole susceptibility. J Clin Microbiol 2005;43:4434–40.

[21] Colombo AL, Perfect J, DiNubile M, et al. Global distribution and outcomes for *Candida* species causing invasive candidiasis: results from an international randomized double-blind study of caspofungin versus amphotericin B for treatment of invasive candidiasis. Eur J Clin Micro 2003;22:470–4.

[22] Hajjeh RA, Sofair AN, Harrison IH, et al. Incidence of bloodstream infections due to *Candida* species and in vitro susceptibilities of isolates collected from 1998 to 2000 in a population-based active surveillance program. J Clin Microbiol 2004;42:1519–27.

[23] Marchetti O, Bille J, Fluckinger U, et al. Epidemiology of candidemia in Swiss tertiary care hospitals: secular trends, 1991–2000. Clin Infect Dis 2004;38:311–20.

[24] Pfaller MA, Messer SA, Boyken L, et al. Geographic variation in the susceptibilities of invasive isolates of *Candida glabrata* to seven systemically active antifungal agents: a global assessment from the ARTEMIS Antifungal Surveillance Program conducted in 2001 and 2002. J Clin Microbiol 2004;42:3142–6.

[25] Richet H, Roux P, Des Champs C, et al. Candidemia in French hospitals: incidence rates and characteristics. Clin Microbiol Infect 2002;8:405–12.

[26] St. Germain G, Laverdieu M, Pelletier R, et al. Prevalence and antifungal susceptibility of 442 *Candida* isolates from blood and other normally sterile sites: results from a 2-year (1996 to 1998) multicenter surveillance study in Quebec, Canada. J Clin Microbiol 2001;39: 949–53.

[27] Tortorano AM, Biraghi E, Astofi A, et al. European Confederation of Medical Mycology (ECMM) prospective survey of candidaemia: report from one Italian region. J Hosp Infect 2002;51:297–304.

[28] Yamamura DLR, Rotstein C, Nicolle LE, et al. Candidemia at selected Canadian sites: results from the Fungal Disease Registry, 1992–1994. CMAJ 1999;160:493–9.

[29] Gudlaugsson O, Gillespie S, Lee K, et al. Attributable mortality of nosocomial candidemia, revisited. Clin Infect Dis 2002;37:1172–7.

[30] Wey SB, Mori M, Pfaller MA, et al. Hospital-acquired candidemia: the attributable mortality and excess length of stay. Arch Intern Med 1988;148:2642–5.

[31] Wenzel RP. Nosocomial candidemia: risk factors and attributable mortality. Clin Infect Dis 1995;20:1531–4.

[32] Blot SI, Vandewoude KH. Estimating attributable mortality of candidemia: clinical judgment vs. matched cohort studies. Eur J Clin Microbiol Infect Dis 2003;22:132–3.

[33] McNeil MM, Nash SL, Hajjeh RA, et al. Trends in mortality due to invasive mycotic diseases in the United States, 1980–1997. Clin Infect Dis 2001;33:641–7.

[34] Fridkin SK. Candidemia is costly-plain and simple. Clin Infect Dis 2005;41:1240–1.

[35] Pfaller MA, Messer SA, Hollis RJ, et al. In vitro activities of ravuconazole and voriconazole compared with those of four approved systemic antifungal agents against 6,970 clinical isolates of *Candida* spp. Antimicrob Agents Chemother 2002;46:1723–7.

[36] Pfaller MA, Diekema DJ. Twelve years of fluconazole in clinical practice: global trends in species distribution and fluconazole susceptibility of bloodstream isolates of *Candida*. Clin Microbiol Infect 2004;10(Suppl 1):11–23.

[37] Pfaller MA, Messer SA, Boyken L, et al. Further standardization of broth microdilution methodology for in vitro susceptibility testing of caspofungin against *Candida* species by

use of an international collection of more than 3,000 clinical isolates. J Clin Microbiol 2004; 42:3117–9.

[38] Pfaller MA, Hazen KC, Messer SA, et al. Comparison of results of fluconazole disk diffusion testing for *Candida* species with results from a central reference laboratory in the ARTEMIS Global Antifungal Surveillance Program. J Clin Microbiol 2004;42: 3607–12.

[39] Pfaller MA, Boyken L, Hollis RJ, et al. In vitro activities of anidulafungin against more than 2,500 clinical isolates of *Candida* spp., including 315 isolates resistant to fluconazole. J Clin Microbiol 2005;43:5425–7.

[40] Pfaller MA, Diekema DJ, Rinaldi MG, et al. Results from the ARTEMIS DISK Global Antifungal Surveillance Study: a 6.5-year analysis of susceptibilities of *Candida* and other yeast species to fluconazole and voriconazole by standardized disk diffusion testing. J Clin Microbiol 2005;43:5848–59.

[41] Wingard JR. Importance of *Candida* species other than *C. albicans* as pathogens in oncology patients. Clin Infect Dis 1995;20:115–25.

[42] Saxen H, Virtanen M, Carlson P, et al. Neonatal *Candida parapsilosis* outbreak with a high case fatality rate. Pediatr Infect Dis J 1995;14:776–81.

[43] Kontoyiannis DP, Vaziri I, Hanna HA, et al. Risk factors for *Candida tropicalis* fungemia in patients with cancer. Clin Infect Dis 2001;33:1676–81.

[44] Gumbo T, Isada CM, Hall G, et al. *Candida glabrata* fungemia: clinical features of 139 patients. Medicine 1999;78:220–7.

[45] Wingard JR, Dick JD, Merz WG, et al. Differences in virulence of clinical isolates of *Candida tropicalis* and *Candida albicans* in mice. Infect Immun 1982;37:833–6.

[46] Blumberg HM, Jarvis WR, Soucie JM, et al. Risk factors for candidal bloodstream infections in surgical intensive care unit patients: The NEMIS Prospective Multicenter Study. Clin Infect Dis 2001;33:177–86.

[47] Eggimann P, Francioli P, Bille J, et al. Fluconazole prophylaxis prevents intra-abdominal candidiasis in high-risk surgical patients. Crit Care Med 1999;27:1066–72.

[48] Pittet D, Monod M, Suter PM, et al. *Candida* colonization and subsequent infections in critically ill surgical patients. Ann Surg 1994;220:751–8.

[49] Saiman L, Ludington E, Pfaller M, et al. Risk factors for candidemia in neonatal intensive care unit patients. Pediatr Infect Dis J 2000;19:319–24.

[50] Shin JH, Kee SJ, Shin MG, et al. Biofilm production by isolates of *Candida* species recovered from nonneutropenic patients: comparison of bloodstream isolates with isolates from other sources. J Clin Microbiol 2002;40:1244–8.

[51] Al-Fattani MA, Douglas LJ. Penetration of *Candida* biofilms by antifungal agents. Antimicrob Agent Chemo 2004;48:3291–7.

[52] Murphy JW, Bistoni F, Deepe GS, et al. Type 1 and type 2 cytokines: from basic science to fungal infections. Med Mycol 1998;36:109–18.

[53] Kirkpatrick CH. Chronic mucocutaneous candidiasis. J Am Acad Dermatol 1994;31(Suppl 2):S14–7.

[54] Roilides E, Uhlig K, Venzon D, et al. Neutrophil oxidative burst in response to blastoconidia and pseudohyphae of *C. albicans*: augmentation by GCSF and interferon gamma. J Infect Dis 1992;166:668–73.

[55] Stevens DA, Walsh TJ, Bistoni F, et al. Cytokines and mycoses. Med Mycol 1998; 36(Suppl 1):S174–82.

[56] Garbino J, Lew DP, Romand JA, et al. Prevention of severe *Candida* infections in nonneutropenic, high-risk, critically ill patients: a randomized, double-blind, placebo-controlled trial in patients treated by selective digestive-decontamination. Intensive Care Med 2002; 28:1708–17.

[57] Pelz RK, Hendrix CW, Swoboda SM, et al. Double-blind placebo-controlled trial of fluconazole to prevent candidal infections in critically ill surgical patients. Ann Surg 2001;233: 542–8.

[58] Charles PE. Multifocal *Candida* species colonization as a trigger for early antifungal therapy in critically ill patients: what about other risk factors for fungal infection? Crit Care Med 2006;34:913–4.

[59] Leon C, Ruiz-Santana S, Saavedra P, et al. A bedside scoring system ("Candida score") for early antifungal treatment in nonneutropenic critically ill patients with *Candida* colonization. Crit Care Med 2006;34:730–7.

[60] Pfaller M, Cabezudo I, Koontz F, et al. Predictive value of surveillance cultures for systemic infection due to *Candida* species. Eur J Clin Microbiol 1987;6:628–33.

[61] Baran J Jr, Buckatira B, Khatib R. Candidemia before and during the fluconazole era: prevalence, types of species and approach to treatment in a tertiary care community hospital. Scand J Infect Dis 2001;33:137–9.

[62] Charlier C, Hart E, Lefort A, et al. Fluconazole for the management of invasive candidiasis: where do we stand after 15 years? J Antimicrob Chemother 2006;57:384–410.

[63] Wingard JR, Merz WG, Rinaldi MG, et al. Increase in *Candida krusei* infection among patients with bone marrow transplantation and neutropenia treated prophylactically with fluconazole. N Engl J Med 1991;325:1274–7.

[64] Wingard JR, Merz WG, Rinaldi MG, et al. Association of *Torulopsis glabrata* infections with fluconazole prophylaxis in neutropenic bone marrow transplant patients. Antimicrob Agents Chemother 1993;37:1847–9.

[65] Fidel PL, Vazquez JA, Sobel JD. *Candida glabrata*: review of epidemiology, pathogenesis, and clinical disease with comparison to *C. albicans*. Clin Microbiol Rev 1999;12:80–96.

[66] Berenguer J, Buck M, Witebsky F, et al. Lysis-centrifugation blood cultures in the detection of proven invasive candidiasis: disseminated versus single organ infection. Diagn Microbiol Infect Dis 1993;17:103–9.

[67] Ostrosky-Zeichner L, Alexander BD, Kett DH, et al. Multicenter clinical evaluation of the (1–3) beta-D-glucan assay as an aid to diagnosis of fungal infections in humans. Clin Infect Dis 2005;41:654–9.

[68] Wilson DA, Joyce MJ, Hall LS, et al. Multicenter evaluation of a *Candida albicans* peptide nucleic acid fluorescent in situ hybridization probe for characterization of yeast isolates from blood cultures. J Clin Microbiol 2005;43(6):2909–12.

[69] Pfaller MA. Antifungal susceptibility testing methods. Curr Drug Targets 2005;6:929–43.

[70] Pfaller MA, Messer SA, Bolmstrom A. Evaluation of Etest for determining in vitro susceptibility of yeast isolates to amphotericin B. Diagn Microbiol Infect Dis 1998;32:223–7.

[71] Pfaller MA, Boyken L, Messer SA, et al. Evaluation of the Etest method using Mueller-Hinton agar with glucose and methylene blue for determining amphotericin B MICs for 4,936 clinical isolates of *Candida* species. J Clin Microbiol 2004;42:4977–9.

[72] Pfaller MA, Boyken L, Hollis RJ, et al. In vitro susceptibilities of *Candida* spp. to caspofungin: four years of global surveillance. J Clin Microbiol 2006;44:760–3.

[73] Pfaller MA, Diekema DJ, Rex JH, et al. Correlation of MIC with outcome for *Candida* species tested against voriconazole: analysis and proposal for interpretive breakpoints. J Clin Microbiol 2006;44:819–26.

[74] Pappas PG, Rex JH, Sobel JD, et al. Guidelines for treatment of candidiasis. Clin Infect Dis 2004;38:161–89.

[75] Spellberg BJ, Filler SG, Edwards JE Jr. Current treatment strategies for disseminated candidiasis. Clin Infect Dis 2006;42:244–51.

[76] Anaissie EJ, Rex JH, Uzen O, et al. Predictors of adverse outcome in cancer patients with candidemia. Am J Med 1998;104:238–45.

[77] Edwards JE, Lehrer RI, Stiehm ER, et al. Severe candidal infections: clinical perspective, immune defense mechanisms, and current concepts of therapy. Ann Intern Med 1978;89:91–106.

[78] Ferra C, Doebbeling BN, Hollis RJ. *Candida tropicalis* vertebral osteomyelitis: a late sequela of fungemia. Clin Infect Dis 1993;19:697–703.

[79] Miller DJ, Mejicano GC. Vertebral osteomyelitis due to *Candida* species: case report and literature review. Clin Infect Dis 2001;33:523–30.

[80] Brooks RG. Prospective study of *Candida* endophthalmitis in hospitalized patients with candidemia. Arch Intern Med 1989;149:2226–8.

[81] Edwards JE, Foos RY, Mongomerie JZ, et al. Ocular manifestations of candida septicemia: review of 26 cases of hematogenous candida endophthalmitis. Medicine 1974;53: 47–75.

[82] Kontoyiannis DP, Luna MA, Samuels BI, et al. Hepatosplenic candidiasis: a manifestation of chronic disseminated candidiasis. Infect Dis Clin North Am 2000;14:721–39.

[83] Murray HW, Fialk MA, Roberts RB. Candida arthritis: a manifestation of disseminated candidiasis. Am J Med 1976;60:587–95.

[84] Nguyen MH, Yu VL. Meningitis caused by *Candida* species: an emerging problem in neurosurgical patients. Clin Infect Dis 1995;21:323–7.

[85] Haron E, Vartivarian S, Anaissie E, et al. Primary candida pneumonia. Medicine 1993;72: 17–42.

[86] Kullberg BJ, Sobel JD, Rhunke M, et al. Voriconazole versus a regimen of amphotericin B followed by fluconazole for candidemia in non-neutropenic patients: a randomized noninferiority trial. Lancet 2005;366:1435–42.

[87] Johnson LB, Kauffman CA. Voriconazole: a new triazoles antifungal agent. Clin Infect Dis 2003;36:630–7.

[88] Pfaller MA, Messer SA, Boyken RJ, et al. In vitro activities of voriconazole, posaconazole, and fluconazole against 4169 clinical isolates of *Candida* spp. and *C. neoformans* collected during 2001 and 2002 in the ARTEMIS global antifungal surveillance program. Diagn Microbiol Infect Dis 2004;48:201–5.

[89] Zaas AK, Alexander BD. Echinocandins: role in antifungal therapy, 2005. Expert Opin Pharmacother 2005;6:1657–68.

[90] Mora-Duarte J, Betts R, Rotstein C, et al. Comparison of caspofungin and amphotericin B for invasive candidiasis. N Engl J Med 2002;347:2020–9.

[91] Runke M, Kuse E, Chetchotisakd P, et al. Comparison of micafungin and liposomal amphotericin B for invasive candidiasis. Proceedings of the 45th Interscience Conference on Antimicrobial Agents and Chemotherapy [abstract M-722C]. Washington, DC, December 17–20, 2005.

[92] Wiederhold NP, Lewis RE. The echinocandin antifungals: an overview of the pharmacology, spectrum, and clinical efficacy. Expert Opin Investig Drugs 2003;12:1313–33.

[93] Moudgal V, Little T, Boikov D, et al. Multiechinocandin- and multiazole-resistant *Candida parapsilosis* isolates serially obtained during therapy for prosthetic valve endocarditis. Antimicrob Agents Chemother 2005;49:767–9.

[94] Krogh-Madsen M, Arendrup MC, Heslet L, et al. Amphotericin B and caspofungin resistance in *Candida glabrata* isolates recovered from a critically ill patient. Clin Infect Dis 2006;42:938–44.

[95] Rex JH, Bennett JE, Sugar AM, et al. A randomized trial comparing fluconazole with amphotericin B for the treatment of candidemia in patients without neutropenia. N Engl J Med 1994;331:1325–30.

[96] Phillips P, Shafran S, Garber G, et al. Multicenter randomized trial of fluconazole versus amphotericin B for treatment of candidemia in non-neutropenic patients. Eur J Clin Microbiol Infect Dis 1997;16:337–45.

[97] Rex JH, Pappas PG, Karchmer AW, et al. A randomized and blinded multicenter trial of high dose fluconazole plus placebo versus fluconazole plus amphotericin B as therapy for candidemia and its consequences in non-neutropenic patients. Clin Infect Dis 2003;36: 1221–8.

[98] Imhof A, Walter RB, Schaffner A. Continuous infusion of escalated doses of amphotericin B deoxycholate: an open-label observational study. Clin Infect Dis 2003;36:943–51.

[99] Able AZ, Blumer NA, Valainis GT. Fluconazole prophylaxis of severe candida infections in trauma and post-surgical patients: prospective, double blind, randomized, placebo controlled trial. Infect Dis Clin Pract 2000;9:169–75.

[100] Ho KM, Lipman J, Dobb GJ, et al. The use of prophylactic fluconazole in immunocompetent high-risk surgical patients: a meta-analysis. Crit Care 2005;9:R710–7.

[101] Ostrosky-Zeichner L. Prophylaxis and treatment of invasive candidiasis in the intensive care setting. Eur J Clin Microbiol Infect Dis 2004;23:739–44.

[102] Lipsett PA. Clinical trials of antifungal prophylaxis among patients in surgical intensive care units: concepts and considerations. Clin Infect Dis 2004;39:S193–9.

[103] Playford EG, Webster AC, Sorrell TC, et al. Antifungal agents for preventing fungal infections in non-neutropenic critically ill and surgical patients: systematic review and meta-analysis of randomized clinical trials. J Antimicrob Chemother 2006;57:628–38.

[104] Piarroux R, Grenouillet F, Balvay P, et al. Assessment of preemptive treatment to prevent severe candidiasis in critically ill surgical patients. Crit Care Med 2004;32:2443–9.

[105] Shorr AF, Chung K, Jackson WL, et al. Fluconazole prophylaxis in critically ill surgical patients: a meta-analysis. Crit Care Med 2005;33:1928–35.

[106] Vardakas KZ, Samonis G, Michalopoulos A, et al. Antifungal prophylaxis with azoles in high-risk, surgical intensive care unit patients: a meta-analysis of randomized, placebo-controlled trials. Crit Care Med 2006;34:1216–24.

ELSEVIER
SAUNDERS

Infect Dis Clin N Am
20 (2006) 507–544

INFECTIOUS
DISEASE CLINICS
OF NORTH AMERICA

Cryptococcosis

Methee Chayakulkeeree, MD[a,b],
John R. Perfect, MD[a,c,*]

[a]*Department of Medicine, Division of Infectious Diseases and International Health,*
Duke University Medical Center, P.O. Box 3353, Durham, NC 27710, USA
[b]*Division of Infectious Diseases and Tropical Medicine, Department of Medicine,*
Faculty of Medicine Siriraj Hospital, Mahidol University, Bangkok, 10700 Thailand
[c]*Department of Microbiology and Molecular Genetics,*
Duke University Medical Center, P.O. Box 3353,
Durham, NC 27710, USA

The encapsulated yeast, *Cryptococcus* spp, has rapidly risen to a worldwide highly recognizable major opportunistic fungal pathogen. Since the epidemic of HIV infections, *C neoformans* has become a critically important opportunistic infection in individuals in all parts of the world who are infected with HIV. Furthermore, *C gattii* has recently caused an impressive localized outbreak of cryptococcosis in apparently immunocompetent humans and animals on Vancouver Island in Canada [1]. Studies into the molecular pathogenesis of these encapsulated fungal pathogens have been elegantly explored and these yeasts have become model fungi to investigate various paradigms in the host–fungus relationships [2]. In fact, the genome of several *C neoformans* strains has been recently sequenced [3]. Thus, genomic studies are advancing the knowledge on cryptococcal evolution and should allow a comprehensive dissection of its virulence composite, which can lead to development of creative and new therapeutic strategies for this life-threatening fungus. A previous complete comprehensive review of cryptococcosis was completed in 2002 [4]. This article builds on this review by adding current issues with cryptococcosis, including its new classification, epidemiology, pathogenesis, and clinical aspects.

* Corresponding author.
E-mail address: perfe001@mc.duke.edu (J.R. Perfect).

0891-5520/06/$ - see front matter © 2006 Elsevier Inc. All rights reserved.
doi:10.1016/j.idc.2006.07.001
id.theclinics.com

Epidemiology

Taxonomic classification and distribution of pathogenic
Cryptococcus *spp*

Although more than 30 species are included in the genus *Cryptococcus*, the pathogenic yeasts of cryptococcosis currently consist of two species: *C neoformans* and *C gattii*, as proposed by Kwon-Chung and colleagues [5]. These species were previously classified as three varieties: *C neoformans* var *neoformans*, *C neoformans* var *grubii*, and *C neoformans* var *gattii* [6,7], which were classified into five capsular serotypes and eight molecular genotypes. The serotype classification is based on the agglutination reactions of the capsular polysaccharide antigens, which can be determined by using absorbed rabbit sera [8] or monoclonal antibodies [9]. The serotype A and D and the hybrid diploid AD strains belong to *C neoformans*, whereas serotype B and C strains have been classified as *C gattii*. Serotype A strains have been named *C neoformans* var *grubii* [6] and serotype D strains named *C neoformans* var *neoformans* based on capsular structural differences, DNA fingerprinting, and complete genome sequencing comparisons between these two serotypes (varieties) [6]. As more molecular information is gathered from genome sequencing and evolutionary studies, the *C neoformans* var *neoformans* and *C neoformans* var *grubii* may be further divided into separate species. In fact, molecular typing using M13 polymerase chain reaction–fingerprinting, orotidine monophosphate pyrophosphorylase (URA5) gene restriction fragment length polymorphism analysis [10], and randomly amplified polymorphic DNA analysis [11] of many clinical and environmental strains has been performed, and further classifying *C neoformans* and *C gattii* into four molecular types for each species: VNI through IV and VGI through IV, respectively (Table 1) [10,11]. Thus, the ability to subdivide cryptococcal strains into several more species remains possible.

The life cycles of *C neoformans* and *C gattii* are composed of asexual and sexual stages. The sexual stage of *C neoformans* has a teleomorph named *Filobasidiella neoformans*, and the teleomorph of *C gattii* was named *F bacillospora* [12,13]. Although the sexual stage exists as basidiospores, basidium, and hyphae with clamp connections, the asexual stage appears as

Table 1
Current taxonomy and classification of pathogenic *Cryptococcus* spp

Species	Varieties	Serotypes	Molecular types
Cryptococcus neoformans	*grubii*	A	VNI, VNII
	neoformans	D	VNIV
	—	AD[a]	VNIII
Cryptococcus gattii	—	B	VGI, VGII, VGIII, VGIV
	—	C	

[a] hybrid diploid

a yeast that has one of two mating types, *alpha* or *a*. Strains of opposite mating type can mate under certain in vitro conditions to form hyphae with clamp connections and produce fertile basidiospores after the meiosis event [14]. In fact, although recombination has occurred in nature, most strains in the environment clearly appear to represent several clonal lineages, and the sexual stage structures of hyphae and basidiospores have yet to be found in nature. Furthermore, the asexual yeast form is the structure found at infection sites. Strains can also haploid fruit, wherein an isolate without sexual crosses can produce hyphae and basidiospores [15]. Recombination can also be observed between two alpha-mating–type strains [16]. These new findings may help explain the prominent bias of alpha-mating–type strains (95%) in patients and the environment [17]. These observations continue to support the possibility that the 1- to 2-μ basidiospores could be the infectious propagule. In the environment, *C neoformans* is primarily found worldwide associated with excreta from certain birds, such as pigeons, and in tree hollows. For years, *C gattii* was found primarily in tropical and subtropical regions. It has been associated primarily with eucalyptus trees, which were considered its primary environmental niche [18]. However, new evidence from the unprecedented emergence of many *C gattii* isolates on Vancouver Island shows that the distribution and ecology of *C gattii* is now changing with its ability to associate with a wide range of trees, such as firs and oaks.

Incidence of human cryptococcosis

Before the HIV epidemic, cryptococcal infection was an uncommon systemic fungal infection that occurred primarily in patients who had impaired immunity, such as those who had hematologic malignancies; those who had undergone solid organ transplantation; and those undergoing systemic corticosteroid therapy or other immunosuppressive treatments [19]. An active surveillance study showed that the incidence of cryptococcosis in patients who did not have AIDS was approximately 0.2 to 0.8 per 100,000, depending on the geographic areas [20]. However, during the past 2 decades of the HIV epidemic, the incidence of cryptococcosis increased dramatically. For instance, HIV infection was found to be associated with more than 80% of cryptococcosis cases worldwide [20,21]. A population-based surveillance study conducted during 1992 through 2000 in Atlanta, Ga, and Houston, Tex, showed that fewer than one-third of patients infected with HIV who had cryptococcosis had undergone highly active antiretroviral therapy (HAART) before being diagnosed with cryptococcosis and, in fact, 6% to 10% of patients who had AIDS who had limited access to HAART developed cryptococcosis [22]. In the pre-HAART era, cryptococcal infection became a major opportunistic infection and a major cause of death in patients infected with HIV as CD4 lymphocyte counts dropped below 100 cells/μL. The average CD4 lymphocyte count in patients who have AIDS and cryptococcosis is $73/\mu L$ [23]. However, after potent antiretroviral treatment became widely available in the United States and other developed countries, the incidence of cryptococcosis decreased significantly, but the incidence of cryptococcal infection in patients not infected with HIV has not changed during this time. The incidence of cryptococcosis in patients who have HIV/AIDS has fallen from 66 per 1000 in 1992 to 7 per 1000 in 2000 in Atlanta, Ga, and from 24 per 1000 in 1993 to 2 per 1000 in 2000 in Houston, Tex [22]. Furthermore, a retrospective study of 1644 HIV-associated crypto-coccosis cases recorded at the National Reference Center for Mycoses in France during 1985 through 2001 showed a 46% decrease of the incidence of cryptococcosis during the post-HAART era (1997–2001, n = 292) com-pared with the pre-HAART era (1985–1996, n = 1352). This study also showed that an increased risk for cryptococcosis in the post-HAART era is related to the failure to be tested or treated for HIV infection [24]. Although the increased use of HAART has been associated with a lower incidence of cryptococcosis cases in medically developed countries [25], the incidence and mortality of cryptococcosis are still extremely high in countries with uncontrolled HIV epidemics and limited access to HAART or health care, such as certain areas within Africa and Asia [26,27].

In medically developed countries, the number of patients who have cryp-tococcal infections has not disappeared because risk groups continue to broaden because of further development in transplantation medicine and the creation of new therapies to manipulate immunity. The increased num-ber of patients undergoing organ transplantation and the use of corticoste-roids and other immunosuppressive agents and monoclonal antibodies, such as alemtuzumab and infliximab, can produce a profoundly immunosup-pressed state and allow reactivation of a cryptococcal infection [28,29]. For instance, cryptococcosis is the third most common invasive fungal infec-tion after candidiasis and aspergillosis in patients who undergo solid organ transplantation [30]. In a study at the University of Pittsburgh Medical Cen-ter during 1989 to 1999, 28 of 5521 patients who underwent transplantation were diagnosed with cryptococcal meningitis. Patients who undergo solid-organ transplantation who develop cryptococcosis include those who un-dergo transplantation of their liver (11 of 2539), heart (8 of 372), kidney (7 of 2122), lung (1 of 432), or small bowel (1 of 56). Furthermore, the cryp-tococcal meningitis–related morbidity and mortality in patients who un-dergo transplantation makes this infection an independent risk factor for poor prognosis [31,32].

As shown in Box 1, in addition to HIV and organ transplantation, risk factors for acquiring cryptococcal infections include other medical condi-tions producing an immunocompromised state and associated with treat-ment with corticosteroids, such as systemic lupus erythematosus, diabetes mellitus, and hematologic malignancies [4,33]. The recent introduction of powerful immunosuppressive monoclonal antibodies, such as alemtuzumab with its ability to produce prolonged $CD4^+$ lymphocytopenia, have produced

Box 1. Predisposing factors of cryptococcosis

HIV infection
Corticosteroids (≥20 mg of prednisone)
Solid organ transplantation[a]
Malignancies[a] (ie, Hodgkin's disease, lymphomas, chronic lymphocytic leukemia)
CD4+ T-cell lymphopenia
Connective tissue diseases or immunologic diseases[a] (ie, sarcoidosis, systemic lupus erythematosus, rheumatoid arthritis, hyper IgM syndrome or hyper IgE syndrome)
Monoclonal antibodies (etanercept, infliximab, alemtuzumab)
Diabetes mellitus
Chronic pulmonary diseases or lung cancer
Renal failure or peritoneal dialysis
Cirrhosis
Pregnancy

___
[a] Immunosuppressive therapies add to the risk.

additional high-risk groups [29]. We have recently observed an example of a new risk group with significant clinical implications. An aggressive chemotherapeutic approach has emerged for managing fatal brain tumors that includes potent immunosuppressive regimens and prolonged survival, causing complicating infections with *Pneumocystis* and *Cryptococcus* to become more common. Cryptococcal meningitis can have a serious delay in diagnosis within this risk group because headaches might be considered to be caused by the underlying disease rather than infection, and lumbar punctures are less attractive to perform in this risk group because of herniation risks.

Among human cases of cryptococcosis, *C neoformans* var *grubii* (serotype A) is the most common isolate found in clinical specimens worldwide [34,35]. This serotype accounts for more than 95% of cryptococcal cases. *C neoformans* var *neoformans* (serotype D) will commonly cause cryptococcal disease in certain European countries, such as Denmark, Germany, Italy, France, Switzerland, and the United States. Until recently, *C gattii* (serotypes B and C) was found to cause cryptococcosis primarily in tropical and subtropical areas, such as Australia, Southeast Asia, Central Africa, and the tropical and subtropical areas of the Americas. For example, a study of cryptococcosis in Australia and New Zealand by Chen and colleagues [36] found that 85% of cryptococcal infections were still caused by serotype A strains, whereas serotype B and C were the etiologic agents in the other 15%. The authors noted that 44% of patients who had cryptococcosis caused by *C gattii* were apparently immunocompetent, whereas 98% of

C neoformans infections occurred in individuals who were immunocompromised. Further evidence to support the high predilection of *C gattii* for causing disease in apparently immunocompetent hosts is the *C gattii* infection outbreak on Vancouver Island, British Columbia, Canada, since 1999 [1]. On the other hand, a recent epidemiologic survey of isolates in Southern California showed that *C gattii* produced disease in a substantial number of individuals infected with HIV [37]. Therefore, reduced frequency of *C gattii* infections observed in patients who are severely immunosuppressed may partially be caused by limited environment exposure or reduced ability of this species to reactivate in the host, rather than a specific tropism or augmented virulence for individuals who are immunocompetent compared with those who are immunosuppressed.

Recent studies on the largest reported outbreak of human cryptococcosis show interesting fungal epidemiologic features and dramatic evolutionary drift. Before 1999, no evidence of *C gattii* infections existed on Vancouver Island, but their sudden emergence since 1999 is well documented [38]. Study of the environment on this island showed a striking change in the environmental niches for this species to a variety of trees in a temperate climate. The incidence of *C gattii* infections on this island was found to be the highest in the world and 37 times greater than that reported in Australia, where *C gattii* is considered endemic [1,36]. The disease was shown to produce substantial morbidity and mortality rates. All of the clinical isolates from Vancouver Island's outbreak were alpha-mating type [1]. Furthermore, using polymerase chain reaction fingerprinting and amplified fragment length polymorphism (AFLP) of the isolates, most cases ($\sim$95%) were shown to be caused by *C gattii* molecular type VG II/AFLP6 and a small number by molecular type VGI/AFLP4 [1]. All of the environmental isolates belonged to molecular type VGII/AFLP6, showing the potential direct link between the environmental and clinical isolates. In fact, further genotypic analysis with multilocus sequencing of the isolates showed that the outbreak strains were clonal and seemed to have descended from two alpha-mating–type parents (same-sex mating) [39]. The minority isolate (VGI/AFLP4) is hypothesized to have mated with another alpha-mating–type isolate to create the outbreak strain VGII/AFLP6. This majority isolate was also found to be much more virulent in an animal model than the parental strain.

This outbreak of disease and molecular studies of isolates may be one of the first examples in medical mycology in which a defined genetic recombinational event in nature has yielded a hypervirulent yeast strain leading to an infectious disease epidemic. Most of the individuals infected with *C gattii* in this outbreak were immunocompetent, and pulmonary cryptococcosis accounted for approximately 70% of cases. Cryptococcomas were also common in the brains of patients who had central nervous system (CNS) involvement [40]. Many of the prominent features that are more common in infections from *C gattii* than in those from *C neoformans* were seen in these patients [7,36,41]. The Vancouver Island's outbreak dramatically high-lighted the potential for rapid, novel change in ecology, clinical manifesta-tions, and molecular virulence characteristics of certain cryptococcal strains. Some researchers have considered that all pathogenic cryptococcal strains produce similar clinical manifestations and prognosis, which to some extent is true. However, increasing evidence suggests some differences between *C neoformans* and *C gattii* strains, and even within these cryptococ-cal species (serotype A vs. serotype D), and these differences may impact clinical disease. The evolution of the ecology and virulence characteristics in these yeasts can occur rapidly and must be watched closely.

Pathogenesis

Well-characterized links exist between environmental sources of *C neo-formans* and cryptococcosis [42,43]. For instance, clinical isolates have been reported to have the same molecular typing to environmental isolates [44,45] and show identical antifungal susceptibility pattern [45,46]. Thus, it is firmly established that *Cryptococcus* infects humans from environmental exposures. The portal of entry of *Cryptococcus* is primarily through inhala-tion of the infectious propagules from the environment. Considering the size, either dehydrated yeast cells or basidiospores are able to be inhaled and deposited in the alveoli ($<$ 5–10 µm), but which structure is actually the primary infectious propagule remains uncertain. Besides through the re-spiratory and gastrointestinal tracts, direct inoculation into tissue from trauma and transplantation of infected tissue can be the portal of entry in occasional cases [4]. After the fungus enters the human body of susceptible hosts, it can either produce latent infection or acute disease. Initial disease manifestations are likely controlled by the inoculum, immune status of the host, or virulence of the strain. Unfortunately, no convincing or precise studies show specific genetic polymorphisms associated with increased sus-ceptibility to cryptococcal disease, although these undoubtedly exist. Latent cryptococcal infection in a lymph node complex is considered similar to the pathophysiology of tuberculosis and can reactivate to produce disease after an asymptomatic initial dormant infection [47]. These latent asymptomatic individuals can be discovered through positive cryptococcal skin testing for delayed hypersensitivity to *Cryptococcus* or through a serologic test for the fungus [48,49], but these laboratory tests are not used in clinical practice, and antibody serology only provides the magnitude of the infection rate [50]. These serologic studies suggest that the rate of asymptomatic crypto-coccal infection is extremely high in certain geographic locales.

Cell-mediated immunity is the most important arm of host defenses against *C neoformans* and *C gattii* and patients who have compromised cell-mediated immunity have the highest risk for acquiring cryptococcosis. A strong cell-mediated immune response is believed to be crucial for con-taining cryptococcal infection and producing granulomatous inflammation

[51,52]. In many circumstances, the yeasts can remain dormant for years in hilar lymph nodes or pulmonary foci of an asymptomatic individual, and then the yeasts may grow and disseminate outside these host immune complexes when the local cellular immunity is suppressed [53]. For example when the fungus enters alveoli, it is processed by alveolar macrophages, and then other inflammatory cells are recruited through cytokines and chemokines, such as interleukin (IL)-12, IL-18, monocyte chemotactic protein (MCP)-1, and macrophage inflammatory protein 1α. Studies by Uicker and colleagues [52] supported this Th1 paradigm in mice, whereby they observed an increased expression of IL-1β, tumor necrosis factor α (TNF-α), interferon γ (IFN-γ), MCP-1, and RANTES in *C neoformans*–infected brains of immune mice compared with control mice. These results suggested that cytokines and chemokines are associated with the protective immune response and correlate with protection against *C neoformans* even in the CNS [52]. Cryptococcal infection primarily involves granulomatous inflammation, which is caused by a helper T-cell (Th1) response with cytokines such as TNF-α, IFN-γ, and IL-2, but reduced Th2 cytokines IL-4 IL-5, and IL-10. In fact, even placing a functional murine gamma interferon gene into a *C neoformans* strain to up-regulate the local Th1 response can at the site of infection aid in its own destruction and, furthermore, create an inflammatory milieu to protect against a second cryptococcal challenge [54].

These basic science studies on immunity are being confirmed as they are transferred to clinical practice. For instance, studies in humans have documented high cerebrospinal fluid (CSF) IL-10 levels in patients who are immunosuppressed who have cryptococcal meningitis, and have shown that a defective production of IFN-γ and TNF-α, but not IL-10, occurs in patients who have cryptococcosis, indicating a predominant Th2 host response [55,56]. However, during treatment at the CNS site of cryptococcal infection, an up-regulated Th1 response occurs, measured by higher CSF IFN-γ levels and lower CSF yeast cell counts, and this cytokine elevation correlated with an improved clinical response [57]. In an illustrative case, antifungal therapy in a patient who was HIV-negative who had cryptococcal meningitis was shown to help change a Th2 to a Th1 inflammatory response in the CNS that was associated initially with an exacerbation of clinical and radiologic signs of infection (immune reconstitution inflammatory syndrome [IRIS]), but the yeast infection was ultimately eradicated [56].

Current studies on the molecular biology of cryptococcal pathogenesis have validated several virulence factors in *C neoformans* and *C gattii* at the gene level. Both *Cryptococcus* spp are attractive for molecular virulence studies because they are primary fungal pathogens that cause invasive mycoses in healthy and immunocompromised hosts. The genome-wide sequencing availability [3], ease of targeted gene deletions in *Cryptococcus* [58], and robust animal models allow insightful study of molecular fungal pathogenesis. The three known classical virulence factors of *Cryptococcus* are capsule formation, melanin pigment production [59,60], and ability to grow well at 37°C [61,62]. The prominent antiphagocytic polysaccharide capsule, which is comprised of glucuronoxylomannan (GXM), is unique to *Cryptococcus* spp and is considered as an essential virulence factor that has multiple effects on host immunity [2]. Capsule formation is controlled by many genes, and creation of null mutants with hypocapsular or acapsular phenotype in *C neoformans* consistently exhibit an attenuated phenotype in animals [63–65]. Although occasionally a natural, poorly encapsulated strain has been observed to cause disease in humans, these strains are rare [66]. Furthermore, phenotypic colony switching has been discovered in *C neoformans* and can occur during chronic infection. The strain alters its polysaccharide capsule and cell wall, which can rapidly affect the yeast's ability to resist phagocytosis through host immunity. Furthermore, a recent study has shown that the mucoid colony variant, but not the smooth variant, can promote increased intracerebral pressure in a rat model of cryptococcal meningitis [67]. Thus, rapid phenotypic variability exists within this yeast in response to changing local environments, which adds greater flexibility to an isolate and likely improves its ability to be a good pathogen [68].

In addition, *C neoformans* possesses an enzyme that catalyzes the conversion of diphenolic compounds to melanin (observed in many pathogenic fungi) to potentially protect the yeasts from host oxidative stresses [2]. Melanin is produced by a laccase enzyme, which is encoded by two paralogs, the *LAC1* and *LAC2* genes, and is an important virulence factor for *Cryptococcus*. Laccase is regulated under various environmental signals, such as nutrient starvation, multivalent cations, and temperature stress, and is mediated through multiple signal transduction pathways [69]. Another classical virulence factor of *C neoformans* and *C gattii* is their ability to grow at human body temperature (37°C), which is a basic part of the virulence composite for most human pathogenic fungi. In *C neoformans*, high-temperature growth has also been shown to be linked with many genes and certain signaling pathways [70]. As understanding increases of how this pathogenic fungus grows at high temperature, knowledge of how it has become a pathogen will also likely increase. Several other virulence factors with identified genes include the alpha-mating–type locus [16,71,72], the secretory phospholipase B [73], urease production [74], and enzymes associated with protection against oxidative stresses [75,76].

Recent studies in molecular pathogenesis of *C neoformans* have begun to study families of genes and genetic linkage groups. Several signal transduction pathways regulating differentiation and virulence in *C neoformans* have been discovered [77,78]. For instance, a conserved G-protein alpha subunit (Gpa1)/cyclic adenosine monophosphate pathway was found to control melanin and capsule production and to sense nutrients during mating and disease production [78]. The conserved multigenic cascade involves genes encoding Gpa1, adenylyl cyclase, protein kinase A catalytic subunit, and the regulatory subunit Pkr1 [79–83], and is regulated by the adenyl cyclase–associated protein, Aca1 [84]. It can be manipulated to decrease and increase the virulence potential of strains. Another signaling cascade is a conserved mitogen-activated protein kinase (MAPK) cascade that senses pheromone during mating, and also regulates haploid fruiting and virulence [78]. Recently, the conserved Pbs2–Hog1 MAPK cascade was found to control morphologic differentiation and virulence factors in serotype A but not serotype D, therefore emphasizing serotype-specific differences in the role of signaling cascades in the pathogenesis of cryptococcosis, even in very closely related species or varieties [85]. High-temperature growth in *C neoformans* is regulated by two other signal transduction pathways, the RAS (Ras1/Ras2) signaling cascade [62,86] and the calcineurin-dependent pathway [87].

The secretory mechanisms of some virulence factors in *C neoformans* have also been studied. For instance, phospholipase B was found to attach the yeast to a lipid raft membrane with a glycosylphosphatidylinositol anchor before it is cleaved [88]. In fact, superoxide dismutase and phospholipase B are concentrated in lipid raft membranes before they are cleaved and secreted, which has raised the hypothesis that lipid raft membranes may cluster certain virulence enzymes at the yeast cell surface and therefore may impact pathogenesis of cryptococcosis [89]. Experts have just begun to understand the regulation and mechanistic behavior of the virulence composite, but the molecular infrastructure and preliminary studies already clearly show great potential for further understanding how this yeast has become a premier pathogen in clinical medicine.

Clinical manifestations

The CNS and respiratory tract are the most common organs involved in *C neoformans* and *C gattii* infections. Other prominent infected organs include skin, prostate, eyes, bone, urinary tract, and blood. In fact, this yeast can cause disease in every organ of the human body, and widely disseminated cryptococcal infection can occur in multiple organs in patients who are severely immunosuppressed [4]. Previously, infections caused by *C neoformans* and *C gattii* were considered to have similar clinical manifestations. However, increasing evidence, including the Vancouver Island outbreak, confirms that different clinical manifestations between these two species may occur [7,36,41]. For example, *C gattii* causes disease primarily in immunocompetent hosts who have prominent inflammatory masses, and commonly produces neurologic sequelae that require surgery or prolonged antifungal therapy [7]. The presentation of cryptococcosis has a few differences among patients infected with HIV compared with those not infected [4]. HIV-associated cryptococcosis produces more CNS and extrapulmonary involvement, higher rate of positive India ink examinations, positive blood cultures, and fewer CSF inflammatory cells. These clinical results suggest that patients infected with HIV present with high burden of organisms and poor inflammatory reactions at the site of infection, and a similar presentation could potentially occur in a severely immunocompromised host from other causes of severe CD4-lymphocytopenia.

Respiratory system

As the most important portal of entry for this fungus, the lung is one of the most common sites of cryptococcal infection, producing several clinical manifestations of pulmonary cryptococcosis. Pulmonary cryptococcosis varies from an asymptomatic infection with yeast colonization of the airway or an abnormal radiograph as a solitary nodule to a life-threatening fungal pneumonia [4,90]. Asymptomatic pulmonary cryptococcosis can occur in approximately one third of normal hosts who have pulmonary cryptococcal infection [91], and patients may present only with an abnormal chest radiograph, even those who are immunocompromised, such as those who have undergone transplantation [92]. Patients who have acute pulmonary cryptococcosis can manifest symptoms such as fever, productive cough, chest pain, and weight loss [91,93]. In a review of 24 patients who had cryptococcosis, cough was the most common symptom, experienced by 83% of patients [94]. However, symptomatic pulmonary cryptococcosis can even present with acute respiratory failure [95], especially in those who have severe immunocompromised conditions. Although clinical and radiologic manifestations of cryptococcal lung infection are nonspecific and usually occur in hosts who are severely immunocompromised (eg, those who have AIDS) [96], fulminant pulmonary cryptococcosis with or without extrapulmonary involvement has also been reported in patients who are apparently immunocompetent [97]. In fact, in the outbreak of *C gattii* infections in Vancouver Island, several cases of severe symptomatic pulmonary cryptococcosis occurred in individuals who were apparently immunocompetent.

Radiographic presentations are varied. Well-defined single or multiple pulmonary nodules are the most frequent radiologic abnormality [94], followed by pulmonary infiltrates. Furthermore, cavitation within nodules and parenchymal consolidation are more common in patients who are immunocompromised than in those who are immunocompetent [94]. Other less frequent radiographic findings include pleural effusions, hilar lymphadenopathy, diffuse reticulonodular opacities [98], endobronchial lesion resulting in airway obstruction with lung collapse [98,99], and findings mimicking pulmonary metastasis [100,101]. Patients who are immunocompromised who have pulmonary cryptococcosis generally have the same chest radiograph findings as patients who are immunocompetent, except that alveolar and interstitial infiltrates tend to be more frequent and can potentially mimic pneumocystis pneumonia. Patients who are immunocompromised who have cryptococcal infection usually present with CNS rather than pulmonary symptoms. In fact, more than 90% of patients who have HIV/AIDS who have pulmonary cryptococcal infection already have CNS cryptococcosis at diagnosis. In contrast, CNS involvement in pulmonary cryptococcosis in patients not infected with HIV is less common. For example, in a retrospective study, CSF examination for cryptococcal meningoencephalitis in 11 patients not infected with HIV who had no CNS symptoms but *C neoformans* isolated from lung all showed negative results [101]. In pulmonary cryptococcosis, if the infection is confined to the lung, serum cryptococcal polysaccharide antigen is usually negative and a positive serum polysaccharide antigen may indicate dissemination of the yeast from the lung. Thus, an asymptomatic patient who is immunocompetent who has cryptococcal lung involvement and negative serum polysaccharide antigen does not necessarily need a screening lumbar puncture to rule out CNS disease. However, a lumbar puncture to rule out CNS disease is generally considered in patients who are immunocompromised who have pulmonary cryptococcosis, regardless of symptoms.

Central nervous system

C neoformans and *C gattii* have a predilection to invade the CNS and can cause a life-threatening meningoencephalitis. Patients can present with acute, subacute or chronic meningitis, or meningoencephalitis. These signs and symptoms are usually present for several weeks and include headache, fever, cranial neuropathy, alteration of consciousness, lethargy, memory loss, meningeal irritation signs, and coma [4,90]. However, occasionally symptoms may occur over only several days or, in contrast, may be chronic with symptoms measured over months. Patients infected with HIV can present with symptoms of acute or intermittent headaches or with an altered mental status without signs of meningeal irritation, even though the burden of fungal organisms in the CNS is high. These patients may have a short onset of signs and symptoms, high CSF polysaccharide antigen titers, high intracranial pressures, and slow CSF sterilization after starting antifungal treatment. However, patients who are less immunosuppressed can present with subacute or chronic complaints of headaches or altered mental status. Without specific risk factors, this presentation can delay diagnosis and potentially lead to a poor prognosis despite the lack of a serious underlying disease [102].

With the use of HAART or a rapid change in immunosuppressive therapies, patients who have cryptococcal meningitis during therapy can present with signs and symptoms that are indistinguishable from progressive cryptococcal meningitis/meningoencephalitis, such as worsening headaches, new lesions noted on MRI scan, and elevated intracranial pressures. However, cultures from clinical specimens are always negative for cryptococci, although the yeasts may be observed under microscopy on a specimen. Identification of IRIS has major implications for treatment strategies because it is not an antifungal treatment failure, but a host immunity issue that must be controlled. Occasionally reports arise of patients who are not infected with HIV in whom cryptococcal meningitis is only mildly symptomatic or asymptomatic [33]. Although individuals who are immunocompetent and those who are immunocompromised can have similar syndromes of CNS cryptococcosis, some differences in etiology, clinical manifestations, and outcomes of CNS cryptococcosis exist between these groups. In a retrospective study of 46 patients who had culture- or histology-confirmed cryptococcosis, 20 were apparently immunocompetent. Among this group, three of eight (37.5%) isolates were caused by *C gattii*, whereas all six culture-positive isolates from patients who were immunocompromised were caused by *C neoformans* var *grubii* [103]. Patients who were immunocompetent and had CNS disease more commonly presented with meningitis (80%) and had a lower rate of fungemia (10%) and mortality (25%). Moreover, cryptococcal meningitis in patients who were immunocompetent also had a longer mean time from illness onset to presentation and more intense inflammatory responses [103].

However, a recent report of cryptococcal meningitis in nine patients who were immunocompetent provided a sobering report on outcome. Death occurred in four patients and significant morbidity was produced by a profound inflammatory response [102]. *C gattii* has a predilection to cause disease in brain parenchyma rather than meninges, resulting in more evidence of cerebral cryptococcomas or hydrocephalus. These patients who have brain parenchymal involvement usually have high intracranial pressure, cranial neuropathies, and a poor response to antifungal therapy [7,41].

Immune reconstitution inflammatory syndrome

An important clinical concept emerged over the past decade that has been associated with the rapid changes in immunity in some patients who have cryptococcosis. It is a consequence of the dramatic swings in immunologic responses in certain patient groups. The condition is IRIS, in which new or worsening of clinical or radiographic manifestations occur that are consistent with an inflammatory process but negative studies for biomarkers or cultures. IRIS has been reported to occur in 30% to 35% of patients infected with HIV who have cryptococcosis in whom HAART was initiated. Usual time to onset of IRIS is 4 to 6 weeks after initiation of HAART and is associated with decreasing viral load and increasing CD4 counts. Patients infected with HIV who have cryptococcal meningitis and IRIS have a greater fungal burden, as indicated by higher CSF antigen titer and the presence of disseminated infection or fungemia. IRIS is most prominently featured in patients undergoing treatment with a combination of protease inhibitor or non-nucleoside reverse transcriptase inhibitors [104–109].

IRIS in cryptococcal meningitis is not limited to HIV and HAART. In fact, it can arise in any situation in which a rapid change in immune status occurs. For instance, in 5% of patients who had cryptococcosis who had undergone solid organ transplantation, IRIS was observed a median of

5.5 weeks (range, 4–12 weeks) after antifungal therapy was initiated. Patients who had IRIS who had undergone transplantation were more likely to have been treated with potent immunosuppressive regimens (a combination of tacrolimus, mycophenolate mofetil, and prednisone) compared with patients who had cryptococcal meningitis but not IRIS [110]. Similar to patients infected with HIV, those who had undergone transplantation and had higher cryptococcal antigen titers and disseminated disease were more likely to develop IRIS after initiation of therapy [110], and graft survival was reduced in these patients [111]. Complications of IRIS are not limited to patients infected with HIV and those who have undergone transplantation, but have been shown in patients who had cryptococcal meningitis during pregnancy and those who experienced postpartum IRIS [56]. It is also likely that management of cryptococcal meningitis in apparently normal hosts is complicated by the occurrence of IRIS as treatment is started [102]. The ability to precisely diagnose this condition and specifically treat it remains a therapeutic challenge for clinicians, but it clearly cannot be ignored in the successful management of some cases. It is a two-edged sword: successful management needs immunity to eradicate fungus, but not too much.

Skin

Cutaneous cryptococcal infections are the third most common clinical site of cryptococcosis. Serotype D strains are reported to be associated with a propensity to cause cutaneous lesions [112]. However, cutaneous cryptococcosis produced by other serotypes have been reported in immunocompromised and immunocompetent hosts [113–116], and this clinical presentation can be either a primary cutaneous infection from direct inoculation or a secondary lesion as part of disseminated disease. A cohort of patients who had undergone solid organ transplantation and were receiving tacrolimus appeared to be more likely to develop skin, soft tissue, or osteoarticular cryptococcal involvement [117]. Tacrolimus has anticryptococcal activity at high temperatures, but loses this activity as environmental temperatures decrease [118], which may explain the frequency of cutaneous cryptococcosis with its lower body temperatures in solid organ transplants. However, despite this series of patients, in our experience, the most common site of disseminated infection in patients who have undergone solid organ transplantation, including those undergoing tacrolimus therapy, is still the CNS.

Primary cutaneous cryptococcosis has been considered a distinct syndrome and is different from cutaneous cryptococcosis secondary to hematogenous dissemination. For instance, review of cryptococcosis cases associated with skin lesions reported in the French National Registry has shown that patients who had primary cutaneous cryptococcosis differed significantly from those who had secondary cutaneous cryptococcosis or other forms of the disease. Patients who have primary cutaneous cryptococcosis are more likely to live in a rural area, are older age, and have no underlying disease. Primary cutaneous cryptococcosis may be associated with a solitary skin lesion presenting as a whitlow or phlegmon, a history of skin injury, participation in outdoor activities, exposure to bird droppings, and isolation of *C neoformans* serotype D [119]. Risk factors for cutaneous *C gattii* infection include exposure to the eucalypt reservoirs in tropical and subtropical areas [120]. Despite these cases of primary cutaneous infection, most skin infections occur in patients who are immunosuppressed as a secondary manifestation of disseminated disease.

In general, patients who have skin cryptococcosis can manifest many types of skin lesions. A common skin lesion for patients infected with HIV is a papule or maculopapule with central ulceration that may be described as a molluscum contagiosum-like lesion. These lesions cannot be distinguished from those found in infections caused by *Histoplasma capsulatum*, *Coccidioides immitis*, or *Penicillium marneffei*. Other cutaneous lesions of cryptococcosis include acneiform lesions, purpura, vesicles, nodules, abscesses, ulcers, granulomas, pustules, plaques, draining sinus, and cellulitis. Because many skin manifestations in cryptococcosis mimic other infections caused by various microorganisms, biopsy of the skin lesion with culture and histopathology is therefore essential for definitive diagnosis, especially in patients who are immunocompromised.

Prostate

Prostatic cryptococcosis is usually asymptomatic and, in fact, the prostate gland is considered a site for yeast sequestration after an occult or treated disseminated infection and protected from the antifungal treatments. It can be an important reservoir for relapse of cryptococcosis in patients who have a high burden of yeasts [121]. A latent *C neoformans* infection of the prostate has even been recognized to spread into the blood during urologic surgery on the prostate [122]. Diagnosis of prostatic cryptococcosis can be achieved by using ultrasound-guided prostatic biopsy with fungal culture or histopathology of prostatic tissue. In fact, high levels of prostate-specific antigen (PSA), which may represent prostatic inflammation, were recognized in prostatic cryptococcosis in a patient who underwent renal transplantation [123]. After initial induction antifungal treatment of cryptococcal meningoencephalitis in patients who have AIDS, urine or seminal fluid cultures may still be positive for yeasts [124]; therefore, the prostate might be an important site for relapsed infections if therapy is discontinued early and immune reconstitution has not occurred.

Eye

Ocular signs and symptoms were noted in approximately 45% of patients in the reports of cryptococcal meningoencephalitis before the HIV/AIDS era [125]. The most common manifestations are ocular palsies and papilledema. However, in the present HIV/AIDS era, several other manifestations of ocular cryptococcosis have been identified, such as bilateral retinal and peripapillary hemorrhages [126] and the presence of extensive retinal lesions with or without vitritis, which can lead to blindness. A study of neuro-ophthalmologic disorders using the visual evoked potential (VEP) in patients infected with HIV showed that 60% of these patients who were neurologically symptomatic had an abnormal neuro-ophthalmologic examination, and that cryptococcosis was one of the most frequently associated pathologies [127]. Furthermore, catastrophic loss of vision without evidence of endophthalmitis has also been reported [128]. Ocular manifestations of cryptococcal infection and vision loss may be caused by two pathogenic processes. The first process is caused by infiltration of the optic nerve by the yeasts and produces a rapid visual loss with few effective treatments. The second process is caused by increased intracranial pressure and leads to a slower visual loss. This process of visual loss can be prevented or slowed down through treatment with ventricular shunts [4].

Other body sites

C neoformans and *C gattii* can cause diseases in all parts of the human body. Cryptococcal infection of bone and joints can present with osteolytic lesions or arthritis. Cryptococcal peritonitis [129] and cryptococcuria are also reported in several case series [130]. Cryptococcemia can occur in patients who are severely immunosuppressed, such as those who have AIDS, but rarely causes endocarditis on either native or prosthetic valves. Manifestations in other organs of cryptococcosis include mycotic aortitis/aneurysm, myositis, genital lesions, hepatitis, thyroiditis, adrenal mass, gingivitis, sinusitis, salivary gland involvement, neck mass, esophagitis, biliary tract involvement, enteritis, mastitis, breast mass, and lymphadenopathy [90].

Laboratory diagnosis

Several laboratory methods for diagnosing cryptococcosis have been established, including direct examination of the fungus in body fluids, cytology or histopathology of infected tissues using several staining techniques, serologic studies, or culture.

Direct examination of specimens

A widely used, low-tech, rapid, and inexpensive diagnostic test for cryptococcal meningitis is direct microscopic examination for the presence of encapsulated yeasts using an India ink preparation of CSF [90]. This technique can be performed immediately after a lumber puncture to visualize the round encapsulated yeast cells that range from 5 to 20 μm in diameter and are rapidly distinguished in a colloidal medium of India ink when mixed with CSF. An India ink examination usually allows detection of yeasts in a CSF specimen when between 10^3 and 10^4 colony-forming units of yeasts are present per milliliter of CSF or greater concentrations. This simple India ink preparation technique is 30% to 50% sensitive in cases of non-AIDS cryptococcal meningitis and up to 80% sensitive in AIDS-related cryptococcal meningitis. Centrifuging the CSF specimen and using the pellet for India ink preparation can improve the sensitivity of the test, but can also cause the production of pseudo-cryptococcal artifacts from lysed lymphocytes [131,132]. Myelin globules, fat droplets, and tissue cells can also cause false-positive results. Another potential false-positive result can be caused by carbon particles in the India ink being repelled by leukocytes in the CSF, forming a halo around the cell that suggests the presence of a capsule that might be misinterpreted as cryptococci. This effect does not seem to occur with nigrosin, which is free from discernible particulate matter [133,134]. The observation that dead yeast cells can remain in the CSF and be seen through India ink examination for varying periods during and after appropriate antifungal treatment and despite negative culture limits the usefulness of direct microscopy of CSF during management of cryptococcal meningitis [135].

Histopathology

Histologic stains of tissues from lungs, skin, bone marrow, brain, or other organs [136–141] can be used to identify cryptococci with their prominent capsule. Furthermore, histopathologic staining of centrifuged CSF sediment has been more sensitive for rapid diagnosis of cryptococcal meningitis than the India ink method [142]. Other body fluids and fine needle aspiration (FNA) specimens obtained from various body sites, such as lymph nodes [143], adrenal glands [144], or vitreous aspiration [145], can also be properly used for cytologic study. Percutaneous transthoracic FNA under real-time ultrasound guidance for pulmonary nodules, masses, or infiltrative lesions can be performed safely and accurately to diagnose pulmonary cryptococcosis [146–148]. Other specimens that can be used for cytologic examination include peritoneal fluid from chronic ambulatory peritoneal dialysis [149], seminal fluid [150], and bronchoalveolar lavage fluid [151,152].

A simple Gram stain is not optimal for identifying this yeast, but may show cryptococci as a poorly stained gram-positive budding yeast [90,149]. However, cryptococci in tissue or fluids can be stained using other methods. The nonspecific stains include Papanicolaou's, hematoxylin-eosin, Diff-Quick, May-Giemsa, and Riu's, and acridine orange preparations. Specific stains are also available for diagnosing cryptococcosis. Fungal chitin can be stained with Calcofluor, and its cell wall can be visualized with Gomori's methenamine silver stain [90,144,146,151,153]. Sensitivity of acridine orange staining followed by fluorescence microscopy is comparable to an India ink examination and detection of cryptococcal capsular polysaccharide antigen using latex agglutination [154]. As a unique component in cryptococci, the polysaccharide capsular material can be stained and visualized using several specific methods to help identify the yeasts. These staining techniques include Mayer's mucicarmine, periodic acid–Schiff, and alcian blue stains [90,155–157]. In rare instances of cryptococcal infections caused by poorly encapsulated cryptococci [158,159], the yeast may be identified only through Gomori's methenamine silver stain or Fontana-Masson silver stain, which identifies melanin in the yeast cell wall [160]. Combinations of Fontana-Masson silver stain and specific polysaccharide stains, such as alcian blue and mucicarmine, will distinctively show the cell wall and capsule of most cryptococci. The alcian blue stain combined with the periodic acid–Schiff reaction is also helpful in identifying cryptococci [161].

Serology

Serum cryptococcal antibodies are not helpful in diagnosing and deciding treatment for cryptococcosis, although some experts suggest that their presence favors a good prognostic sign [135,162] and a better response to therapy [163]. Problems with the serum cryptococcal antibodies test include its poor sensitivity and specificity performance. For instance, an indirect fluorescent antibody test for serum cryptococcal antibodies can be falsely positive in patients undergoing a cryptococcal skin test and in those infected with *Blastomyces dermatitidis* and *H capsulatum* [163]. Furthermore, sensitivity and specificity of the immunodiffusion test for serum cryptococcal antibodies can vary widely depending on the method of antigen preparation and several other factors [164]. Using cryptococcal antibodies in diagnosing cryptococcal infection was further complicated by the type of cryptococcal infection and timing of antibody presence. Apparently, the antibody test was often positive in the absence of overt disease and therefore has been devalued as a test for diagnosing acute cryptococcal infections [165]. Moreover, considering the immunologically paralyzed status of patients infected with HIV and those who are severely immunosuppressed, these antibody tests have limited usefulness for diagnosing cryptococcosis in such patients who have high burdens of yeasts.

However, detection of cryptococcal capsular polysaccharide antigen in serum or body fluids has performed robustly for many years and is one of the most useful serologic tests in mycology. The test uses latex particles coated with polyclonal cryptococcal capsular antibodies. In general, all commercially available kits for cryptococcal (latex agglutination) antigen tests can detect at least 10 ng of polysaccharide per milliliter of biologic fluids [166]. Correlation has been seen between initial CSF antigen titer and burden of yeast at the CNS site through quantitative cultures [167]. The sensitivity and specificity of these latex agglutination kits for cryptococcal antigen depend on the commercial kits and type of specimens, but overall sensitivities and specificities were found to be 93% to 100% and 93% to 98%, respectively [168–173], and false-positive results of the tests are approximately 0% to 0.4% [170,171].

Rheumatoid factor is one of the most common causes of false-positive results of latex agglutination tests of cryptococcal polysaccharide antigen and has been found more frequently in serum specimens [174–176] than in CSF specimens [177]. However, false-positive results caused by rheumatoid factor and other interference factors can be eliminated through heating serum specimens at 56°C for 30 minutes [174] and CSF specimens at 100°C for 10 minutes [162], or pretreating with dithiothreitol [175,177], 2-β-mercaptoethanol [178,179], or a protease enzyme. Other factors that cause false-positive results include infections with *Trichosporon beigelii* [180,181], *Stomatococcus mucilaginosus* [182], *Capnocytophaga canimorsus* [183], and *Klebsiella pneumoniae* [184], and contamination by syneresis fluid transferred from agar plates through pipetting that was heat stable [168,185]. However, most of the false-positive results had initial reciprocal titers of less than or equal to 8 [169] except in patients who had *T beigelii* infections, who can have titers as high as 1000 [180,181]. Therefore, results of these low titers must be carefully interpreted within the clinical context [162,186].

Prozone effect was described as a cause of false-negative results in a latex cryptococcal polysaccharide antigen agglutination test of CSF [174,187]. Thus, experts recommended that a CSF specimen with positive findings on India ink examination but negative results with the cryptococcal polysaccharide antigen test should be diluted and retested [187]. Furthermore, a low fungal burden, such as in chronic "low-grade" cryptococcal meningitis or very early stages of cryptococcal infection, can also cause apparent false-negative results in cryptococcal polysaccharide antigen tests [174].

Enzyme immunoassay for detecting and quantifying cryptococcal polysaccharide antigen of all four serotypes of *C neoformans* in sera and CSF is also commercially available. This test detects the major component of the polysaccharide capsule, GXM [188], and possesses sensitivities and specificities of 85.2% to 99% and 97%, respectively [169,189], with 84.6% to 97.8% agreement with latex cryptococcal polysaccharide antigen agglutination tests [169,190,191]. Enzyme immunoassay for cryptococcal polysaccharide antigen did not provide discrepant results with rheumatoid factor, syneresis fluid, or serum macroglobulins, and therefore specimens did not need to be pretreated with pronase [189,192].

Although using latex agglutination tests to detect cryptococcal polysaccharide antigen in other fluids, such as bronchoalveolar lavage fluid, is not as well studied, detecting cryptococcal antigen in CSF or serum is rapid, specific, noninvasive, and virtually diagnostic of meningoencephalitic or disseminated cryptococcosis at high titer even when the India ink examination or culture is negative [193–195]. The term *isolated cryptococcal polysaccharidemia* describes a condition in very high-risk patients who have a positive cryptococcal antigen titer and no positive cultures or prominent symptoms [90,188,196]. A study of patients infected with HIV in Uganda found that the frequency of asymptomatic isolated cryptococcal antigenemia among patients who had positive serum cryptococcal polysaccharide antigen was

38.1% (8 of 21), and that all were extremely immunosuppressed [196]. Follow-up studies suggest that an isolated positive latex agglutination assay of four or more in serum or CSF in patients who have AIDS should be regarded as an early sign of invasive cryptococcosis and likely requires prompt treatment if the patient is known to be at high-risk for disease. Therefore, patients who have isolated cryptococcal antigenemia who are in a high-risk group for disease would probably benefit from antifungal therapy for preventing or delaying development of overt cryptococcosis [188].

Baseline cryptococcal polysaccharide antigen titers in serum and CSF have been shown to be useful in predicting outcome in patients who have cryptococcal meningitis [163] and can be correlated with burden of yeasts, but serum cryptococcal polysaccharide antigen titers may have less correlation with infection outcome in patients who have AIDS and others who are severely immunosuppressed [197]. On the other hand, initial CSF cryptococcal polysaccharide antigen may be more precise in predicting outcome in patients infected with HIV who have cryptococcal meningitis. A study in HIV-related acute cryptococcal meningitis indicated that a baseline titer of CSF cryptococcal polysaccharide antigen of 1:1024 or more was a predictor of death during systemic antifungal treatment [198]. After initiation of systemic antifungal therapy, most patients whose infection responded to treatment experienced falling titers of cryptococcal polysaccharide antigen [195]. Some correlation occurred between unchanged or increased titers (titers rise by at least two dilutions or by fourfold) of CSF cryptococcal polysaccharide antigen and a higher risk for clinical and microbiologic failure to respond to treatment. This correlation was especially strong among patients whose baseline CSF cryptococcal polysaccharide antigen titers were eight or more. Also, a rise in CSF cryptococcal polysaccharide antigen titers during suppressive therapy has been associated with cryptococcal meningitis relapse [197]. However, using changing antigen titers to make decisions during therapy is not precise. The kinetics of polysaccharide antigen elimination remains unclear, and despite the accuracy of commercial kits for diagnosis, the accuracy of titers can vary among kits even with the same specimen, and therefore serial antigen titer changes should probably not be used to make antifungal decisions during therapy.

Culture and identification

C neoformans and *C gattii* can be grown easily from biologic samples on routine standard fungal and bacterial culture media, and its colonies can usually be observed on solid agar plates after 48 to 72 hours incubation at 30°C to 35°C in aerobic conditions. *C neoformans* and *C gattii* are consistently able to grow at 37°C. The growth rates of *C neoformans* strains are significantly reduced at temperatures between 39°C and 40°C, and the more temperature-sensitive strains of *C gattii* will die when temperatures exceed 40°C. In fact, *C neoformans* var *grubii* generally tends to be more thermotolerant than *C neoformans* var *neoformans* and *C gattii* [199]. The yeasts, however, do not grow in the presence of cycloheximide at the concentration used in selective isolation media. Notably, in patients undergoing systemic antifungal therapy, cryptococci may require more time to produce visible colonies (ie, more than 1 week). On the other hand, negative cultures may occur despite positive India ink examinations because of nonviable yeast cells that may have prolonged persistence at the infection site. The radiometric methods, such as the BACTEC system (Becton-Dickinson), are limited in that they may not identify positive cultures when the numbers of yeasts in the blood are very low [200]. Therefore, subculture of blood culture bottles from high-risk patients, despite the low radiometric readings, is occasionally recommended. Continuous agitation of BACTEC blood culture bottles for the full incubation time can significantly improve detection and recovery of cryptococci [201]. Negative cultures of CSF in patients who have cryptococcal meningitis may be caused by a low burden of yeasts, such as occurs in some cases of chronic cryptococcal meningitis. Because only a few cryptococcal cells may be present at the infection site, some have suggested culturing pellets from centrifuged CSF, blood, and other body fluids. Furthermore, bronchial secretions and urine, especially from patients who have AIDS, are often contaminated by many microorganisms, including *Candida* spp, whose rapid growth may mask the growth of cryptococci.

Yeasts within genus *Cryptococcus* spp do not produce hyphae or pseudohyphae, but are able to assimilate inositol, and hydrolyze urea. A rapid test to identify *C neoformans* urease activity was developed based on its ability to produce urease [202]. *C neoformans* will become urease-positive within 15 minutes, whereas other urease-positive species of yeasts from clinical specimens require more than 3 hours, and *Candida* spp, which do not produce urease, will be negative [202]. Other formal biochemical profiles of *C neoformans* and *C gattii* show that they are unable to assimilate nitrate, but can use galactose, maltose, and sucrose. They will not assimilate lactose and melibiose, and growth is strain-variable with erythritol. Many micromethod systems are commercially available for identifying *C neoformans* using carbohydrate assimilation, generally requiring 24-hour incubation. Commercial multitest identification systems, based on detection of preformed enzymes that can identify yeasts with chromogenic substrates within 4 hours of inoculation, are also available [203]. A DNA probe for ribosomal RNA (rRNA) can confirm or identify a yeast isolate as *C neoformans* with 100% sensitivity and specificity and is also commercially available [204].

Management

Management of cryptococcosis has been well studied, resulting in some general agreements about recommendations for treatment. The Infectious Diseases Society of America proposed the 2000 Practice Guidelines for the Management of Cryptococcal Disease, which are summarized in Box 2

Box 2. Treatments of cryptococcal disease

Cryptococcal disease in patients who are HIV-negative
Pulmonary
  Mild-to-moderate symptoms or asymptomatic with culture
  positive from the lungs:
  • Fluconazole, 200 to 400 mg/d, for 6 to 12 months
  • Itraconazole, 200 to 400 mg/d, for 6 to 12 months
  • Amphotericin B, 0.5 to 1 mg/kg/d (total 1 to 2 g)
  Severe symptoms and immunocompromised hosts:
  • Treat like CNS disease
Central nervous system
  Induction/consolidation or clearance therapy:
  • Amphotericin B, 0.7 to 1 mg/kg/d (preferably 0.7 mg/kg/d), plus
    flucytosine, 100 mg/kg/d (assuming normal renal function), for
    2 weeks, then fluconazole, 400-800 mg/d, for minimum 10 weeks
  Alternative regimens:
  • Amphotericin B, 0.3 mg/kg/d, plus flucytosine, 100 mg/kg/d,
    for 6 to 10 weeks
  • Amphotericin B, 0.4 to 1 mg/kg/d, for 6 to 10 weeks
  • Lipid formulation of amphotericin B, 4 to 6 mg/kg/d, for 6 to
    10 weeks, with or without 2 weeks of flucytosine (100 mg/kg/d)
  Suppressive therapy:
  • Fluconazole 200 to 400 mg/d, for completion of 1 year of
    therapy.

Cryptococcal disease in patients infected with HIV
Pulmonary
  Mild-to-moderate symptoms or asymptomatic with culture
  positive from the lungs:
  • Fluconazole, 200 to 400 mg/d, for 1 to 2 years (depending on
    response to HAART)
  Alternative regimen:
  • Itraconazole, 200 to 400 mg/d, for 1 to 2 years (depending on
    response to HAART)
  • Fluconazole, 200 to 400 mg/d, and flucytosine, 100 to
    150 mg/kg/d, for 10 weeks
  Severe symptoms:
  • Treat like CNS disease
Central nervous system[a]
  Induction/consolidation or clearance therapy:
  • Amphotericin B, 0.7 to 1 mg/kg/d (preferably 0.7 mg/kg/d),
    plus flucytosine,100 mg/kg/d, for 2 weeks, then fluconazole,
    400 to 800 mg/d, for minimum 10 weeks

Alternatives regimens:
- Fluconazole, 400 to 800 mg/d, for 10 to 12 weeks
- Fluconazole, 400 to 800 mg/d, plus flucytosine, 100 to 150 mg/kg/d, for 6 to 10 weeks
- Lipid formulation of amphotericin B, 4 to 6 mg/kg/d, for 6 to 10 weeks, with or without flucytosine

Maintenance or suppressive therapy:
- 1 to 2 years and may consider stopping if response to HAART
- Fluconazole, 200 to 400 mg/d

Alternatives regimens:
- Itraconazole, 200 mg/d

Amphotericin B, 1 mg/kg intravenously, one to three times per week

---

Control IRIS with corticosteroids.
[a] Start HAART 8 to 10 weeks after beginning antifungal regimen.
Data from Saag MS, Graybill RJ, Larsen RA, et al. Practice guidelines for the management of cryptococcal disease. Infectious Diseases Society of America. Clin Infect Dis 2000;30(4):710–8.

[205]. These guidelines provide insights for clinicians and can be used at the beginning of treatment to guide clinical decision in caring for patients who have cryptococcosis. Adherence to these guidelines has been shown to generally improve outcome [206]. However, these guidelines are not absolute, and specific clinical situations may dictate creative management plans.

Asymptomatic individuals in whom cryptococci have been isolated from respiratory secretions have been observed without treatment and no clinical relapse has occurred. Approximately 20% of patients who have positive pulmonary cultures do not undergo treatment [207]. Recent reports have shown that 92% of patients who were not immunocompromised who had pulmonary cryptococcosis experienced disease resolution with no treatment, surgical resection only, or antifungal therapy [91]. Therefore, some experts suggest that an initial period of observation without administering antifungal therapy is a reasonable option for these patients who have no systemic symptoms or evidence of dissemination, and after surgical resection for focal cryptococcal pneumonia [91]. However, if viable yeasts are grown from pulmonary specimens, we will generally treat patients with 3 to 6 months of fluconazole, with or without symptoms. This practice is based on the safety of fluconazole and the difficulty in predicting patients' future immune status, but these recommendations can be questioned. We believe that all patients who are immunosuppressed should be treated regardless of symptoms. In symptomatic patients who have limited pulmonary cryptococcosis with or without HIV infection, treatment with an oral regimen of fluconazole is warranted. However, in those who have severe symptoms, treatment similar to that for cryptococcal meningitis is recommended [205].

In cryptococcal meningitis, which can still have poor prognosis and a high mortality rate, and in disseminated cryptococcosis, amphotericin B deoxycholate remains the preferred drug. Cryptococcosis is one of few infections in clinical mycology for which this former gold-standard drug is the first consideration for treatment. It combines excellent direct fungicidal activity and host immunostimulation to produce consistent anticryptococcal activity. Obtaining fungicidal activity is essential in patients who have a high burden of organisms, poor nutritional status, and profound immunosuppression. A standard induction dose for amphotericin B is 0.7 mg/kg/d. Liposomal amphotericin B (AmBisome) at 4 mg/kg/d or amphotericin B lipid complex (ABLC) at 5 mg/kg/d can be used as alternative treatments with a similar outcome and less nephrotoxicity [208,209]. Flucytosine (5-FC) is primarily used in combination therapy with amphotericin B for first-line therapy in cryptococcal meningitis or severe pulmonary cryptococcosis at 100 mg/kg/d in divided doses in patients who have normal renal function [210,211]. The combination of amphotericin B and 5-FC represents the most potent available fungicidal regimen that produces consistently negative CSF cultures at 2 weeks of treatment in patients who do not have AIDS. In fact, an elegant study comparing quantitative CSF yeast counts over 2 weeks using several antifungal regimens showed that this combination was more fungicidal than amphotericin B, amphotericin B plus fluconazole, or all three drugs together [212]. Our goal is to efficiently reduce the burden of yeasts in the CSF, and this combination is very effective.

Patients infected with HIV who have cryptococcal meningitis undergo three stages of treatment, a strategy that can also be followed in patients not infected with HIV [207,210]. Induction treatment usually begins with amphotericin B plus 5-FC for 2 weeks and is followed by a clearance stage with fluconazole, 400 to 800 mg/d, for a minimum of 10 weeks. Finally, a long-term suppressive/maintenance therapy or secondary prophylaxis usually begins with fluconazole, 200 to 400 mg, once daily for at least 1 year. Other azoles, such as voriconazole, posaconazole, and itraconazole, have been used successfully in cryptococcosis for patients who are intolerant or refractory to treatment [213,214] and could be used as alternatives to fluconazole, although itraconazole has been shown to be inferior during clearance phase [215]. However, fluconazole is currently the primary azole that is used routinely. Secondary prophylaxis can be discontinued in patients whose infection responds to HAART with a rise in CD4 counts greater than 100 cells/μL and an undetectable HIV RNA level for at least 3 months and after 2 years of suppressive therapy [216,217].

Patients who do not have AIDS can be treated similarly to those who do, but criteria for stopping treatment in those who do not have AIDS who have cryptococcal meningitis include resolution of symptoms, negative CSF cultures, normal CSF glucose, and generally at least 1 year of suppressive therapy. However, very good results in organ transplantations occurred with stopping drug at 6 months [218]. Patients may have a prolonged positive CSF or serum cryptococcal polysaccharide antigen or slightly abnormal cellular or chemistry findings in CSF for several months during successful therapy. There are still very few cases of drug-resistant strains (azole/polyene) of *C neoformans* [219]. The present echinocandins do not have clinical activity against cryptococcal infections.

In patients infected with HIV, HAART has a major impact on long-term prognosis in cryptococcosis. However, treatment with HAART during antifungal therapy can cause cryptococcal IRIS. Limited data are available for formal recommendations to prevent and treat cryptococcal IRIS in AIDS, but with potent antiretrovirals, IRIS commonly occurs within the first 1 to 2 months after starting HAART. Therefore, after starting antifungal therapy for cryptococcal diseases, an 8- to 10-week delay in initiating HAART is generally recommended to reduce the complexities of dealing with IRIS and the increased intracranial pressure that might occur during induction therapy in patients who have a high burden of yeasts in CSF. In fact, despite retrospective data suggesting poor outcome with corticosteroid therapy for increased intracranial pressure [220], corticosteroid treatment may be necessary to control symptoms if severe cryptococcal IRIS occurs. One study showed that patients who had cryptococcal IRIS had higher CSF opening pressures, CSF glucose levels, and CSF white blood cell counts compared with patients who had typical HIV-associated cryptococcal meningitis. Although development of IRIS did not impact overall survival, it could substantially add to costs and morbidity of infections [109]. IRIS in cryptococcosis is not limited to HIV and HAART, although it has been reported in up to 30% of patients [109]. However, it can occur in any patient whose immune status changes rapidly, and IRIS has been reported in 5% of patients who have undergone solid organ transplantation who have cryptococcosis [110]. Therefore, the reduction in immune suppression, which is an important goal during therapy, must be carefully controlled in its rapid decline. However, for patients in whom sterilizing CSF is difficult, the additional use of IFN-γ with antifungal therapy to increase Th1 response could be considered. When used in primary therapy, it was shown to have a trend toward more rapid clearance of viable yeasts from CSF [221].

In general, symptoms and signs of patients who have cryptococcal meningitis should resolve within 2 weeks after start of initial treatment. More than 80% of all patients, including those who have AIDS who are undergoing treatment, have a sterile CSF at 2 weeks, but the cryptococcal polysaccharide antigen is usually still high. Patients who do not have negative CSF cultures by day 14 have a five times higher risk for treatment failure at week 10 than those whose cultures are negative [222]. A recent study showed that CSF cryptococcal colony-forming unit counts can serve as an alternative measure of organism load in cryptococcal meningitis and can be used in follow-up after cryptococcal treatment. CSF cryptococcal colony-forming unit counts and CSF cryptococcal antigen titers have a high correlation at baseline before treatment, and CSF cryptococcal colony-forming unit counts decreased readily during the first 2 weeks of treatment. However, no correlation occurred between the rate of decline in CSF cryptococcal colony-forming unit counts and drop in CSF cryptococcal antigen titers [167].

Managing increased intracranial pressure is equally important as using direct antifungal therapy. An opening pressure of 250 mm H_2O or more is considered an elevated intracranial pressure. A study showed that high intracranial pressure after 2 weeks of treatment predicted a poorer clinical response in patients infected with HIV who had cryptococcal meningitis [205]. However, a recent retrospective study of 26 patients who had cryptococcal meningitis showed that CSF opening pressure had been measured for only 13 (50%) of 26 patients, and major deviations from the cryptococcal guidelines with respect to intracranial pressure management were observed in the care of more than half the patients. Of the patients for which guidelines were not followed, 7 of 13 developed neuropathies during therapy compared with 1 of 5 patients whose care had minor or no deviations from the guidelines [206]. Some bias may exist in this study for not measuring pressures, but the finding emphasizes that a potential problem exists with increased intracranial pressure during therapy and that it requires a management strategy.

Control of increased intracranial pressure is generally needed with symptom development (eg, increasing headache, mental status changes, new neurologic findings), and a precise opening pressure for treatment is not yet established. As listed in Box 3, treatment options recommended for managing an acute elevated intracranial pressure include repeated lumbar punctures, lumbar drain insertion [223], ventriculostomy, or ventriculoperitoneal shunt. Medical treatments such as corticosteroids (unless a component of IRIS is linked to the increased opening pressures), mannitol, or acetazolamide have some clinical experience and are generally unsuccessful, and therefore their use is not recommended for managing increased intracranial pressure in cryptococcal meningitis [224]. However, in patients who have clear symptoms of IRIS, corticosteroids are necessary to control symptoms. With CNS disease and IRIS, we recommend using dexamethasone and a steroid taper for 6 weeks to 2 months, but more definitive management studies are needed for treating this inflammatory condition. During the first 1 to 2 years of treatment or at presentation, some patients may develop symptoms of obstructive hydrocephalus (eg, headaches, confusion, various neurologic symptoms), which require a permanent ventriculoperitoneal shunt. The shunt can be placed when the patient is undergoing appropriate antifungal therapy; if it is placed before antifungal therapy is started, it may need to be removed and replaced under antifungal coverage [4].

Prognosis in cryptococcal meningitis is primarily based on underlying disease, burden of organisms, symptoms at presentation, and host

> **Box 3. Management of elevated intracranial pressure in patients infected with HIV who have cryptococcosis, based on the 2000 IDSA Practice Guideline for the Management of Cryptococcal Diseases**
>
> *Before treatment*
> *Focal neurologic signs, obtunded*
> - Radiographic imaging before lumbar puncture to exclude contraindications
>
> *Normal opening pressure*
> - Initiate medical therapy, with follow-up lumbar puncture at 2 weeks
>
> *Opening pressure 250 mm H_2O or more with signs or symptoms*
> - Lumbar drainage sufficient to achieve closing pressure less than 200 mm H_2O or 50% of initial opening pressure[a]
>
> *Follow-up for elevated pressure*
> - Repeated drainage daily until opening pressure and symptoms/signs are stable
>
> *If elevated pressure persists*
> - Lumbar drain
> - Ventriculoperitoneal shunt
>
> _____
> [a] This is not an evidence-based recommendation and is used as a guide only.
> *Data from* Saag MS, Graybill RJ, Larsen RA, et al. Practice guidelines for the management of cryptococcal disease. Infectious Diseases Society of America. Clin Infect Dis 2000;30(4):710–8.

inflammatory reactions. Factors for poor prognosis include (1) comatose state, (2) high cryptococcal antigen titers or concentrations of yeasts, (3) low number of CSF inflammatory cells, and (4) symptomatic elevated increased intracranial pressure. For us and others, a serious consideration for successful outcome is serious underlying liver disease and its stage [225]. In patients who have undergone transplantation, prognosis has ranged from very poor to relatively good in the literature [32,207], and likely reflects the ability to save the graft and manage complexities of drugs and immune suppression in this fragile patient population.

Prevention

Cryptococcal diseases can be prevented in patients infected with HIV by using HAART to improve their immunity. Fluconazole prophylaxis has been shown to be effective for preventing cryptococcosis in patients who have AIDS who have persistently low CD4 counts below 100 cells/μL [226], but HAART remains the best prevention strategy during HIV infection. Furthermore, high-risk patients should avoid high-risk environmental factors, such as bird droppings or certain trees in endemic areas.

Currently, a GXM-protein conjugate vaccine synthesized as a heptasaccharide oligosaccharide representing the putative dominant motif of the serotype A cryptococcal GXM showed that it is recognized by some monoclonal antibodies generated to GXM and might be a potential synthetic oligosaccharide vaccine against *C neoformans* [227]. Although a cryptococcal GXM-protein conjugate vaccine and specific monoclonal antibodies to cryptococci have been developed, only early clinical trials with a monoclonal antibody have been initiated in humans and this study was a phase I toxicity and dose-ranging study [228]. Either passive or active immunologic strategies will require further studies on product development and efficacy, risk–patient assessment, and cost–benefit analysis.

References

[1] Kidd SE, Hagen F, Tscharke RL, et al. A rare genotype of *Cryptococcus gattii* caused the cryptococcosis outbreak on Vancouver Island (British Columbia, Canada). Proc Natl Acad Sci USA 2004;101(49):17258–63.

[2] Perfect JR. *Cryptococcus neoformans*: a sugar-coated killer with designer genes. FEMS Immunol Med Microbiol 2005;45(3):395–404.

[3] Loftus BJ, Fung E, Roncaglia P, et al. The genome of the basidiomycetous yeast and human pathogen *Cryptococcus neoformans*. Science 2005;307(5713):1321–4.

[4] Perfect JR, Casadevall A. Cryptococcosis. Infect Dis Clin North Am 2002;16(4):837–74.

[5] Kwon-Chung KJ, Boekhout T, Fell JW, et al. Proposal to conserve the name *Cryptococcus gattii* against *C. hondurianus* and *C. bacillisporus*. Taxon 2002;51:804–6.

[6] Franzot SP, Salkin IF, Casadevall A. *Cryptococcus neoformans* var. *grubii*: separate varietal status for *Cryptococcus neoformans* serotype A isolates. J Clin Microbiol 1999;37(3): 838–40.

[7] Speed B, Dunt D. Clinical and host differences between infections with the two varieties of *Cryptococcus neoformans*. Clin Infect Dis 1995;21(1):28–34 [discussion 5–6].

[8] Ikeda R, Shinoda T, Fukazawa Y, et al. Antigenic characterization of *Cryptococcus neoformans* serotypes and its application to serotyping of clinical isolates. J Clin Microbiol 1982; 16(1):22–9.

[9] Dromer F, Gueho E, Ronin O, et al. Serotyping of *Cryptococcus neoformans* by using a monoclonal antibody specific for capsular polysaccharide. J Clin Microbiol 1993;31(2): 359–63.

[10] Meyer W, Castaneda A, Jackson S, et al. Molecular typing of IberoAmerican *Cryptococcus neoformans* isolates. Emerg Infect Dis 2003;9(2):189–95.

[11] Meyer W, Marszewska K, Amirmostofian M, et al. Molecular typing of global isolates of *Cryptococcus neoformans* var. *neoformans* by polymerase chain reaction fingerprinting and randomly amplified polymorphic DNA-a pilot study to standardize techniques on which to base a detailed epidemiological survey. Electrophoresis 1999;20(8):1790–9.

[12] Kwon-Chung KJ. A new species of *Filobasidiella*, the sexual state of *Cryptococcus neoformans* B and C serotypes. Mycologia 1976;68(4):943–6.

[13] Kwon-Chung KJ. A new genus, filobasidiella, the perfect state of *Cryptococcus neoformans*. Mycologia 1975;67(6):1197–200.

[14] Kwon-Chung KJ. Morphogenesis of *Filobasidiella neoformans*, the sexual state of *Cryptococcus neoformans*. Mycologia 1976;68(4):821–33.

[15] Wickes BL, Mayorga ME, Edman U, et al. Dimorphism and haploid fruiting in *Cryptococcus neoformans*: association with the alpha-mating type. Proc Natl Acad Sci USA 1996; 93(14):7327–31.

[16] Lin X, Hull CM, Heitman J. Sexual reproduction between partners of the same mating type in *Cryptococcus neoformans*. Nature 2005;434(7036):1017–21.

[17] Kwon-Chung KJ, Bennett JE. Distribution of alpha and alpha mating types of *Cryptococcus neoformans* among natural and clinical isolates. Am J Epidemiol 1978;108(4): 337–40.

[18] Hull CM, Heitman J. Genetics of *Cryptococcus neoformans*. Annu Rev Genet 2002;36: 557–615.

[19] Mitchell TG, Perfect JR. Cryptococcosis in the era of AIDS–100 years after the discovery of *Cryptococcus neoformans*. Clin Microbiol Rev 1995;8(4):515–48.

[20] Hajjeh RA, Conn LA, Stephens DS, et al. Cryptococcosis: population-based multistate active surveillance and risk factors in human immunodeficiency virus-infected persons. Cryptococcal Active Surveillance Group. J Infect Dis 1999;179(2):449–54.

[21] Dromer F, Mathoulin S, Dupont B, et al. Epidemiology of cryptococcosis in France: a 9-year survey (1985–1993). French Cryptococcosis Study Group. Clin Infect Dis 1996; 23(1):82–90.

[22] Mirza SA, Phelan M, Rimland D, et al. The changing epidemiology of cryptococcosis: an update from population-based active surveillance in 2 large metropolitan areas, 1992–2000. Clin Infect Dis 2003;36(6):789–94.

[23] Crowe SM, Carlin JB, Stewart KI, et al. Predictive value of CD4 lymphocyte numbers for the development of opportunistic infections and malignancies in HIV-infected persons. J Acquir Immune Defic Syndr 1991;4(8):770–6.

[24] Dromer F, Mathoulin-Pelissier S, Fontanet A, et al. Epidemiology of HIV-associated cryptococcosis in France (1985–2001): comparison of the pre- and post-HAART eras. AIDS 2004;18(3):555–62.

[25] Friedman GD, Jeffrey Fessel W, Udaltsova NV, et al. Cryptococcosis: the 1981–2000 epidemic. Mycoses 2005;48(2):122–5.

[26] French N, Gray K, Watera C, et al. Cryptococcal infection in a cohort of HIV-1-infected Ugandan adults. AIDS 2002;16(7):1031–8.

[27] Anekthananon T, Ratanasuwan W, Techasathit W, et al. HIV infection/acquired immunodeficiency syndrome at Siriraj Hospital, 2002: time for secondary prevention. J Med Assoc Thai 2004;87(2):173–9.

[28] Nath DS, Kandaswamy R, Gruessner R, et al. Fungal infections in transplant recipients receiving alemtuzumab. Transplant Proc 2005;37(2):934–6.

[29] Hage CA, Wood KL, Winer-Muram HT, et al. Pulmonary cryptococcosis after initiation of anti-tumor necrosis factor-alpha therapy. Chest 2003;124(6):2395–7.

[30] Vilchez RA, Fung J, Kusne S. Cryptococcosis in organ transplant recipients: an overview. Am J Transplant 2002;2(7):575–80.

[31] Wu G, Vilchez RA, Eidelman B, et al. Cryptococcal meningitis: an analysis among 5,521 consecutive organ transplant recipients. Transpl Infect Dis 2002;4(4):183–8.

[32] Husain S, Wagener MM, Singh N. *Cryptococcus neoformans* infection in organ transplant recipients: variables influencing clinical characteristics and outcome. Emerg Infect Dis 2001;7(3):375–81.

[33] Kiertiburanakul S, Wirojtananugoon S, Pracharktam R, et al. Cryptococcosis in human immunodeficiency virus-negative patients. Int J Infect Dis 2006;10(1):72–8.

[34] Bennett JE, Kwon-Chung KJ, Howard DH. Epidemiologic differences among serotypes of *Cryptococcus neoformans*. Am J Epidemiol 1977;105(6):582–6.

[35] Kwon-Chung KJ, Bennett JE. Epidemiologic differences between the two varieties of *Cryptococcus neoformans*. Am J Epidemiol 1984;120(1):123–30.

[36] Chen S, Sorrell T, Nimmo G, et al. Epidemiology and host- and variety-dependent characteristics of infection due to *Cryptococcus neoformans* in Australia and New Zealand. Australasian Cryptococcal Study Group. Clin Infect Dis 2000;31(2):499–508.

[37] Chaturvedi S, Dyavaiah M, Larsen RA, et al. *Cryptococcus gattii* in AIDS patients, southern California. Emerg Infect Dis 2005;11(11):1686–92.

[38] Kidd SE, Guo H, Bartlett KH, et al. Comparative gene genealogies indicate that two clonal lineages of *Cryptococcus gattii* in British Columbia resemble strains from other geographical areas. Eukaryot Cell 2005;4(10):1629–38.

[39] Fraser JA, Giles SS, Wenink EC, et al. Same-sex mating and the origin of the Vancouver Island *Cryptococcus gattii* outbreak. Nature 2005;437(7063):1360–4.

[40] Hoang LM, Maguire JA, Doyle P, et al. *Cryptococcus neoformans* infections at Vancouver Hospital and Health Sciences Centre (1997–2002): epidemiology, microbiology and histopathology. J Med Microbiol 2004;53(Pt 9):935–40.

[41] Mitchell DH, Sorrell TC, Allworth AM, et al. Cryptococcal disease of the CNS in immunocompetent hosts: influence of cryptococcal variety on clinical manifestations and outcome. Clin Infect Dis 1995;20(3):611–6.

[42] Nosanchuk JD, Shoham S, Fries BC, et al. Evidence of zoonotic transmission of *Cryptococcus neoformans* from a pet cockatoo to an immunocompromised patient. Ann Intern Med 2000;132(3):205–8.

[43] Garcia-Hermoso D, Mathoulin-Pelissier S, Couprie B, et al. DNA typing suggests pigeon droppings as a source of pathogenic *Cryptococcus neoformans* serotype D. J Clin Microbiol 1997;35(10):2683–5.

[44] Sorrell TC, Chen SC, Ruma P, et al. Concordance of clinical and environmental isolates of *Cryptococcus neoformans* var. *gattii* by random amplification of polymorphic DNA analysis and PCR fingerprinting. J Clin Microbiol 1996;34(5):1253–60.

[45] Delgado AC, Taguchi H, Mikami Y, et al. Human cryptococcosis: relationship of environmental and clinical strains of *Cryptococcus neoformans* var. *neoformans* from urban and rural areas. Mycopathologia 2005;159(1):7–11.

[46] Souza LK, Fernandes Ode F, Kobayashi CC, et al. Antifungal susceptibilities of clinical and environmental isolates of *Cryptococcus neoformans* in Goiania city, Goias, Brazil. Rev Inst Med Trop Sao Paulo 2005;47(5):253–6.

[47] Garcia-Hermoso D, Janbon G, Dromer F. Epidemiological evidence for dormant *Cryptococcus neoformans* infection. J Clin Microbiol 1999;37(10):3204–9.

[48] Schimpff SC, Bennett JE. Abnormalities in cell-mediated immunity in patients with *Cryptococcus neoformans* infection. J Allergy Clin Immunol 1975;55(6):430–41.

[49] Chen LC, Goldman DL, Doering TL, et al. Antibody response to *Cryptococcus neoformans* proteins in rodents and humans. Infect Immun 1999;67(5):2218–24.

[50] Goldman DL, Khine H, Abadi J, et al. Serologic evidence for *Cryptococcus neoformans* infection in early childhood. Pediatrics 2001;107(5):E66.

[51] Goldman D, Lee SC, Casadevall A. Pathogenesis of pulmonary *Cryptococcus neoformans* infection in the rat. Infect Immun 1994;62(11):4755–61.

[52] Uicker WC, Doyle HA, McCracken JP, et al. Cytokine and chemokine expression in the central nervous system associated with protective cell-mediated immunity against *Cryptococcus neoformans*. Med Mycol 2005;43(1):27–38.

[53] Perfect JR. *Cryptococcus neoformans*. In: Mandell GL, Bennett JE, Dolin R, editors. Mandell, Douglas, and Bennett's principles and practice of infectious diseases, Vol 2. 6th edition. Philadelphia: Elsevier Churchill Livingstone; 2005. p. 2997–3012.

[54] Wormley Jr FL, Perfect JR, Cox GM. Protection against cryptococcosis using cytokine secreting *Cryptococcus neoformans* [abstract S7.1Oral]. In: Programs and abstracts of the 6th International Conference of Cryptococcus and Cryptococcosis. Boston: 2005. p. 50.

[55] Chaka W, Heyderman R, Gangaidzo I, et al. Cytokine profiles in cerebrospinal fluid of human immunodeficiency virus-infected patients with cryptococcal meningitis: no leukocytosis despite high interleukin-8 levels. University of Zimbabwe Meningitis Group. J Infect Dis 1997;176(6):1633–6.

[56] Einsiedel L, Gordon DL, Dyer JR. Paradoxical inflammatory reaction during treatment of *Cryptococcus neoformans* var. *gattii* meningitis in an HIV-seronegative woman. Clin Infect Dis 2004;39(8):e78–82.

[57] Siddiqui AA, Brouwer AE, Wuthiekanun V, et al. IFN-gamma at the site of infection determines rate of clearance of infection in cryptococcal meningitis. J Immunol 2005; 174(3):1746–50.

[58] Kwon-Chung K. Gene disruption to evaluate the role of fungal candidate virulence genes. Curr Opin Microbiol 1998;1(4):381–9.

[59] Casadevall A, Rosas AL, Nosanchuk JD. Melanin and virulence in *Cryptococcus neoformans*. Curr Opin Microbiol 2000;3(4):354–8.

[60] Salas SD, Bennett JE, Kwon-Chung KJ, et al. Effect of the laccase gene *CNLAC1*, on virulence of *Cryptococcus neoformans*. J Exp Med 1996;184(2):377–86.

[61] Kraus PR, Boily MJ, Giles SS, et al. Identification of *Cryptococcus neoformans* temperature-regulated genes with a genomic-DNA microarray. Eukaryot Cell 2004;3(5):1249–60.

[62] Alspaugh JA, Cavallo LM, Perfect JR, et al. *RAS1* regulates filamentation, mating and growth at high temperature of *Cryptococcus neoformans*. Mol Microbiol 2000;36(2): 352–65.

[63] Chang YC, Penoyer LA, Kwon-Chung KJ. The second capsule gene of *Cryptococcus neoformans*, CAP64, is essential for virulence. Infect Immun 1996;64(6):1977–83.

[64] Chang YC, Kwon-Chung KJ. Isolation of the third capsule-associated gene, CAP60, required for virulence in *Cryptococcus neoformans*. Infect Immun 1998;66(5):2230–6.

[65] Chang YC, Kwon-Chung KJ. Complementation of a capsule-deficient mutation of *Cryptococcus neoformans* restores its virulence. Mol Cell Biol 1994;14(7):4912–9.

[66] Bottone EJ, Toma M, Johansson BE, et al. Capsule-deficient *Cryptococcus neoformans* in AIDS patients. Lancet 1985;1(8425):400.

[67] Guerrero A, Jain N, Goldman DL, et al. Phenotypic switching in *Cryptococcus neoformans*. Microbiol 2006;152(Pt 1):3–9.

[68] Jain N, Guerrero A, Fries BC. Phenotypic switching and its implications for the pathogenesis of *Cryptococcus neoformans*. FEMS Yeast Res 2006;6(4):480–8.

[69] Zhu X, Williamson PR. Role of laccase in the biology and virulence of *Cryptococcus neoformans*. FEMS Yeast Res 2004;5(1):1–10.

[70] Perfect JR. *Cryptococcus neoformans*: the yeast that likes it hot. FEMS Yeast Res 2006;6(4): 463–8.

[71] Nielsen K, Cox GM, Litvintseva AP, et al. *Cryptococcus neoformans* {alpha} strains preferentially disseminate to the central nervous system during coinfection. Infect Immun 2005; 73(8):4922–33.

[72] Nielsen K, Cox GM, Wang P, et al. Sexual cycle of *Cryptococcus neoformans* var. *grubii* and virulence of congenic a and alpha isolates. Infect Immun 2003;71(9):4831–41.

[73] Cox GM, McDade HC, Chen SC, et al. Extracellular phospholipase activity is a virulence factor for *Cryptococcus neoformans*. Mol Microbiol 2001;39(1):166–75.

[74] Cox GM, Mukherjee J, Cole GT, et al. Urease as a virulence factor in experimental cryptococcosis. Infect Immun 2000;68(2):443–8.

[75] Giles SS, Batinic-Haberle I, Perfect JR, et al. *Cryptococcus neoformans* mitochondrial superoxide dismutase: an essential link between antioxidant function and high-temperature growth. Eukaryot Cell 2005;4(1):46–54.

[76] Wormley FL Jr, Heinrich G, Miller JL, et al. Identification and characterization of an *SKN7* homologue in *Cryptococcus neoformans*. Infect Immun 2005;73(8):5022–30.

[77] Lengeler KB, Davidson RC, D'Souza C, et al. Signal transduction cascades regulating fungal development and virulence. Microbiol Mol Biol Rev 2000;64(4):746–85.

[78] Wang P, Heitman J. Signal transduction cascades regulating mating, filamentation, and virulence in *Cryptococcus neoformans*. Curr Opin Microbiol 1999;2(4):358–62.

[79] Alspaugh JA, Perfect JR, Heitman J. *Cryptococcus neoformans* mating and virulence are regulated by the G-protein alpha subunit GPA1 and cAMP. Genes Dev 1997;11(23): 3206–17.

[80] Alspaugh JA, Pukkila-Worley R, Harashima T, et al. Adenylyl cyclase functions downstream of the Galpha protein Gpa1 and controls mating and pathogenicity of *Cryptococcus neoformans*. Eukaryot Cell 2002;1(1):75–84.

[81] Pukkila-Worley R, Gerrald QD, Kraus PR, et al. Transcriptional network of multiple capsule and melanin genes governed by the *Cryptococcus neoformans* cyclic AMP cascade. Eukaryot Cell 2005;4(1):190–201.

[82] D'Souza CA, Alspaugh JA, Yue C, et al. Cyclic AMP-dependent protein kinase controls virulence of the fungal pathogen *Cryptococcus neoformans*. Mol Cell Biol 2001;21(9): 3179–91.

[83] Hicks JK, D'Souza CA, Cox GM, et al. Cyclic AMP-dependent protein kinase catalytic subunits have divergent roles in virulence factor production in two varieties of the fungal pathogen *Cryptococcus neoformans*. Eukaryot Cell 2004;3(1):14–26.

[84] Bahn YS, Hicks JK, Giles SS, et al. Adenylyl cyclase-associated protein Aca1 regulates virulence and differentiation of *Cryptococcus neoformans* via the cyclic AMP-protein kinase A cascade. Eukaryot Cell 2004;3(6):1476–91.

[85] Bahn YS, Kojima K, Cox GM, et al. Specialization of the HOG pathway and its impact on differentiation and virulence of *Cryptococcus neoformans*. Mol Biol Cell 2005;16(5): 2285–300.

[86] Waugh MS, Nichols CB, DeCesare CM, et al. Ras1 and Ras2 contribute shared and unique roles in physiology and virulence of *Cryptococcus neoformans*. Microbiol 2002;148(Pt 1): 191–201.

[87] Kraus PR, Nichols CB, Heitman J. Calcium- and calcineurin-independent roles for calmodulin in *Cryptococcus neoformans* morphogenesis and high-temperature growth. Eukaryot Cell 2005;4(6):1079–87.

[88] Djordjevic JT, Del Poeta M, Sorrell TC, et al. Secretion of cryptococcal phospholipase B1 (PLB1) is regulated by a glycosylphosphatidylinositol (GPI) anchor. Biochem J 2005; 389(Pt 3):803–12.

[89] Siafakas AR, Wright LC, Sorrell TC, et al. Lipid rafts in *Cryptococcus neoformans* concentrate the virulence determinants phospholipase B1 and Cu/Zn superoxide dismutase. Eukaryot Cell 2006;5(3):488–98.

[90] Casadevall A, Perfect JR. *Cryptococcus neoformans*. Washington (DC): ASM Press; 1998.

[91] Nadrous HF, Antonios VS, Terrell CL, et al. Pulmonary cryptococcosis in nonimmunocompromised patients. Chest 2003;124(6):2143–7.

[92] Mueller NJ, Fishman JA. Asymptomatic pulmonary cryptococcosis in solid organ transplantation: report of four cases and review of the literature. Transpl Infect Dis 2003;5(3): 140–3.

[93] Warr W, Bates JH, Stone A. The spectrum of pulmonary cryptococcosis. Ann Intern Med 1968;69(6):1109–16.

[94] Chang WC, Tzao C, Hsu HH, et al. Pulmonary cryptococcosis: comparison of clinical and radiographic characteristics in immunocompetent and immunocompromised patients. Chest 2006;129(2):333–40.

[95] Vilchez RA, Linden P, Lacomis J, et al. Acute respiratory failure associated with pulmonary cryptococcosis in non-AIDS patients. Chest 2001;119(6):1865–9.

[96] Lortholary O, Nunez H, Brauner MW, et al. Pulmonary cryptococcosis. Semin Respir Crit Care Med 2004;25(2):145–57.

[97] Nunez M, Peacock JE Jr, Chin R Jr. Pulmonary cryptococcosis in the immunocompetent host. Therapy with oral fluconazole: a report of four cases and a review of the literature. Chest 2000;118(2):527–34.

[98] Piyavisetpat N, Chaowanapanja P. Radiographic manifestations of pulmonary cryptococ-cosis. J Med Assoc Thai 2005;88(11):1674–9.
[99] Chang YS, Chou KC, Wang PC, et al. Primary pulmonary cryptococcosis presenting as endobronchial tumor with left upper lobe collapse. J Chin Med Assoc 2005;68(1):33–6.
[100] Endo S, Saito N, Hasegawa T, et al. Pulmonary cryptococcosis mimicking pulmonary metastases in a patient treated with Tegafur-uracil after lung cancer surgery. Jpn J Thorac Cardiovasc Surg 2005;53(7):369–71.
[101] Su CT, Chen LK, Tsai YF, et al. Disseminated cryptococcosis with pulmonary and marrow involvement mimicking radiological features of malignancy. J Chin Med Assoc 2004;67(2): 89–92.
[102] Ecevit IZ, Clancy CJ, Schmalfuss IM, et al. The poor prognosis of central nervous system cryptococcosis among nonimmunosuppressed patients: a call for better disease recognition and evaluation of adjuncts to antifungal therapy. Clin Infect Dis 2006; 42(10):1443–7.
[103] Lui G, Lee N, Ip M, et al. Cryptococcosis in apparently immunocompetent patients. QJM 2006;99(3):143–51.
[104] Jenny-Avital ER, Abadi M. Immune reconstitution cryptococcosis after initiation of successful highly active antiretroviral therapy. Clin Infect Dis 2002;35(12):e128–33.
[105] Lortholary O, Fontanet A, Memain N, et al. Incidence and risk factors of immune recon-stitution inflammatory syndrome complicating HIV-associated cryptococcosis in France. AIDS 2005;19(10):1043–9.
[106] King MD, Perlino CA, Cinnamon J, et al. Paradoxical recurrent meningitis following therapy of cryptococcal meningitis: an immune reconstitution syndrome after initiation of highly active antiretroviral therapy. Int J STD AIDS 2002;13(10):724–6.
[107] Boelaert JR, Goddeeris KH, Vanopdenbosch LJ, et al. Relapsing meningitis caused by persistent cryptococcal antigens and immune reconstitution after the initiation of highly active antiretroviral therapy. AIDS 2004;18(8):1223–4.
[108] Cattelan AM, Trevenzoli M, Sasset L, et al. Multiple cerebral cryptococcomas associated with immune reconstitution in HIV-1 infection. AIDS 2004;18(2):349–51.
[109] Shelburne SA III, Darcourt J, White AC Jr, et al. The role of immune reconstitution inflam-matory syndrome in AIDS-related *Cryptococcus neoformans* disease in the era of highly ac-tive antiretroviral therapy. Clin Infect Dis 2005;40(7):1049–52.
[110] Singh N, Lortholary O, Alexander BD, et al. An immune reconstitution syndrome-like ill-ness associated with Cryptococcus neoformans infection in organ transplant recipients. Clin Infect Dis 2005;40(12):1756–61.
[111] Singh N, Lortholary O, Alexander BD, et al. Allograft loss in renal transplant recipients with *Cryptococcus neoformans* associated immune reconstitution syndrome. Transplanta-tion 2005;80(8):1131–3.
[112] Dromer F, Mathoulin S, Dupont B, et al. Individual and environmental factors associated with infection due to *Cryptococcus neoformans* serotype D. French Cryptococcosis Study Group. Clin Infect Dis 1996;23(1):91–6.
[113] Baumgarten KL, Valentine VG, Garcia-Diaz JB. Primary cutaneous cryptococcosis in a lung transplant recipient. South Med J 2004;97(7):692–5.
[114] Joshi S, Wattal C, Duggal L, et al. Cutaneous cryptococcosis. J Assoc Physicians India 2004;52:242–3.
[115] Franca AV, Carneiro M, dal Sasso K, et al. Cryptococcosis in cirrhotic patients. Mycoses 2005;48(1):68–72.
[116] Pasqualotto AC, Bittar AE, de Quadros M, et al. Cryptococcal cellulitis in a renal trans-plant patient. Nephrol Dial Transplant 2005;20(9):2007–8.
[117] Singh N, Gayowski T, Wagener MM, et al. Clinical spectrum of invasive cryptococcosis in liver transplant recipients receiving tacrolimus. Clin Transplant 1997;11(1):66–70.
[118] Odom A, Muir S, Lim E, et al. Calcineurin is required for virulence of *Cryptococcus neofor-mans*. EMBO J 1997;16(10):2576–89.

[119] Neuville S, Dromer F, Morin O, et al. Primary cutaneous cryptococcosis: a distinct clinical entity. Clin Infect Dis 2003;36(3):337–47.

[120] Dora JM, Kelbert S, Deutschendorf C, et al. Cutaneous cryptococcosis due to *Cryptococcus gattii* in immunocompetent hosts: case report and review. Mycopathologia 2006;161(4): 235–8.

[121] Larsen RA, Bozzette S, McCutchan JA, et al. Persistent *Cryptococcus neoformans* infection of the prostate after successful treatment of meningitis. California Collaborative Treatment Group. Ann Intern Med 1989;111(2):125–8.

[122] Allen R, Barter CE, Chachoua LL, et al. Disseminated cryptococcosis after transurethral resection of the prostate. Aust N Z J Med 1982;12(4):296–9.

[123] Siddiqui TJ, Zamani T, Parada JP. Primary cryptococcal prostatitis and correlation with serum prostate specific antigen in a renal transplant recipient. J Infect 2005;51(3): e153–7.

[124] Staib F, Seibold M, L'Age M. Persistence of *Cryptococcus neoformans* in seminal fluid and urine under itraconazole treatment. The urogenital tract (prostate) as a niche for *Cryptococcus neoformans*. Mycoses 1990;33(7–8):369–73.

[125] Okun E, Butler WT. Ophthalmologic complications of cryptococcal meningitis. Arch Ophthalmol 1964;71:52–7.

[126] Battu RR, Biswas J, Jayakumar N, et al. Papilloedema with peripapillary retinal haemorrhages in an acquired immunodeficiency syndrome (AIDS) patient with cryptococcal meningitis. Indian J Ophthalmol 2000;48(1):47–9.

[127] Mwanza JC, Nyamabo LK, Tylleskar T, et al. Neuro-ophthalmological disorders in HIV infected subjects with neurological manifestations. Br J Ophthalmol 2004;88(11):1455–9.

[128] Rex JH, Larsen RA, Dismukes WE, et al. Catastrophic visual loss due to *Cryptococcus neoformans* meningitis. Medicine (Baltimore) 1993;72(4):207–24.

[129] Albert-Braun S, Venema F, Bausch J, et al. *Cryptococcus neoformans* peritonitis in a patient with alcoholic cirrhosis: case report and review of the literature. Infection 2005;33(4):282–8.

[130] Kiertiburanakul S, Sungkanuparph S, Buabut B, et al. Cryptococcuria as a manifestation of disseminated cryptococcosis and isolated urinary tract infection. Jpn J Infect Dis 2004; 57(5):203–5.

[131] Merz WG, Roberts GD. Detection and recovery of fungi from clinical specimens. In: Balows A, editor. Manual of clinical microbiology. Washington (DC): American Society for Microbiology; 1991. p. 550.

[132] Thiruchelvan N, Wuu KY, Arseculeratne SN, et al. A pseudo-cryptococcal artefact derived from leucocytes in wet India ink mounts of centrifuged cerebrospinal fluid. J Clin Pathol 1998;51(3):246–8.

[133] Portnoy D, Richards GK. Cryptococcal meningitis: misdiagnosis with india ink. Can Med Assoc J 1981;124(7):891–2.

[134] Dolan CT, Woodward MR. Identification of *Cryptococcus* species in the diagnostic laboratory. Am J Clin Pathol 1971;55(5):591–5.

[135] Diamond RD, Bennett JE. Prognostic factors in cryptococcal meningitis. A study in 111 cases. Ann Intern Med 1974;80(2):176–81.

[136] Davies SF. Diagnosis of pulmonary fungal infections. Semin Respir Infect 1988;3(2): 162–71.

[137] Cunha BA. Central nervous system infections in the compromised host: a diagnostic approach. Infect Dis Clin North Am 2001;15(2):567–90.

[138] Shibuya K, Coulson WF, Wollman JS, et al. Histopathology of cryptococcosis and other fungal infections in patients with acquired immunodeficiency syndrome. Int J Infect Dis 2001;5(2):78–85.

[139] Picon L, Vaillant L, Duong T, et al. Cutaneous cryptococcosis resembling molluscum contagiosum: a first manifestation of AIDS. Acta Derm Venereol 1989;69(4):365–7.

[140] Pantanowitz L, Omar T, Sonnendecker H, et al. Bone marrow cryptococcal infection in the acquired immunodeficiency syndrome. J Infect 2000;41(1):92–4.

[141] Ferry JA, Pettit CK, Rosenberg AE, et al. Fungi in megakaryocytes. An unusual manifestation of fungal infection of the bone marrow. Am J Clin Pathol 1991;96(5):577–81.

[142] Sato Y, Osabe S, Kuno H, et al. Rapid diagnosis of cryptococcal meningitis by microscopic examination of centrifuged cerebrospinal fluid sediment. J Neurol Sci 1999; 164(1):72–5.

[143] Alfonso F, Gallo L, Winkler B, et al. Fine needle aspiration cytology of peripheral lymph node cryptococcosis. A report of three cases. Acta Cytol 1994;38(3):459–62.

[144] Powers CN, Rupp GM, Maygarden SJ, et al. Fine-needle aspiration cytology of adrenal cryptococcosis: a case report. Diagn Cytopathol 1991;7(1):88–91.

[145] O'Dowd GJ, Frable WJ. Cryptococcal endophthalmitis: diagnostic vitreous aspiration cytology. Am J Clin Pathol 1983;79(3):382–5.

[146] Hsu CY. Cytologic diagnosis of pulmonary cryptococcosis in immunocompetent hosts. Acta Cytol 1993;37(5):667–72.

[147] Kuo TH, Hsu WH, Chiang CD, et al. Ultrasound-guided fine needle aspiration biopsy in the diagnosis of pulmonary cryptococcosis. J Formos Med Assoc 1998;97(3):197–203.

[148] Lee LN, Yang PC, Kuo SH, et al. Diagnosis of pulmonary cryptococcosis by ultrasound guided percutaneous aspiration. Thorax 1993;48(1):75–8.

[149] Morris B, Chan YF, Reddy J, et al. Cryptococcal peritonitis in a CAPD patient. J Med Vet Mycol 1992;30(4):309–15.

[150] Staib F, Seibold M, L'Age M, et al. *Cryptococcus neoformans* in the seminal fluid of an AIDS patient. A contribution to the clinical course of cryptococcosis. Mycoses 1989; 32(4):171–80.

[151] Kanjanavirojkul N, Sripa C, Puapairoj A. Cytologic diagnosis of *Cryptococcus neoformans* in HIV-positive patients. Acta Cytol 1997;41(2):493–6.

[152] Malabonga VM, Basti J, Kamholz SL. Utility of bronchoscopic sampling techniques for cryptococcal disease in AIDS. Chest 1991;99(2):370–2.

[153] Lee CH, Lan RS, Tsai YH, et al. Riu's stain in the diagnosis of pulmonary cryptococcosis. Introduction of a new diagnostic method. Chest 1988;93(3):467–70.

[154] Cohen J. Comparison of the sensitivity of three methods for the rapid identification of *Cryptococcus neoformans*. J Clin Pathol 1984;37(3):332–4.

[155] Vance AM. The use of the mucicarmine stain for a rapid presumptive identification of *Cryptococcus* from culture. Am J Med Technol 1961;27:125–8.

[156] Lopez JF, Lebron RF. *Cryptococcus neoformans*: their identification in body fluids and cultures by mucicarmine stain (Mayer). Bol Asoc Med P R 1972;64(8):203–5.

[157] Monteil RA, Hofman P, Michiels JF, et al. Oral cryptococcosis: case report of salivary gland involvement in an AIDS patient. J Oral Pathol Med 1997;26(1):53–6.

[158] Bottone EJ, Wormser GP. Poorly encapsulated *Cryptococcus neoformans* from patients with AIDS. II. Correlation of capsule size observed directly in cerebrospinal fluid with that after animal passage. AIDS Res 1986;2(3):219–25.

[159] Harding SA, Scheld WM, Feldman PS, et al. Pulmonary infection with capsule-deficient *Cryptococcus neoformans*. Virchows Arch A Pathol Anat Histol 1979;382(1):113–8.

[160] Ro JY, Lee SS, Ayala AG. Advantage of Fontana-Masson stain in capsule-deficient cryptococcal infection. Arch Pathol Lab Med 1987;111(1):53–7.

[161] Lazcano O, Speights VO Jr, Strickler JG, et al. Combined histochemical stains in the differential diagnosis of *Cryptococcus neoformans*. Mod Pathol 1993;6(1):80–4.

[162] Gordon MA, Vedder DK. Serologic tests in diagnosis and prognosis of cryptococcosis. JAMA 1966;197(12):961–7.

[163] Bindschadler DD, Bennett JE. Serology of human cryptococcosis. Ann Intern Med 1968; 69(1):45–52.

[164] Widra A, McMillen S, Rhodes HJ. Problems in serodiagnosis of cryptococcosis. Mycopathol Mycol Appl 1968;36(3):353–8.

[165] Gordon MA, Lapa E. Charcoal particle agglutination test for detection of antibody to *Cryptococcus neoformans*: a preliminary report. Am J Clin Pathol 1971;56(3):354–9.

[166] Viviani MA, Tortorano AM, Ajello L. *Cryptococcus*. In: Anaissie EJ, McGinnis MR, Pfaller MA, editors. Clinical mycology, Vol. 1. 1st edition. Philadelphia: Churchill Livingstone; 2003. p. 240–59.

[167] Brouwer AE, Teparrukkul P, Pinpraphaporn S, et al. Baseline correlation and comparative kinetics of cerebrospinal fluid colony-forming unit counts and antigen titers in cryptococcal meningitis. J Infect Dis 2005;192(4):681–4.

[168] Boom WH, Piper DJ, Ruoff KL, et al. New cause for false-positive results with the cryptococcal antigen test by latex agglutination. J Clin Microbiol 1985;22(5):856–7.

[169] Tanner DC, Weinstein MP, Fedorciw B, et al. Comparison of commercial kits for detection of cryptococcal antigen. J Clin Microbiol 1994;32(7):1680–4.

[170] Kauffman CA, Bergman AG, Severance PJ, et al. Detection of cryptococcal antigen. Comparison of two latex agglutination tests. Am J Clin Pathol 1981;75(1):106–9.

[171] Prevost E, Newell R. Commercial cryptococcal latex kit: clinical evaluation in a medical center hospital. J Clin Microbiol 1978;8(5):529–33.

[172] Wu TC, Koo SY. Comparison of three commercial cryptococcal latex kits for detection of cryptococcal antigen. J Clin Microbiol 1983;18(5):1127–30.

[173] Kiska DL, Orkiszewski DR, Howell D, et al. Evaluation of new monoclonal antibody-based latex agglutination test for detection of cryptococcal polysaccharide antigen in serum and cerebrospinal fluid. J Clin Microbiol 1994;32(9):2309–11.

[174] Bloomfield N, Gordon MA, Elmendorf DF Jr. Detection of *Cryptococcus neoformans* antigen in body fluids by latex particle agglutination. Proc Soc Exp Biol Med 1963; 114:64–7.

[175] Gordon MA, Lapa EW. Elimination of rheumatoid factor in the latex test for cryptococcosis. Am J Clin Pathol 1974;61(4):488–94.

[176] Bennett JE, Bailey JW. Control for rheumatoid factor in the latex test for cryptococcosis. Am J Clin Pathol 1971;56(3):360–5.

[177] Hay RJ, Mackenzie DW. False positive latex tests for cryptococcal antigen in cerebrospinal fluid. J Clin Pathol 1982;35(2):244–5.

[178] Whittier S, Hopfer RL, Gilligan P. Elimination of false-positive serum reactivity in latex agglutination test for cryptococcal antigen in human immunodeficiency virus-infected population. J Clin Microbiol 1994;32(9):2158–61.

[179] Sachs MK, Huang CM, Ost D, et al. Failure of dithiothreitol and pronase to reveal a false-positive cryptococcal antigen determination in cerebrospinal fluid. Am J Clin Pathol 1991; 96(3):381–4.

[180] Campbell CK, Payne AL, Teall AJ, et al. Cryptococcal latex antigen test positive in patient with *Trichosporon beigelii* infection. Lancet 1985;2(8445):43–4.

[181] McManus EJ, Bozdech MJ, Jones JM. Role of the latex agglutination test for cryptococcal antigen in diagnosing disseminated infections with *Trichosporon beigelii*. J Infect Dis 1985; 151(6):1167–9.

[182] Chanock SJ, Toltzis P, Wilson C. Cross-reactivity between *Stomatococcus mucilaginosus* and latex agglutination for cryptococcal antigen. Lancet 1993;342(8879):1119–20.

[183] Westerink MA, Amsterdam D, Petell RJ, et al. Septicemia due to DF-2. Cause of a false-positive cryptococcal latex agglutination result. Am J Med 1987;83(1):155–8.

[184] MacKinnon S, Kane JG, Parker RH. False-positive cryptococcal antigen test and cervical prevertebral abscess. JAMA 1978;240(18):1982–3.

[185] Heelan JS, Corpus L, Kessimian N. False-positive reactions in the latex agglutination test for *Cryptococcus neoformans* antigen. J Clin Microbiol 1991;29(6):1260–1.

[186] Snow RM, Dismukes WE. Cryptococcal meningitis: diagnostic value of cryptococcal antigen in cerebrospinal fluid. Arch Intern Med 1975;135(9):1155–7.

[187] Stamm AM, Polt SS. False-negative cryptococcal antigen test. JAMA 1980;244(12): 1359.

[188] Feldmesser M, Harris C, Reichberg S, et al. Serum cryptococcal antigen in patients with AIDS. Clin Infect Dis 1996;23(4):827–30.

[189] Gade W, Hinnefeld SW, Babcock LS, et al. Comparison of the PREMIER cryptococcal antigen enzyme immunoassay and the latex agglutination assay for detection of cryptococcal antigens. J Clin Microbiol 1991;29(8):1616–9.

[190] Sekhon AS, Garg AK, Kaufman L, et al. Evaluation of a commercial enzyme immunoassay for the detection of cryptococcal antigen. Mycoses 1993;36(1–2):31–4.

[191] Frank UK, Nishimura SL, Li NC, et al. Evaluation of an enzyme immunoassay for detection of cryptococcal capsular polysaccharide antigen in serum and cerebrospinal fluid. J Clin Microbiol 1993;31(1):97–101.

[192] Engler HD, Shea YR. Effect of potential interference factors on performance of enzyme immunoassay and latex agglutination assay for cryptococcal antigen. J Clin Microbiol 1994;32(9):2307–8.

[193] Shih CC, Chen YC, Chang SC, et al. Cryptococcal meningitis in non-HIV-infected patients. QJM 2000;93(4):245–51.

[194] Chuck SL, Sande MA. Infections with *Cryptococcus neoformans* in the acquired immunodeficiency syndrome. N Engl J Med 1989;321(12):794–9.

[195] Goodman JS, Kaufman L, Koenig MG. Diagnosis of cryptococcal meningitis. Value of immunologic detection of cryptococcal antigen. N Engl J Med 1971;285(8):434–6.

[196] Tassie JM, Pepper L, Fogg C, et al. Systematic screening of cryptococcal antigenemia in HIV-positive adults in Uganda. J Acquir Immune Defic Syndr 2003;33(3):411–2.

[197] Powderly WG, Cloud GA, Dismukes WE, et al. Measurement of cryptococcal antigen in serum and cerebrospinal fluid: value in the management of AIDS-associated cryptococcal meningitis. Clin Infect Dis 1994;18(5):789–92.

[198] Saag MS, Powderly WG, Cloud GA, et al. Comparison of amphotericin B with fluconazole in the treatment of acute AIDS-associated cryptococcal meningitis. The NIAID Mycoses Study Group and the AIDS Clinical Trials Group. N Engl J Med 1992;326(2):83–9.

[199] Martinez LR, Garcia-Rivera J, Casadevall A. *Cryptococcus neoformans* var. *neoformans* (serotype D) strains are more susceptible to heat than *C. neoformans* var. *grubii* (serotype A) strains. J Clin Microbiol 2001;39(9):3365–7.

[200] Robinson PG, Sulita MJ, Matthews EK, et al. Failure of the Bactec 460 radiometer to detect *Cryptococcus neoformans* fungemia in an AIDS patient. Am J Clin Pathol 1987; 87(6):783–6.

[201] Prevost-Smith E, Hutton N. Improved detection of *Cryptococcus neoformans* in the BACTEC NR 660 blood culture system. Am J Clin Pathol 1994;102(6):741–5.

[202] Zimmer BL, Roberts GD. Rapid selective urease test for presumptive identification of *Cryptococcus neoformans*. J Clin Microbiol 1979;10(3):380–1.

[203] Buesching WJ, Kurek K, Roberts GD. Evaluation of the modified API 20C system for identification of clinically important yeasts. J Clin Microbiol 1979;9(5):565–9.

[204] Huffnagle KE, Gander RM. Evaluation of Gen-Probe's *Histoplasma capsulatum* and *Cryptococcus neoformans* AccuProbes. J Clin Microbiol 1993;31(2):419–21.

[205] Saag MS, Graybill RJ, Larsen RA, et al. Practice guidelines for the management of cryptococcal disease. Infectious Diseases Society of America. Clin Infect Dis 2000;30(4):710–8.

[206] Shoham S, Cover C, Donegan N, et al. *Cryptococcus neoformans* meningitis at 2 hospitals in Washington, D.C.: adherence of health care providers to published practice guidelines for the management of cryptococcal disease. Clin Infect Dis 2005;40(3):477–9.

[207] Pappas PG, Perfect JR, Cloud GA, et al. Cryptococcosis in human immunodeficiency virus-negative patients in the era of effective azole therapy. Clin Infect Dis 2001;33(5):690–9.

[208] Leenders AC, Reiss P, Portegies P, et al. Liposomal amphotericin B (AmBisome) compared with amphotericin B both followed by oral fluconazole in the treatment of AIDS-associated cryptococcal meningitis. AIDS 1997;11(12):1463–71.

[209] Baddour LM, Perfect JR, Ostrosky-Zeichner L. Successful use of amphotericin B lipid complex in the treatment of cryptococcosis. Clin Infect Dis 2005;40(Suppl 6):S409–13.

[210] van der Horst CM, Saag MS, Cloud GA, et al. Treatment of cryptococcal meningitis associated with the acquired immunodeficiency syndrome. National Institute of Allergy and

Infectious Diseases Mycoses Study Group and AIDS Clinical Trials Group. N Engl J Med 1997;337(1):15–21.

[211] Dismukes WE, Cloud G, Gallis HA, et al. Treatment of cryptococcal meningitis with combination amphotericin B and flucytosine for four as compared with six weeks. N Engl J Med 1987;317(6):334–41.

[212] Brouwer AE, Rajanuwong A, Chierakul W, et al. Combination antifungal therapies for HIV-associated cryptococcal meningitis: a randomised trial. Lancet 2004;363(9423):1764–7.

[213] Pitisuttithum P, Negroni R, Graybill JR, et al. Activity of posaconazole in the treatment of central nervous system fungal infections. J Antimicrob Chemother 2005;56(4):745–55.

[214] Perfect JR, Marr KA, Walsh TJ, et al. Voriconazole treatment for less-common, emerging, or refractory fungal infections. Clin Infect Dis 2003;36(9):1122–31.

[215] Saag MS, Cloud GA, Graybill JR, et al. A comparison of itraconazole versus fluconazole as maintenance therapy for AIDS-associated cryptococcal meningitis. National Institute of Allergy and Infectious Diseases Mycoses Study Group. Clin Infect Dis 1999;28(2):291–6.

[216] Vibhagool A, Sungkanuparph S, Mootsikapun P, et al. Discontinuation of secondary prophylaxis for cryptococcal meningitis in human immunodeficiency virus-infected patients treated with highly active antiretroviral therapy: a prospective, multicenter, randomized study. Clin Infect Dis 2003;36(10):1329–31.

[217] Mussini C, Pezzotti P, Miro JM, et al. Discontinuation of maintenance therapy for cryptococcal meningitis in patients with AIDS treated with highly active antiretroviral therapy: an international observational study. Clin Infect Dis 2004;38(4):565–71.

[218] Singh N, Lortholary O, Alexander BD, et al. Antifungal management practices and evolution of infection in organ transplant recipients with *Cryptococcus neoformans* infection. Transplantation 2005;80(8):1033–9.

[219] Perfect JR, Cox GM. Drug resistance in *Cryptococcus neoformans*. Drug Resist Updat 1999;2(4):259–69.

[220] Graybill JR, Sobel J, Saag M, et al. Diagnosis and management of increased intracranial pressure in patients with AIDS and cryptococcal meningitis. The NIAID Mycoses Study Group and AIDS Cooperative Treatment Groups. Clin Infect Dis 2000;30(1):47–54.

[221] Pappas PG, Bustamante B, Ticona E, et al. Recombinant interferon- gamma 1b as adjunctive therapy for AIDS-related acute cryptococcal meningitis. J Infect Dis 2004;189(12): 2185–91.

[222] Robinson PA, Bauer M, Leal MA, et al. Early mycological treatment failure in AIDS-associated cryptococcal meningitis. Clin Infect Dis 1999;28(1):82–92.

[223] Macsween KF, Bicanic T, Brouwer AE, et al. Lumbar drainage for control of raised cerebrospinal fluid pressure in cryptococcal meningitis: case report and review. J Infect 2005; 51(4):e221–4.

[224] Newton PN, Thai le H, Tip NQ, et al. A randomized, double-blind, placebo-controlled trial of acetazolamide for the treatment of elevated intracranial pressure in cryptococcal meningitis. Clin Infect Dis 2002;35(6):769–72.

[225] Singh N, Husain S, De Vera M, et al. *Cryptococcus neoformans* infection in patients with cirrhosis, including liver transplant candidates. Medicine (Baltimore) 2004;83(3):188–92.

[226] Powderly WG, Finkelstein D, Feinberg J, et al. A randomized trial comparing fluconazole with clotrimazole troches for the prevention of fungal infections in patients with advanced human immunodeficiency virus infection. NIAID AIDS Clinical Trials Group. N Engl J Med 1995;332(11):700–5.

[227] Oscarson S, Alpe M, Svahnberg P, et al. Synthesis and immunological studies of glycoconjugates of *Cryptococcus neoformans* capsular glucuronoxylomannan oligosaccharide structures. Vaccine 2005;23(30):3961–72.

[228] Larsen RA, Pappas PG, Perfect J, et al. Phase I evaluation of the safety and pharmacokinetics of murine-derived anticryptococcal antibody 18B7 in subjects with treated cryptococcal meningitis. Antimicrob Agents Chemother 2005;49(3):952–8.

ELSEVIER
SAUNDERS

Infect Dis Clin N Am
20 (2006) 545–561

INFECTIOUS
DISEASE CLINICS
OF NORTH AMERICA

Aspergillosis: Spectrum of Disease, Diagnosis, and Treatment

Penelope D. Barnes, MBBS, PhD[a,b],
Kieren A. Marr, MD[a,b,*]

[a]*Program in Infectious Diseases, Fred Hutchinson Cancer Research Center,
1100 Fairview Avenue, N. D3-100, Seattle, WA 98109, USA*
[b]*University of Washington, Seattle, WA 98195, USA*

Aspergillus species are ubiquitous environmental molds that grow on organic matter and aerosolize conidia [1]. Humans inhale hundreds of conidia per day without adverse consequences except for a small minority of people for whom infection with *Aspergillus* spp causes significant morbidity. The clinical manifestations of aspergillosis are determined by the host immune response to *Aspergillus* spp with the spectrum ranging from a local inappropriate inflammatory response, causing allergy, to local saprophytic lung disease with mycelial balls, to catastrophic failure of the immune response to contain pulmonary disease and resultant systemic *Aspergillus* spp dissemination. For the clinician, *Aspergillus* spp infection presents a diagnostic and management challenge. Only by understanding the immune status of the host and the resultant risk of allergic versus local versus potentially invasive disease can the clinician attempt to make an appropriate diagnosis and management plan.

Mycology and pathogenesis of disease

In the environment *Aspergillus* spp are present as the mold form with formation of aerial hyphal stalks [1]. The conidia formed by asexual reproduction are small (2–10 μm in diameter) and hydrophobic, which aids aerosolization

Kieren A. Marr has been a consultant for Pfizer, Inc.; Merck and Company, Inc.; Enzon Pharmaceuticals; Astellas Pharma Inc.; Nektar Therapeutics; Basilea Pharmaceuticals; and Schering Plough.

* Corresponding author. D3-100, 1100 Fairview Ave North, Seattle, WA 98109.

E-mail address: kmarr@fhcrc.org (K.A. Marr).

[2]. After inhalation by the host, uncontrolled germination of conidia into hyphae in the lung results in the potentially angioinvasive form of the mold [2].

The *Aspergillus* genus comprises approximately 180 species, of which 34 have been associated with human disease. Historically, *A fumigatus* caused 90% of aspergillosis syndromes. Increasingly, disease is caused by non-fumigatus species, however [3–5]. In a recent study the *Aspergillus* spp associated with infections occurring after hematopoietic stem cell transplantation (HSCT) included *A fumigatus* (56% of cases), *A flavus* (18.7%), *A terreus* (16%), *A niger* (8%), and *A versicolor* (1.3%) [3]. Of particular concern is *A terreus*; the prognosis of invasive disease is especially poor, and the organism is resistant to amphotericin in vitro [4]. In addition, other species with variable susceptibilities to antifungal agents are being described [5,6].

Although *A fumigatus* is recognized as the most common cause of invasive infection, few virulence genes have been identified, probably, in part, because of difficulties in disruption of gene candidates and redundancies in cellular functions [2]. Recently, however, the expressed transcriptional regulator; LaeA, which coordinates multiple gene clusters of *A fumigatus*, was demonstrated to be important to allow the organism to establish invasive infection in the murine host [7]. The size, hydrophobicity, and cell wall pigments of conidia are thought to be important in conidia dissemination and interaction with the host immune response [2,7,8]. As reviewed elsewhere, proteases secreted from hyphae mediate tissue destruction, hinder the immune response, and also are important in the allergic manifestations of aspergillosis [2].

Both the acquired and innate immune systems have vital roles in defense against *Aspergillus* spp. As conidia enter the lung, resident pulmonary macrophages are ideally placed to phagocytose and destroy the conidia [9], presumably with little local cytokine response, because people inhale hundreds of conidia per day with no evident inflammation. Germination of conidia into the more invasive form hyphae, however, exposes β-glucans, and possibly other *Aspergillus* ligands, which interact with pattern recognition receptors (Toll-like receptors and Dectin) on macrophages, with the resultant production of proinflammatory cytokines [10,11]. Animal studies of invasive aspergillosis (IA) show a profound pulmonary neutrophil response to *A fumigatus* followed by a lymphocytic infiltrate, probably attracted by macrophage cytokines [12]. The vital role of neutrophils is demonstrated in animal models, in which neutropenic rabbits rapidly develop invasive disease [12], and in humans, for whom neutropenia is an independent risk factor for IA [13]. The development of a CD4 Th-1 lymphocyte response seems to be protective in animal studies of IA [14]. A CD4 Th-2 response in humans is associated with the allergic forms of aspergillosis, however [15,16]. The reasons some people develop a Th-2 rather than a Th-1 response to *Aspergillus* spp are not yet well described.

Clinical syndromes, epidemiology, diagnosis, and treatment

Allergy

The immune system of some individuals reacts inappropriately to *Aspergillus* spp and causes symptomatic local "allergic" disease that can be manifest by asthma, allergic bronchopulmonary aspergillosis (ABPA), and allergic sinusitis [16–18]. The risk of invasive disease is very low in these individuals.

Asthma

There is accumulating evidence to implicate fungi, including *Aspergillus* spp, as a cause of severe asthma [17]. Mold sensitivity has been associated with increased asthma severity and death [19].

Allergic bronchopulmonary aspergillosis

ABPA may be an extreme form of *Aspergillus* spp–driven asthma. The disease manifests as a vigorous CD4 Th-2 response in the lungs and production of *Aspergillus* spp–specific serum IgE [16,17,20]. The consequent inflammatory and obstructive bronchopulmonary injury produces steroid-dependent asthma, with the unusual symptoms of fever and hemoptysis, bronchiectasis, airway destruction, and, if inadequately treated, permanent lung injury with fibrosis [16,17,20]. The prevalence of ABPA is between 6% and 25% in people who have cystic fibrosis [16] and between 1% and 2% in asthmatic patients [17]. The underlying pathogenesis may be related to the host genetics of *Aspergillus* antigen presentation to the immune system, in particular with HLA-DR restriction [21]. Patients who have ABPA have been shown to have an increased frequency of the cystic fibrosis gene mutation, but a causative role of the gene has not yet been well described [22].

The diagnosis of ABPA is by a combination of clinical, radiologic, and laboratory parameters. Radiographic evidence includes pulmonary infiltrates that resolve with corticosteroids and central bronchiectasis (although infiltrates may not be evident in early disease) [17]. Detection of specific serum IgE against recombinant antigens of *A fumigatus* is sensitive and specific for ABPA, with levels of at least 500 IU/mL thought to be diagnostic [17,23]. This technique also has shown promise in the follow-up of patients after steroid therapy and the early detection of recurrences [23]. Other suggested criteria for diagnosis include detection of IgG specific for *Aspergillus* spp and a positive *Aspergillus* skin prick test, in the absence of response to other fungi [17].

Current treatment for ABPA is oral corticosteroids during an acute phase or exacerbation and itraconazole for antifungal therapy, but there is little evidence to suggest benefit from prolonged use of itraconazole [16,24,25]. Voriconazole and other currently investigational azole drugs probably have a future therapeutic role. In a small study, 13 children who had definitive ABPA were treated with voriconazole, with or without immunomodulatory agents, and all demonstrated significant and sustained improvements in clinical and serologic parameters for up to 13 months [26].

Allergic sinusitis

Allergic fungal sinusitis is a noninvasive but recurrent inflammatory sinusitis that occurs as an allergic response to local *A fumigatus* infection [27]. Patients typically are young (in their early 30s) with a history of atopy and initially present with hypertrophic sinus disease and nasal polyps [18]. Diagnosis depends on the findings of type I hypersensitivity, nasal polyps, and mucus containing fungal elements and Charcot-Leyden crystals (allergic mucin) [27]. CT scan is almost always abnormal with evidence of destructive pansinusitis [18], but histology reveals no fungal invasion, only a local hyperinflammatory response [18,27]. Treatment centers on endoscopic removal of debris and hyperplastic tissue [18]. The role of antifungal agents is unclear, although systemic therapy with itraconazole and topical application of amphotericin have been attempted [28,29]. In a large retrospective review, corticosteroids showed some benefit, as assessed by symptoms [30].

Local saprophytic disease: mycelial balls without allergy or invasion

Aspergillomas are mycelial balls that grow in areas of devitalized lung such as a damaged bronchial tree, a pulmonary cyst, or from the cavities of patients who have underlying cavitary lung diseases [31]. They may manifest as asymptomatic radiographic abnormalities or lead to hemoptysis that can be life threatening [31]. Upper lobes are the most frequently involved sites, perhaps because of the prevalence of tuberculosis cavities [31]. Definitive treatment is surgical resection, but these patients often have inadequate lung function to tolerate thoracic surgery, which can carry a significant mortality (5% in one study) [31]. Other treatment options include azoles and percutaneous instillation of antifungal agents [32].

Mycelial balls can also be found in sinuses [18], and endoscopic removal is required. There is no established role for antifungal agents.

Semi-invasive disease

On the borderline between saprophytic and invasive disease is a group of diseases in which mycelial balls are present, but with progressive fibrosis and minimal fungal invasion [33]. The nomenclature of the disease is currently changing [33], and three distinct entities are suggested based on radiologic appearance [33]. The formation and expansion of multiple cavities, some containing fungus balls, has been termed "chronic cavitary pulmonary aspergillosis" (CCPA) [33]. Patients who have CCPA have positive aspergillus precipitins and raised inflammatory markers. In some cases, this condition progresses to marked and extensive pulmonary fibrosis, termed "chronic fibrosing pulmonary aspergillosis" (CFPA; second category) [33]. Pleural involvement may occur, either as direct invasion of the pleural cavity or as fibrosis. The third category is the progressive enlargement of a single cavity occurring slowly over months or rapidly within weeks, with slowly progressive IA [33]. These patients differ slightly from those who have CCPA and CFPA because they usually have minor or moderate degrees of immune dysfunction, such as diabetes or corticosteroid use [33]. Treatment is with antifungal agents and surgery. Voriconazole is proving efficacious [34]. It may be difficult clinically to differentiate semi-invasive disease from noninvasive saprophytic aspergilloma, however. Factors that always must be considered are whether the patient is immunosuppressed (ie, at higher risk of invasive disease), whether the disease is progressing, and whether hyphae (signalling invasive disease) are seen in tissue on biopsy, if available [33].

Invasive sinopulmonary aspergillosis and disseminated disease

Epidemiology

Invasive sinopulmonary aspergillosis and disseminated aspergillosis represent a direct failure of the immune system to control local infection. With recent historical mortality rates approaching 100% in severely immunosuppressed populations, it is a deservedly feared infection.

In recipients of HSCT, the incidence of IA increased during the 1990s (Table 1). Suggested reasons include changes in conditioning chemotherapy regimens, changes in prophylaxis strategies for cytomegalovirus infection, the introduction of different sources of stem cells, and the use of therapeutic monoclonal antibodies [35,50]. In addition some centers report a much higher incidence than others, suggesting geographic influence or variability in diagnosis between institutions [3,51]. This difference should be considered when assessing incidence of IA disease. In contrast, the incidence of IA in patients receiving lung transplants may be declining, possibly because of effective prophylaxis with nebulized amphotericin [38,40].

The interval between transplantation and the development of IA has increased, particularly in recipients of allogeneic HSCT [13,35,36] and recipients of liver or heart transplants (see Table 1) [43,44]. Clinicians must have a high suspicion of IA long after transplantation, especially in patients who have long-term immunosuppression associated with graft-versus-host disease, organ rejection, or other posttransplantation complications such as cytomegalovirus (Table 2).

At highest risk from IA are recipients of allogeneic HSCT and persons who have hematologic cancer or neutropenia, especially if prolonged. At lower risk are recipients of autologous HSCT and solid-organ transplants. Also at risk are persons who are malnourished, recipients of corticosteroids, and patients who have HIV, diabetes, underlying pulmonary disease, and solid-organ cancer. At low risk, although often colonized with *Aspergillus* spp, are persons who have cystic fibrosis and connective tissue disease

Table 1
Epidemiology of invasive aspergillosis after transplantation

Type of transplant	HSCT Autologous	HSCT Allogeneic	Lung	Heart	Liver	Kidney
Incidence (%)	0.5–4 [3,13,35]	2.3–11 [3,13,35]	2.4–6 [3,38,39]	0.3–6 [3,38,42]	1–8 [38]	0.1–4 [3,38]
Median time to onset after transplantation	78 days –102 days [13,36,37]	78 days –102 days [13,36,37]	TRB = 3 months IA = 5–10 months [40]	75% of cases occur within 90 days [38,43]	17 days [44]	
Survival 3 months after diagnosis of IA (%)	47 [3]	15 [3] Probability of survival by time from transplantation[a] Early IA 0.35 Late IA 0.38 Very late IA 0.4 [35]	IA 18–33 TRB = 80 [3,40,41]	10–50 [3,3]	15–40 [40,45,46–48]	25–33 [3,38,49]

Abbreviations: HSCT, hematopoietic stem cell transplantation; IA, invasive aspergillosis; TRB, tracheobronchitis.

a Early IA, < 40 days after transplantation; late IA, 40 days to 6 months after transplantation; very late IA, > 6 months after transplantation.

[49,51]. In addition, specific factors affect the risk of IA within the cohorts of patients receiving HSCT and solid-organ transplants. These factors are summarized in Table 2.

The understanding of diseases that place a person at particular risk for IA is also changing. Multiple myeloma has emerged as a significant risk factor for IA, even in the absence of neutropenia [35]. In addition, IA is emerging as a devastating infection in ICU patients previously considered immunocompetent. Isolation of *Aspergillus* spp from these patients therefore must be regarded with a higher degree of clinical suspicion for IA than was previously thought necessary [60].

Survival in patients who have IA, particularly HSCT recipients [35], seems to be improving slowly (Box 1). The mortality of HSCT recipients was greater than 95% in 1990 [61] and was between 55% and 80% in recent studies [3,35,50]. This improvement probably reflects better antifungal agents (in particular voriconazole) and increased diagnostic capabilities.

Clinical manifestations of infectious aspergillosis

Invasive pulmonary aspergillosis manifests as pulmonary parenchymal invasion, inflammation, and the possibility of hematogenous spread of the fungus. Invasive pulmonary aspergillosis is the most common manifestation of *Aspergillus* spp infection in immunosuppressed patients.

There are also distinct bronchial diseases. *Aspergillus* tracheobronchitis (ATB) is an uncommon clinical presentation of pulmonary aspergillosis. Patients who have neutropenia and AIDS, and have received lung transplants are at risk. There are three recognized forms of ATB [64]. Obstructive ATB, described initially in patients who had AIDS and heart transplant recipients, is characterized by noninflammatory thick mucous plugs full of *Aspergillus* spp (demonstrated on CT scan in Fig. 1C) [65]. Pseudomembranous ATB shows extensive inflammation of the tracheobronchial tree, with a membrane overlying the mucosa containing *Aspergillus* spp [65]. Ulcerative ATB manifests as limited involvement of the tracheobronchial tree, usually at the suture line in lung transplant recipients [64,65]. Bilateral lung and right lung transplants are particularly susceptible to these infections [66]. The focus of infection is probably a nidus of *Aspergillus* infection in the native diseased lung [41,67]. Amphotericin prophylaxis and surveillance bronchoscopy, with surgery and antifungal therapy, have resulted in favorable outcomes for ulcerative ATB [65]. In contrast, for obstructive and pseudomembranous ATB the prognosis remains very poor [65].

Invasive sinus disease may present with headache, stuffiness, or nonspecifically with fever. In more advanced cases, proptosis and cranial nerve palsies become evident as *Aspergillus* spp invades the skull and neural tissue. The disease is very aggressive [45]. Systemic dissemination may present with infection of any organ, particularly the eyes and the skin [45].

Table 2
Factors reported to increase risk of invasive aspergillosis in hematopoietic stem cell and solid-organ transplantation

Transplant	Factors that increase risk of developing invasive aspergillosis
All HSCT	Type of transplant: allogeneic unrelated > allogeneic HLA matched > autologous
Allogeneic HSCT: early IA (within 40 days of transplantation)	Underlying disease: Hematologic malignancy in other than first remission [13], aplastic anemia, myelodysplastic syndrome, multiple myeloma [35]
	Cells from cord blood [35]
	Development of cytomegalovirus disease [35]
	Transplantation not done in room with laminar air flow [13]
	Transplantation done in summer [13]
Allogeneic HSCT: late IA (41–80 days after transplantation)	Unrelated donor transplant [13]
	Acute GVHD [13,35,36]
	Corticosteroids [13,35,36]
	Increased age [13,35]
	Transplant done at the time of building construction [13]
	Prolonged neutropenia [13,35]
	Delayed engraftment of T cells [35]
	Transplantation with T-cell–depleted or CD34-selected stem cells [35]
	Multiple myeloma [35]
	CMV+ donor /recipient, patients [35]
	Patients who developed CMV disease after day 40 [35,36].
	Respiratory virus infections after day 40; parainfluenza 3 and RSV [35]
HSCT 180+ days after transplantation	Neutropenia [35]
	Clinically extensive chronic GVHD [35]
	Receipt of unrelated or HLA-mismatched PBSCs [35]
	CMV disease [35]
Liver	Renal dysfunction [38,46]
	Retransplantation [38,46]
	Indications for transplant: fulminant hepatic failure [52] or HCV [44]
	CMV infection [53]
Lung	Single lung transplant [40,41]
	History of Aspergillus spp colonization before transplantation (eg, in COPD [40,38,54,55] except in patients who have cystic fibrosis [38]).
	CMV disease [56]
	Steroid therapy [6]
Heart	Reoperation [57]
	CMV disease [57]
	Posttransplantation hemodialysis [57]

Table 2 (*continued*)

Transplant	Factors that increase risk of developing invasive aspergillosis
Kidney	Existence of an episode of invasive aspergillosis in the institution's heart transplant program 2 months before or after the transplantation [57]
	High-dose and prolonged corticosteroids [58]
	Graft failure requiring hemodialysis,
	Potent immunosuppressive therapy [59,49]

Abbreviations: CMV, cytomegalovirus; COPD, chronic obstructive pulmonary disease; GVHD, graft-versus-host disease; HCV, hepatitis C virus; HSCT, hematopoietic stem cell transplantation; IA, invasive aspergillosis; PBSC, peripheral blood stem cell; RSV, respiratory syncytial virus.

Diagnosis of invasive aspergillosis

The clinical symptoms and signs associated with invasive pulmonary aspergillosis are notoriously vague but may be associated with fever, cough, pleuritic pain, and hemoptysis [45]. Early intervention in the high-risk patient is life saving. An ideal diagnostic test for IA would have very high sensitivity for early disease but would be sufficiently specific to allow a reduction in the use of empiric antifungal agents. In addition the test could be used to follow response to therapy. Current diagnostic methods have yet to reach this goal. Diagnosis is based on a combination of clinical risks, symptoms and signs, culture, histopathology, and detection of the fungal components such as the antigen galactomannan. These tests must be interpreted in the context of the patient's individual risk of infection to obtain a realistic probability of IA.

Radiology plays an important role in diagnosis and follow-up. Early findings on CT of invasive pulmonary aspergillosis are ground-glass attenuation surrounding a pulmonary nodule, the halo sign [68]. Although this sign is not specific to IA, use of CT for preemptive screening has been shown to improve early diagnosis and outcome [69]. Lesions may become bigger in the first 10 days of therapy and with neutrophil engraftment. This enlargement should not be taken as a sign of treatment failure [70]. Eventually nodules cavitate (Fig. 1A, B) and can produce the CT air-crescent sign [70]. None of the early CT signs seems to predict outcome of infection [70]. Radiographic presentation of IA in non-neutropenic patients, such as allogeneic HSCT recipients who have graft-versus-host disease, are less well described and may be more variable. The authors have seen cases in this setting diagnosed after appearance of isolated or multiple nodules, lobar infiltrates, and very diffuse ground glass opacities.

Bronchial aspergillosis can present radiographically with an obstructive pneumonia (Fig. 1C). Hence significant *Aspergillus* spp infection should be considered in immunocompromised patients, regardless of the radiographic presentation.

Box 1. Factors reported to affect risk of death from invasive aspergillosis

After hematopoietic stem cell transplantation
Graft-versus-host disease [13,62]
Neutropenia [13]
Cytomegalovirus seropositivity [13]
Prolonged use of corticosteroids [13,62,63]
Prolonged immunosuppression [63]
Disseminated invasive aspergillosis [63]
Fungal load [63]
Presence of pleural effusion [62]
Monocyte count of less than 120 cells/mm^3 [62]

After heart, lung, liver, and kidney transplantation
Hyper immunosuppression
Renal failure
More complicated postoperative course
Repeated bacterial infection
Older age [42]

The culture of *Aspergillus* spp is becoming increasingly important, given the emergence of antifungal drug–resistant non-fumigatus *Aspergillus* spp and a growing incidence of other molds causing invasive disease [3,50]. Growth from a sterile site is diagnostic of disease. A respiratory culture must be interpreted in the context of the risk for the patient, however. The positive predictive value for IA of a respiratory sample growing *Aspergillus* spp increases with rising immunosuppression [51,71]. One study showed a positive predictive value of 77% for respiratory cultures from patients who had hematologic malignancies, granulocytopenia, or HSCT, of 58% for patients who had received solid-organ transplants or steroids, and of 14% from patients who had HIV [71]. In HSCT recipients, the positive predictive value of a respiratory culture of 77% [71] makes preemptive screening for IA using respiratory cultures feasible in this cohort; however, the low negative predictive value raises questions regarding resource use.

Histology is being undertaken less frequently because biopsy is invasive. Identification of dichotomous acute-angle branching hyphae in a tissue section is definitive for fungal infection, however, and often is the only positive indication of etiology, although it is not specific for *Aspergillus* spp [1]. In situ hybridization and polymerase chain reaction (PCR) of fungi from histologic specimens are being analyzed for clinical utility when fungi are not cultured or the morphology is unclear [72,73].

The galactomannan assay (GM) is increasingly used as an aid for detecting IA. GM is the polysaccharide component cell wall of *Aspergillus* spp and is

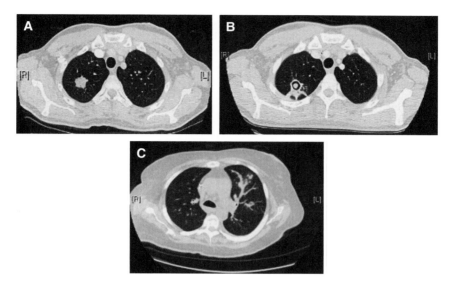

Fig. 1. CT appearances of invasive aspergillosis. (*A*) A 37-year-old man developed fever 40 days after allogeneic HSCT. His serum galactomannan (GM) EIA was positive. CT scan revealed a nodule. BAL was positive for *A fumigatus* by GM EIA and by PCR. No organisms grew. He was treated with voriconazole. (*B*) Fourteen days later the lesion had cavitated. (*C*) A 56-year-old woman with prolonged neutropenia after chemotherapy for multiple myeloma developed fever, wheeze, and cough. CT scan showed obstructive bronchial disease. Bronchoscopy revealed obstructing mucus plugs that grew *A fumigatus*.

released by growing hyphae [74]. A double-sandwich ELISA (EIA) is currently cleared by the Food and Drug Administration [74]. Recent studies suggest that the GM EIA has a sensitivity of 89% and specificity of 92% for detection of IA in the serum of HSCT recipients [74]. The sensitivity and specificity of the GM assay have been reported to be 55.6% and 93.9% to 98.5%, respectively, in liver transplant recipients [75,76] and 95% and 30%, respectively, in lung transplant recipients [77]. In lung transplant recipients, however, the GM EIA detected none of the cases of *Aspergillus* spp tracheobronchitis [77], and false positives have been reported in up to 20% of persons [77], particularly in patients with the underlying diagnosis of cystic fibrosis and chronic obstructive pulmonary disease [77]. Use of the GM EIA in bronchoalveolar lavage (BAL) fluid is less well defined, but studies demonstrate a BAL fluid sensitivity of 76% and specificity of 94% [78].

In addition to diagnosis in high-risk patients, use of the GM EIA is likely to have an increasing role for decreasing empiric antifungal therapy. A recent study examining regular serum screening for GM EIA and CT changes showed that empiric antifungal therapy could be reduced by at least 78% without apparent differences in clinical outcomes [79].

The GM EIA has important caveats, however. The antibiotic piperacillin-tazobactam produces false-positive results, probably because of GM in the product [80]. In addition, concomitant use of GM screening with anti-fungal therapy produces false-negative results [81].

The β-glucan assay detects β-glucans located in the cell wall of multiple fungi, including *Candida, Fusarium, Acremonium, Aspergillus* spp, and *Pneumocystis jiroveci* [82]. Preliminary studies have reported sensitivity of 62% and specificity of 94% for diagnosing invasive fungal infections, although few IA cases were included in the studies [82].

Detection of *Aspergillus* spp nucleic acid by PCR is being used increasingly, and recent studies suggest that in HSCT recipients in combination with GM, sensitivity of IA using BAL fluid is 85% [78]. PCR methods and reagents are not standardized among centers, however, resulting in widely different reports of sensitivity and specificity. PCR also is being analyzed for use for preemptive screening, with promising initial results [83].

Therapeutic options for invasive aspergillosis

Until recently, amphotericin and itraconazole were the standard treatments for IA. In a landmark trial, voriconazole was found to be more effective than amphotericin B in treating IA, with patients having better survival and fewer toxic side effects [84].

Echinocandins inhibit the synthesis of cell wall β-glucan [85]. No large studies have been published for first-line therapy, although caspofungin is approved for use as a salvage agent in progressive infection or intolerance to other agents. There is evidence that dual therapy for IA including the echinocandins may be better than single-drug therapy. One report of experiences with amphotericin and caspofungin suggests a favorable outcome in 40% to 60% of patients [86]. In another retrospective report of outcomes, survival was higher with a combination of caspofungin and voriconazole than with voriconazole alone [87]. In addition, prospectively collected cases in which caspofungin and voriconazole were used for treatment of IA in patients who had received solid-organ transplants demonstrated that combination therapy improved survival, especially in patients who had renal failure [88]. Randomized, controlled trials are currently in development comparing single and double therapies for IA.

The duration of therapy for IA has not been established. In practice, patients are treated until immunosuppression is reduced and there is radiographic resolution. Treatment usually lasts several months but varies among patient cohorts.

There has been growing interest in accelerating or boosting immune reconstitution as an adjunct to antifungal therapy. Theoretically the use of granulocyte macrophage colony-stimulating factor should boost neutrophil counts and help clear *Aspergillus* spp. There is no evidence of improved outcome of IA, however. Likewise, granulocyte infusions have been used, but with no proven benefit. Large studies are currently in development.

Surgery in the severely immunosuppressed patient is a very high-risk option, and there are no controlled trials for its efficacy. In less severely ill patients, surgery is a therapeutic option, particularly using improved minimally invasive surgery techniques. Resection of isolated lesions seems to be particularly important in patients who have lesions next to large blood vessels and possibly in those who will receive additional courses of chemotherapy [89].

The future

Better preemptive methods for early diagnosis and intervention are mandatory to improve patient outcomes. With the availability of the galactomannan EIA, β-glucan test, and improvements in PCR this goal has become reasonable. New drugs are becoming available. In particular, posaconazole is effective in treating aspergillosis, fusariosis, and the emerging zygomycosis [90]. Broader antifungal activity is especially important in settings in which specific mycologic diagnoses remain elusive. Current antifungal agents continue to have limitations, which include drug interactions, toxicities, and cost. A better understanding of patient risks and immunity to these fungi is necessary to develop more rational strategies to prevent and treat diseases caused by *Aspergillus* spp.

References

[1] Hope WW, Walsh TJ, Denning DW. Laboratory diagnosis of invasive aspergillosis. Lancet Infect Dis 2005;5(10):609–22.
[2] Rementeria A, Lopez-Molina N, Ludwig A, et al. Genes and molecules involved in *Aspergillus fumigatus* virulence. Rev Iberoam Micol 2005;22(1):1–23.
[3] Morgan J, Wannemuehler KA, Marr KA, et al. Incidence of invasive aspergillosis following hematopoietic stem cell and solid organ transplantation: interim results of a prospective multicenter surveillance program. Med Mycol 2005;43(Suppl 1):S49–58.
[4] Steinbach WJ, Benjamin DK Jr, Kontoyiannis DP, et al. Infections due to *Aspergillus terreus*: a multicenter retrospective analysis of 83 cases. Clin Infect Dis 2004;39(2):192–8.
[5] Balajee SA, Gribskov JL, Hanley E, Nickle D, et al. *Aspergillus lentulus* sp. *nov.*, a new sibling species of *A. fumigatus*. Eukaryot Cell 2005;4(3):625–32.
[6] Balajee SA, Gribskov J, Brandt M, et al. Mistaken identity: *Neosartorya pseudofischeri* and its anamorph masquerading as *Aspergillus fumigatus*. J Clin Microbiol 2005;43(12):5996–9.
[7] Bok JW, Balajee SA, Marr KA, et al. *LaeA*, a regulator of morphogenetic fungal virulence factors. Eukaryot Cell 2005;4(9):1574–82.
[8] Jahn B, Boukhallouk F, Lotz J, et al. Interaction of human phagocytes with pigmentless *Aspergillus* conidia. Infect Immun 2000;68(6):3736–9.
[9] Ibrahim-Granet O, Philippe B, Boleti H, et al. Phagocytosis and intracellular fate of *Aspergillus fumigatus* conidia in alveolar macrophages. Infect Immun 2003;71(2):891–903.
[10] Steele C, Rapaka RR, Metz A, et al. The beta-glucan receptor Dectin-1 recognizes specific morphologies of *Aspergillus fumigatus*. PLoS Pathog 2005;1(4):e42.
[11] Gersuk GM, Underhill DM, Zhu L, et al. Dectin-1 and TLRs permit macrophages to distinguish between different *Aspergillus fumigatus* cellular states. J Immunol 2006;176(6):3717–24.

[12] Berenguer J, Allende MC, Lee JW, et al. Pathogenesis of pulmonary aspergillosis. Granulo-cytopenia versus cyclosporine and methylprednisolone-induced immunosuppression. Am J Respir Crit Care Med 1995;152(3):1079–86.

[13] Wald A, Leisenring W, van Burik JA, et al. Epidemiology of *Aspergillus* infections in a large cohort of patients undergoing bone marrow transplantation. J Infect Dis 1997;175(6):1459–66.

[14] Cenci E, Mencacci A, Fe d'Ostiani C, et al. Cytokine- and T helper-dependent lung mucosal immunity in mice with invasive pulmonary aspergillosis. J Infect Dis 1998;178(6):1750–60.

[15] Chauhan B, Knutsen A, Hutcheson PS, et al. T cell subsets, epitope mapping, and HLA-restriction in patients with allergic bronchopulmonary aspergillosis. J Clin Invest 1996;97(10): 2324–31.

[16] Stevens DA, Moss RB, Kurup VP, et al. Allergic bronchopulmonary aspergillosis in cystic fibrosis—state of the art: Cystic Fibrosis Foundation Consensus Conference. Clin Infect Dis 2003;37(Suppl 3):S225–64.

[17] Denning DW, O'Driscoll BR, Hogaboam CM, et al. The link between fungi and severe asthma: a summary of the evidence. Eur Respir J 2006;27(3):615–26.

[18] Schubert MS. Allergic fungal sinusitis: pathogenesis and management strategies. Drugs 2004;64(4):363–74.

[19] O'Driscoll BR, Hopkinson LC, Denning DW. Mold sensitization is common amongst patients with severe asthma requiring multiple hospital admissions. BMC Pulm Med 2005; 5(1):4.

[20] Tillie-Leblond I, Tonnel AB. Allergic bronchopulmonary aspergillosis. Allergy 2005;60(8): 1004–13.

[21] Chauhan B, Hutcheson PS, Slavin RG, et al. MHC restriction in allergic bronchopulmonary aspergillosis. Front Biosci 2003;8:S140–8.

[22] Marchand E, Verellen-Dumoulin C, Mairesse M, et al. Frequency of cystic fibrosis trans-membrane conductance regulator gene mutations and 5T allele in patients with allergic bronchopulmonary aspergillosis. Chest 2001;119(3):762–7.

[23] Knutsen AP, Noyes B, Warrier MR, et al. Allergic bronchopulmonary aspergillosis in a patient with cystic fibrosis: diagnostic criteria when the IgE level is less than 500 IU/mL. Ann Allergy Asthma Immunol 2005;95(5):488–93.

[24] Stevens DA, Schwartz HJ, Lee JY, et al. A randomized trial of itraconazole in allergic bronchopulmonary aspergillosis. N Engl J Med 2000;342(11):756–62.

[25] Wark P. Pathogenesis of allergic bronchopulmonary aspergillosis and an evidence-based review of azoles in treatment. Respir Med 2004;98(10):915–23.

[26] Hilliard T, Edwards S, Buchdahl R, et al. Voriconazole therapy in children with cystic fibrosis. J Cyst Fibros 2005;4(4):215–20.

[27] Singh N, Bhalodiya NH. Allergic fungal sinusitis (AFS)—earlier diagnosis and management. J Laryngol Otol 2005;119(11):875–81.

[28] Andes D, Proctor R, Bush RK, et al. Report of successful prolonged antifungal therapy for refractory allergic fungal sinusitis. Clin Infect Dis 2000;31(1):202–4.

[29] Ponikau JU, Sherris DA, Kita H, et al. Intranasal antifungal treatment in 51 patients with chronic rhinosinusitis. J Allergy Clin Immunol 2002;110(6):862–6.

[30] Schubert MS, Goetz DW. Evaluation and treatment of allergic fungal sinusitis. II. Treatment and follow-up. J Allergy Clin Immunol 1998;102(3):395–402.

[31] Lee SH, Lee BJ, Jung do Y, et al. Clinical manifestations and treatment outcomes of pulmonary aspergilloma. Korean J Intern Med 2004;19(1):38–42.

[32] Judson MA. Noninvasive *Aspergillus* pulmonary disease. Semin Respir Crit Care Med 2004; 25(2):203–19.

[33] Denning DW, Riniotis K, Dobrashian R, et al. Chronic cavitary and fibrosing pulmonary and pleural aspergillosis: case series, proposed nomenclature change, and review. Clin Infect Dis 2003;37(Suppl 3):S265–80.

[34] Jain LR, Denning DW. The efficacy and tolerability of voriconazole in the treatment of chronic cavitary pulmonary aspergillosis. J Infect, in press.

[35] Marr KA, Carter RA, Boeckh M, et al. Invasive aspergillosis in allogeneic stem cell transplant recipients: changes in epidemiology and risk factors. Blood 2002;100(13):4358–66.

[36] Grow WB, Moreb JS, Roque D, et al. Late onset of invasive *aspergillus* infection in bone marrow transplant patients at a university hospital. Bone Marrow Transplant 2002;29(1): 15–9.

[37] Baddley JW, Stroud TP, Salzman D, et al. Invasive mold infections in allogeneic bone marrow transplant recipients. Clin Infect Dis 2001;32(9):1319–24.

[38] Singh N. Invasive aspergillosis in organ transplant recipients: new issues in epidemiologic characteristics, diagnosis, and management. Med Mycol 2005;43(Suppl 1):S267–70.

[39] Gavalda J, Len O, San Juan R, et al. Risk factors for invasive aspergillosis in solid-organ transplant recipients: a case-control study. Clin Infect Dis 2005;41(1):52–9.

[40] Singh N, Husain S. *Aspergillus* infections after lung transplantation: clinical differences in type of transplant and implications for management. J Heart Lung Transplant 2003;22(3): 258–66.

[41] Westney GE, Kesten S, De Hoyos A, et al. *Aspergillus* infection in single and double lung transplant recipients. Transplantation 1996;61(6):915–9.

[42] Grossi P, Farina C, Fiocchi R, Dalla Gasperina D. Prevalence and outcome of invasive fungal infections in 1,963 thoracic organ transplant recipients: a multicenter retrospective study. Italian Study Group of Fungal Infections in Thoracic Organ Transplant Recipients. Transplantation 2000;70(1):112–6.

[43] Montoya JG, Chaparro SV, Celis D, et al. Invasive aspergillosis in the setting of cardiac transplantation. Clin Infect Dis 2003;37(Suppl 3):S281–92.

[44] Singh N, Avery RK, Munoz P, et al. Trends in risk profiles for and mortality associated with invasive aspergillosis among liver transplant recipients. Clin Infect Dis 2003;36(1):46–52.

[45] Denning DW. Invasive aspergillosis. Clin Infect Dis 1998;26(4):781–803 [quiz; 804–5].

[46] Fortun J, Martin-Davila P, Moreno S, et al. Risk factors for invasive aspergillosis in liver transplant recipients. Liver Transpl 2002;8(11):1065–70.

[47] Fortun J, Martin-Davila P, Moreno S, et al. Prevention of invasive fungal infections in liver transplant recipients: the role of prophylaxis with lipid formulations of amphotericin B in high-risk patients. J Antimicrob Chemother 2003;52(5):813–9.

[48] Husain S, Tollemar J, Dominguez EA, et al. Changes in the spectrum and risk factors for invasive candidiasis in liver transplant recipients: prospective, multicenter, case-controlled study. Transplantation 2003;75(12):2023–9.

[49] Paterson DL, Singh N. Invasive aspergillosis in transplant recipients. Medicine (Baltimore) 1999;78(2):123–38.

[50] Marr KA, Carter RA, Crippa F, et al. Epidemiology and outcome of mould infections in hematopoietic stem cell transplant recipients. Clin Infect Dis 2002;34(7):909–17.

[51] Perfect JR, Cox GM, Lee JY, et al. The impact of culture isolation of *Aspergillus* species: a hospital-based survey of aspergillosis. Clin Infect Dis 2001;33(11):1824–33.

[52] Collins LA, Samore MH, Roberts MS, et al. Risk factors for invasive fungal infections complicating orthotopic liver transplantation. J Infect Dis 1994;170(3):644–52.

[53] George MJ, Snydman DR, Werner BG, et al. The independent role of cytomegalovirus as a risk factor for invasive fungal disease in orthotopic liver transplant recipients. Boston Center for Liver Transplantation CMVIG-Study Group. Cytogam, MedImmune, Inc. Gaithersburg, Maryland. Am J Med 1997;103(2):106–13.

[54] Patterson JE, Peters J, Calhoon JH, et al. Investigation and control of aspergillosis and other filamentous fungal infections in solid organ transplant recipients. Transpl Infect Dis 2000; 2(1):22–8.

[55] Cahill BC, Hibbs JR, Savik K, et al. *Aspergillus* airway colonization and invasive disease after lung transplantation. Chest 1997;112(5):1160–4.

[56] Ruffini E, Baldi S, Rapellino M, et al. Fungal infections in lung transplantation. Incidence, risk factors and prognostic significance. Sarcoidosis Vasc Diffuse Lung Dis 2001;18(2): 181–90.

[57] Munoz P, Rodriguez C, Bouza E, et al. Risk factors of invasive aspergillosis after heart trans-plantation: protective role of oral itraconazole prophylaxis. Am J Transplant 2004;4(4): 636–43.

[58] Gustafson TL, Schaffner W, Lavely GB, et al. Invasive aspergillosis in renal transplant re-cipients: correlation with corticosteroid therapy. J Infect Dis 1983;148(2):230–8.

[59] Panackal AA, Dahlman A, Keil KT, et al. Outbreak of invasive aspergillosis among renal transplant recipients. Transplantation 2003;75(7):1050–3.

[60] Vandewoude KH, Blot SI, Depuydt P, et al. Clinical relevance of *Aspergillus* isolation from respiratory tract samples in critically ill patients. Crit Care 2006;10(1):R31.

[61] Denning DW, Stevens DA. Antifungal and surgical treatment of invasive aspergillosis: review of 2,121 published cases. Rev Infect Dis 1990;12(6):1147–201.

[62] Cordonnier C, Ribaud P, Herbrecht R, et al. Prognostic factors for death due to invasive aspergillosis after hematopoietic stem cell transplantation: a 1-year retrospective study of consecutive patients at French transplantation centers. Clin Infect Dis 2006;42(7):955–63.

[63] Ribaud P, Chastang C, Latge JP, et al. Survival and prognostic factors of invasive aspergil-losis after allogeneic bone marrow transplantation. Clin Infect Dis 1999;28(2):322–30.

[64] Denning DW. Commentary: unusual manifestations of aspergillosis. Thorax 1995;50(7):812–3.

[65] Tasci S, Glasmacher A, Lentini S, et al. Pseudomembranous and obstructive *Aspergillus* tracheobronchitis—optimal diagnostic strategy and outcome. Mycoses 2006;49(1):37–42.

[66] Hadjiliadis D, Howell DN, Davis RD, et al. Anastomotic infections in lung transplant recip-ients. Ann Transplant 2000;5(3):13–9.

[67] Brenier-Pinchart MP, Lebeau B, Devouassoux G, et al. *Aspergillus* and lung transplant re-cipients: a mycologic and molecular epidemiologic study. J Heart Lung Transplant 1998; 17(10):972–9.

[68] Kuhlman JE, Fishman EK, Siegelman SS. Invasive pulmonary aspergillosis in acute leukemia: characteristic findings on CT, the CT halo sign, and the role of CT in early diag-nosis. Radiology 1985;157(3):611–4.

[69] Caillot D, Casasnovas O, Bernard A, et al. Improved management of invasive pulmonary aspergillosis in neutropenic patients using early thoracic computed tomographic scan and surgery. J Clin Oncol 1997;15(1):139–47.

[70] Caillot D, Couaillier JF, Bernard A, et al. Increasing volume and changing characteristics of invasive pulmonary aspergillosis on sequential thoracic computed tomography scans in patients with neutropenia. J Clin Oncol 2001;19(1):253–9.

[71] Horvath JA, Dummer S. The use of respiratory-tract cultures in the diagnosis of invasive pulmonary aspergillosis. Am J Med 1996;100(2):171–8.

[72] Bialek R, Konrad F, Kern J, et al. PCR based identification and discrimination of agents of mucormycosis and aspergillosis in paraffin wax embedded tissue. J Clin Pathol 2005; 58(11):1180–4.

[73] Rickerts V, Just-Nubling G, Konrad F, et al. Diagnosis of invasive aspergillosis and mucor-mycosis in immunocompromised patients by seminested PCR assay of tissue samples. Eur J Clin Microbiol Infect Dis 2006;25(1):8–13.

[74] Marr KA, Balajce SA, McLaughlin L, et al. Detection of galactomannan antigenemia by enzyme immunoassay for the diagnosis of invasive aspergillosis: variables that affect per-formance. J Infect Dis 2004;190(3):641–9.

[75] Fortun J, Martin-Davila P, Alvarez ME, et al. Aspergillus antigenemia sandwich-enzyme immunoassay test as a serodiagnostic method for invasive aspergillosis in liver transplant recipients. Transplantation 2001;71(1):145–9.

[76] Kwak EJ, Husain S, Obman A, et al. Efficacy of galactomannan antigen in the Platelia *Aspergillus* enzyme immunoassay for diagnosis of invasive aspergillosis in liver transplant recipients. J Clin Microbiol 2004;42(1):435–8.

[77] Husain S, Kwak EJ, Obman A, et al. Prospective assessment of Platelia *Aspergillus* galacto-mannan antigen for the diagnosis of invasive aspergillosis in lung transplant recipients. Am J Transplant 2004;4(5):796–802.

[78] Musher B, Fredricks D, Leisenring W, et al. *Aspergillus* galactomannan enzyme immunoassay and quantitative PCR for diagnosis of invasive aspergillosis with bronchoalveolar lavage fluid. J Clin Microbiol 2004;42(12):5517–22.

[79] Maertens J, Theunissen K, Verhoef G, et al. Galactomannan and computed tomography-based preemptive antifungal therapy in neutropenic patients at high risk for invasive fungal infection: a prospective feasibility study. Clin Infect Dis 2005;41(9):1242–50.

[80] Machetti M, Furfaro E, Viscoli C. Galactomannan in piperacillin-tazobactam: how much and to what extent? Antimicrob Agents Chemother 2005;49(9):3984–5.

[81] Marr KA, Laverdiere M, Gugel A, et al. Antifungal therapy decreases sensitivity of the *Aspergillus* galactomannan enzyme immunoassay. Clin Infect Dis 2005;40(12):1762–9.

[82] Ostrosky-Zeichner L, Alexander BD, Kett DH, et al. Multicenter clinical evaluation of the $(1 \rightarrow 3)$ beta D-glucan assay as an aid to diagnosis of fungal infections in humans. Clin Infect Dis 2005;41(5):654–9.

[83] Halliday C, Hoile R, Sorrell T, et al. Role of prospective screening of blood for invasive aspergillosis by polymerase chain reaction in febrile neutropenic recipients of haematopoietic stem cell transplants and patients with acute leukaemia. Br J Haematol 2006;132(4):478–86.

[84] Herbrecht R, Denning DW, Patterson TF, et al. Voriconazole versus amphotericin B for primary therapy of invasive aspergillosis. N Engl J Med 2002;347(6):408–15.

[85] Deresinski SC, Stevens DA. Caspofungin. Clin Infect Dis 2003;36(11):1445–57.

[86] Nivoix Y, Zamfir A, Lutun P, et al. Combination of caspofungin and an azole or an amphotericin B formulation in invasive fungal infections. J Infect 2006;52(1):67–74.

[87] Marr KA, Boeckh M, Carter RA, et al. Combination antifungal therapy for invasive aspergillosis. Clin Infect Dis 2004;39:797–802.

[88] Singh N, Limaye AP, Forrest G, et al. Combination of voriconazole and caspofungin as primary therapy for invasive aspergillosis in solid organ transplant recipients: a prospective, multicenter, observational study. Transplantation 2006;81(3):320–6.

[89] Offner F, Cordonnier C, Ljungman P, et al. Impact of previous aspergillosis on the outcome of bone marrow transplantation. Clin Infect Dis 1998;26(5):1098–103.

[90] Torres HA, Hachem RY, Chemaly RF, et al. Posaconazole: a broad-spectrum triazole antifungal. Lancet Infect Dis 2005;5(12):775–85.

ELSEVIER
SAUNDERS

Infect Dis Clin N Am
20 (2006) 563–579

INFECTIOUS
DISEASE CLINICS
OF NORTH AMERICA

Emerging Fungi

Marcio Nucci, MD[a], Elias Anaissie, MD[b],*

[a]Hematology Service, Department of Internal Medicine, Hospital Universitário Clementino
Fraga Filho, Universidade Federal do Rio de Janeiro, Avenue Brigadeiro Trompovsky
s/n 21941-590, Rio de Janeiro, Brazil
[b]Division of Supportive Care, Myeloma Institute for Research and Therapy, University
of Arkansas for Medical Sciences, 4301 West Markham,
Slot 776, Little Rock, AR 72205, USA

The epidemiology of invasive fungal infections has changed during the past 20 years. Their incidence has increased, and the population of patients at risk has expanded to include a broad list of medical conditions, such as solid-organ transplantation and hematopoietic stem cell transplantation (HSCT), cancer, immunosuppressive therapy, AIDS, premature birth, advanced age, and major surgery. Furthermore, the etiology of these infections has changed. In the 1980s, yeasts (particularly *Candida albicans*) were the most frequent agents of invasive mycoses. In recent years, molds have become more frequent in certain groups of patients, such as HSCT recipients, whereas in those patients in whom candidiasis is still the most frequent invasive mycosis, non-*albicans Candida* species account for more than 50% of cases [1]. Among mold infections, aspergillosis caused by non-*fumigatus* species [2], zygomycosis [3], fusariosis [4], and infection caused by black molds (phaeohyphomycosis) have been increasingly reported [5]. The exact reasons for these changes are not completely clear. In some circumstances they may be related to specific medical interventions, such as antifungal prophylaxis and the use of medical devices. In most cases, however, they seem to be a consequence of changes in the host, with more severe immunosuppression or different types of immunosuppression impacting both risk periods and the infections that occur [6]. Because zygomycosis and phaeohyphomycosis are discussed in other articles in this issue, this article focuses on fusariosis, providing an up-to-date clinical review on its clinical spectrum, diagnosis, and management.

Dr. Nucci has received CNPq grant 300235/93-3.
* Corresponding author.
E-mail address: anaissieeliasj@uams.edu (E. Anaissie).

Hyalohyphomycoses

Hyalohyphomycosis is a term used to designate invasive fungal infections caused by hyaline-septated hyphae in tissue. This term is clinically useful when hyaline septate fungi are observed on histopathology without recovery of a pathogen. When the causative agent (eg, *Fusarium solani*) is recovered, a more specific term (eg, fusariosis or infection by *Fusarium* spp) should be used. Hyalohyphomycosis is caused by a large list of fungi, including *Fusarium* spp, *Scedosporium* spp, *Acremonium* spp, and *Paecilomyces* spp.

Microbiology

Fusarium is a plant and human pathogen readily recovered from soil and water and is part of water biofilms [7]. The most frequent species causing infection in humans are *F solani*, *F oxysporum*, and *F moniliforme* [8]. *Fusarium* species grow easily and rapidly in most media without cycloheximide. Although the genus *Fusarium* can be identified by the production of hyaline, banana-shaped, multicellular macroconidia with a foot cell at the base, species identification is difficult and may require molecular methods. In tissue, the hyphae are similar to those of *Aspergillus* species, with hyaline and septate filaments that typically dichotomize in acute and right angles. In the absence of microbial growth, the differential diagnosis between fusariosis and other hyalohyphomycoses is difficult and requires the use of in situ hybridization in paraffin-embedded tissue specimens [9].

The genus *Scedosporium* contains two medically important species: *S apiospermum* and *S prolificans*. *S apiospermum* is an asexual form of *Pseudallesceria boydii* [10]. There is some controversy regarding the classification of *S prolificans* as an agent of hyalohyphomycosis [11] or phaeohyphomycosis [5]. *Scedosporium* spp are commonly isolated from rural soils, polluted waters, composts, and from manure of cattle and fowl.

Paecilomyces spp are isolated from soil and decaying plant material. The two most common species of *Paecilomyces*, *P lilacinus* and *P variotii*, are rarely pathogenic in humans. Species of *Acremonium* also are found commonly in soil, decaying vegetation, and in decaying food. Species reported to cause infections in humans include *A alabamensis*, *A falciforme*, *A kiliensis*, *A roseogriseum*, *A strictum*, *A potroni*, and *A recifei*.

Fusariosis

Epidemiology and clinical spectrum of fusariosis

Fusarium spp cause a broad spectrum of infections in humans, including superficial (eg, keratitis and onychomycosis), locally invasive, and disseminated infection, with the last occurring almost exclusively in severely immunocompromised patients [12].

The most common infections in immunocompetent individuals are keratitis and onychomycosis. Less frequently, the infection may occur as a result of skin breakdown, such as burns and wounds [12], or the presence of foreign bodies, such as keratitis in contact lens wearers [13], peritonitis in patients receiving continuous ambulatory peritoneal dialysis [14–16], and catheter-associated fungemia [17–19]. Other infections in immunocompetent patients include pneumonia [20,21], septic arthritis [22], sinusitis [23], thrombophlebitis [24], fungemia with or without organ involvement [12,25], endophthalmitis [26,27], and osteomyelitis [28].

Immunocompromised patients at high risk for fusariosis are those who have prolonged neutropenia and T-cell immunodeficiency. Unlike infection in the normal host, fusariosis in the immunocompromised population is typically invasive and disseminated. In a review of 259 cases of fusariosis including both immunocompromised and immunocompetent patients, 79% had a diagnosis of cancer [12]. In a study of 84 patients who had hematologic diseases, the infection occurred more frequently in patients who had acute leukemia (56%), and most patients (83%) were neutropenic at diagnosis [29]. On the other hand, HSCT recipients may develop late fusariosis weeks or months after neutrophil recovery. In the allogeneic HSCT population, the infection has a trimodal pattern of occurrence: a first peak of incidence in the early posttransplantation period (during neutropenia), a second peak at a median of 70 days after transplantation (in patients who have graft-versus-host disease receiving corticosteroids), and a later peak more than 1 year after transplantation, usually in the setting of treatment of chronic extensive graft-versus-host disease. Severe T-cell immunodeficiency, not neutropenia, is the major risk factor for fusariosis in these patients [4].

The overall incidence of fusariosis per 1000 HSCT recipients is 5.97 cases. The incidence is lowest (1.4–2.0/1000) among autologous HSCT recipients, intermediate (2.28–5.0/1000) in matched-related and matched unrelated allogeneic HSCT recipients, and highest (20/1000) among mismatched related donor allogeneic HSCT recipients [4].

The principal portal of entry for *Fusarium* spp is the airways, followed by the skin at site of tissue breakdown, and possibly the mucosal membranes. Airborne fusariosis is thought to be acquired by the inhalation of aerosols of fusarial conidia. Recently it was shown that the hospital water system may be a reservoir for *Fusarium* spp [30]. Showering seems to be an efficient mechanism for the dispersion of airborne fusarial conidia and transmission to the immunosuppressed host [30]. Another means of transmission is direct contact at sites of skin breakdown, such as onychomycosis [31]. Molecular studies showed a close relationship between water and patients' isolates [30]. This association also has been observed recently in an outbreak of invasive fusariosis at a HSCT center in Brazil (data not shown).

Clinical manifestations of fusariosis

Eye infections: keratitis and endophthalmitis

Fusarium is a frequent cause of fungal keratitis, with an incidence ranging from a low of 8% in India to a high of 75% in Tanzania [13]. This variable range also was observed in two studies from the United States: 25% in Pennsylvania [32] versus 63% in Florida [33]. These differences may be related to climate, with the highest rates observed in tropical and subtropical areas and lower rates in temperate areas [13]. The most frequent predisposing factor for fungal keratitis is corneal trauma by plants, animal matter, dust, and soil [13]. The presence of an underlying corneal disease or the concomitant use of topical corticosteroids, antibiotics, and contaminated contact lens or leans paraphernalia also seem to increase the risk of fusarial keratitis. The clinical manifestations of fusarial keratitis are nonspecific, and the diagnosis requires culture of scrapings or tissue biopsy.

In immunocompetent individuals, endophthalmitis caused by *Fusarium* spp may occur as a complication of advanced keratitis [34] or ocular surgery, such as cataract extraction [35]. By contrast, fusarial endophthalmitis in the immunosuppressed host results from hematogenous seeding in the setting of disseminated infection [36,37].

Sinusitis

Disease related to *Fusarium* spp may manifest as allergic [38] and chronic noninvasive sinusitis in the immunocompetent host [39] and as invasive sinusitis in both immunocompetent [23] and immunocompromised hosts [40–42]. In immunocompromised hosts, sinusitis can serve as the port for disseminated fusariosis [43].

In a literature review of 259 cases of fusariosis [12], updated with 35 additional cases published between 2001 and 2005 (Table 1) [24,36,37,44–71], involvement of the sinuses was reported in 54 cases (18%). Sinusitis was more frequently reported in the setting of immunosuppression (52/262, 20%) than among immunocompetent patients (2/32 [6%]; $P = .06$). The two immunocompetent patients who had sinusitis presented with chronic invasive infection: one patient had a 3-year history of purulent nasal discharge, and the other presented with a 1-year history of swelling of the right cheek and nasal discharge, headache, and otalgia for 2 months [23].

Among immunocompromised patients, fusarial sinusitis is more common in patients who have cancer (22% versus 7.5%; $P = .03$), especially acute myeloid leukemia (28% versus 16%, $P = .02$), and in neutropenic patients (23% versus 10%; $P = .05$). Sinusitis occurred typically in the context of disseminated fusariosis (70%), but sinuses were the main source of diagnosis in 11% of cases, usually by means of sinus biopsy or aspirate [29].

The clinical manifestations of fusarial sinusitis are indistinguishable from those caused by *Aspergillus*: nasal discharge and obstruction. Necrosis of the

Table 1
Clinical characteristics of fusariosis according to the immune status of the host[a]

Site of infection		Immune status of the host		P value
		Normal: n = 32 (%)	Compromised: n = 262 (%)	
Skin	Total	19 (59)	186 (71)	.18
	Extent of skin lesion			
	Localized	18	26	<.001
	Disseminated	1	160	
	Type of lesion			
	Ulcer	4 (21)	4 (2)	.003
	Periungueal cellulitis	3 (16)	9 (5)	.09
	Papular, nodular	4 (21)	160 (86)	<.001
	Subcutaneous abscess	2 (10.5)	3 (2)	.07
	Cellulitis with necrosis	5 (26)	10 (5)	.006
	Phlebitis	1 (5)	0	.09
	Major risk factors	Trauma	Acute leukemia, neutropenia, HSCT	
Sinuses	Total involving sinuses	2 (6)	52 (20)	.06
	Sinusitis only	2 (100)	4 (8)	.01
	Risk	None described	Cancer, acute leukemia, neutropenia	
Pneumonia	Total	5 (16)	109 (42)	.004
	Isolated pneumonia	3 (60)	11 (10)	.01
	Radiological findings[b]			
	Alveolar	3	50	.66
	Interstitial	0	11	1.0
	Nodular, cavitary	0	24	.58
	Risk factors	None described	Acute leukemia, neutropenia, HSCT	
Positive blood cultures	Total	2 (6)	117 (45)	<.001
	Isolated fungemia	1 (3)	27 (10)	.33
Disseminated infection	Total	1 (3)	187 (71)	<.001
	Risk factors	None described	Acute leukemia, neutropenia, HSCT	

Abbreviation: HSCT, hematopoietic stem cell transplantation.

[a] 294 reported cases; keratitis and onychomycosis not included.

[b] Radiologic findings not described in 27 cases.

mucosa is a hallmark and is a consequence of the angioinvasive nature of these mycoses. Periorbital and paranasal cellulitis may be present.

Pneumonia

Lung involvement is common in invasive fusariosis. In a series of 84 patients who had fusariosis and an underlying hematologic disease, lung infiltrates (presumed to be caused by fusariosis) were present in 54% of patients and, as in aspergillosis, consisted of nonspecific alveolar or interstitial infiltrates, nodules, and cavities. The clinical presentation was nonspecific, with some patients presenting with a clinical picture similar to invasive aspergillosis, with dry cough, pleuritic chest pain, and shortness of breath [29].

Among 294 reported cases of fusariosis, lung involvement was present in 114 (39%) and was more common among immunocompromised patients (109 cases [42%]) than immunocompetent patients (five cases [16%]; $P =$ .004). Risk factors for fusarial pneumonia include a diagnosis of acute leukemia, prolonged neutropenia, and HSCT. Pneumonia as the sole manifestation of fusariosis was reported in 14 cases (11 in immunocompromised patients). The most frequent radiologic pattern was alveolar infiltrates (46%), pulmonary nodules and interstitial infiltrates (9% each), and cavities (4%). Nodular and cavitary lesions were more common among patients who had isolated lung involvement (6 of 14 [43%] versus 18 of 100 [18%]; $P = .04$). A confirmation of lung involvement was obtained in 60 cases (53%). The most frequent pulmonary material that contributed to the diagnosis was lung tissue obtained from autopsy (63%), followed by sputum (17%), bronchial aspirate (8%), lung biopsy (7%), and bronchoalveolar lavage (5%). Patients who had fusarial pneumonia were more likely to die than those who did not have lung involvement (77% versus 59%; $P < .001$), even after controlling for status of the host defenses and neutropenia (Table 2).

Fusarium also may be associated with allergic bronchopulmonary disease [72], similar to allergic bronchopulmonary aspergillosis.

Skin involvement

A common feature of infection by *Fusarium* is the development of skin lesions, which frequently are the only source of diagnostic material. In a review of 259 published cases of fusariosis (232 immunocompromised and 27 immunocompetent patients) [12], skin involvement by fusariosis was present in 181 patients (70%). Skin lesions were localized in 13 of the 14 immunocompetent patients and followed a recent history of skin breakdown at the site of the fusarial infection in 10 patients, either as a result of trauma (7 patients who had cellulitis and necrosis) or of a preexisting onychomycosis (3 patients). Three additional patients presented with ulcerated lesions

Table 2
Predictors of death in 294 published cases of fusariosis[a]

Variable	Odds Ratio (95% confidence interval)	
	Univariate	Multivariate
HSCT	5.65 (2.55–12.87)	4.54 (2.03–10.15)
Neutropenia	5.53 (3.09–9.96)	3.10 (1.59–6.05)
Disseminated fusariosis	5.37 (3.10–9.31)	2.54 (1.36–.5)
Lung involvement	3.39 (1.94–5.94)	2.23 (1.24–4.02)

Abbreviation: HSCT, hematopoietic stem cell transplantation.

[a] Variables analyzed: underlying disease, HSCT, solid-organ transplantation, immune status of the host, presence of neutropenia, positive blood cultures, skin lesions, extent of skin lesions (localized or disseminated), pneumonia, and sinusitis.

resembling chromoblastomycosis. The single case of disseminated meta-static skin lesion occurred in a child who had no apparent underlying disease, who developed fever, pulmonary infiltrates, multiple erythematous papules and nodules, and several blood cultures yielding *Fusarium sp*. Two cases of mycetoma caused by *Fusarium* spp have been reported recently [49,58].

In the authors' review of fusarial skin lesions [12], most immunocompromised patients had disseminated skin lesions. Only 20 (12%) presented with primary cellulitis, following a recent history of skin breakdown in 11 (most commonly at the site of preexisting onychomycosis [8 patients]). Onychomycosis and nail paronychia seem to be important risk factors for subsequent disseminated infection, particularly in highly immunosuppressed patients, and can be an important clue to the diagnosis of this infection [12]. Other cutaneous presentations include periorbital cellulitis in patients who have sinusitis or primary ulcerative lesions. Patients who have disseminated disease typically have multiple erythematous papular or nodular and painful lesions, frequently with central necrosis giving the lesions an appearance resembling ecthyma gangrenosum. Target lesions (a thin rim of erythema 1–3 cm in diameter surrounding the papular or nodular lesions) were reported in 16 patients; bullae developed in one patient. Fusarial skin lesions can involve practically any site, with predominance for the extremities, and evolve rapidly, usually over a few days (range, 1–5 days). Lesions at different stages of evolution (papules, nodules, and necrotic lesions) have been reported in 51 patients, and concomitant myalgias (suggesting muscle involvement) have been described in 23. Among 16 patients who had metastatic skin lesions, recent histories of cellulitis at the site of onychomycosis (11 patients), local trauma (3 patients), or an insect bite (2 patients) were reported, suggesting that skin was the primary site of disseminated infection. Skin lesions were the single source of diagnosis of fusarial infection in most patients who had such lesions (100/181; 55%). Diagnosis was based on culture in 2 patients) and on both culture and histopathology in 68 patients. Patients who have skin lesions have a high mortality rate (129/184 [70%] versus 41/75 [55%]; $P = .02$), especially when the lesions are disseminated (114/149 [76%] versus 15/35 [43%]; $P < .001$). A stratified analysis of patients who have metastatic cutaneous lesions according to neutrophil count, however, revealed that the higher mortality rate remained significant only among those who had an adequate neutrophil count throughout the course of their illness.

Fungemia, a common manifestation of disseminated fusariosis

A striking characteristic of fusariosis, as opposed to aspergillosis and most other invasive mold infections, is the high frequency of positive blood cultures, mostly in the context of disseminated disease. Among 294 reported cases, blood cultures yielded the organism in 119 (40.5%). Fungemia as the only manifestation of fusariosis occurred in 28 patients (9.5%): in 1 of 32 immunocompetent patients (3%), and in 27 of 262 immunocompromised patients (10%). Fungemia was more frequent in the absence of neutropenia in immunocompromised patients (10/52 [19%]) than in neutropenic patients (17/210 [8%]; P = .02). In patients who had fungemia, the mortality rate was lower non-neutropenic patients than in neutropenic patients (12/28 [43%] versus 167/266 [63%]; P = .04), probably because of the significant proportion of isolated fungemia among the former group, some of whom had venous catheter-related infection, which seems to have a better prognosis. Ten cases of catheter-related fusarial infection were reported [17–19, 73–76], all with a favorable outcome following antifungal treatment and catheter removal.

Disseminated infection

Disseminated disease is the most frequent clinical form of fusariosis in immunocompromised patients and was reported in 79% of 84 patients who had hematologic diseases [29], in 75% of 61 HSCT recipients [4], and in 64% of all 294 published cases. Except for one patient, who did not have an underlying disease [12], all cases of disseminated fusariosis occurred in the setting of immunosuppression, usually among patients who had acute leukemia (124/155 [80%] versus 64/139 [46%]; P < .001), HSCT recipients (53/67 [79%] versus 135/227 [59.5%]; P = .003), and in neutropenic patients (168/210 [80%] versus 20/84 [24%]; P < .001). As expected, the death rate is higher among patients who have disseminated disease (141/188 [75%] versus 38/106 [36%]; P < .001), and this association remained statistically significant even after controlling for the presence of neutropenia, HSCT, underlying disease, and organ involvement (see Table 2).

The most frequent pattern of disseminated disease is a combination of cutaneous lesions and positive blood cultures, with or without lung or sinus involvement. The typical clinical presentation is a patient who has prolonged (> 10 days) and profound (< $100/mm^3$) neutropenia who is persistently febrile and develops disseminated and characteristic skin lesions with a positive blood culture for a mold.

Prognosis and treatment

Prognosis

An analysis of 84 patients who had hematologic diseases revealed 30- and 90-day survival rates of 50% and 21%, respectively [29]. Multivariate predictors of poor outcome were persistent neutropenia (hazard ratio, 5.43; 95% confidence interval, 2.64–11.11) and recent therapy with corticosteroids (hazard ratio, 2.18; 95% confidence interval, 1.98–3.96). The actuarial survival of patients was 0 for patients who had both unfavorable prognostic factors and 4% for those who had persistent neutropenia only. By contrast, patients who had neither of these two risk factors had a survival rate of

67%, with a survival of 30% for recipients of corticosteroids who had adequate neutrophils counts ($P < .0001$). Among the HSCT recipients, 90-day survival after diagnosis was only 13%, and the single predictor of poor outcome was persistent neutropenia (hazard ratio, 12.05; 95% confidence interval, 1.46–100) [4]. Finally, HSCT, neutropenia, disseminated disease, and lung involvement predicted death among the 294 reported cases of fusariosis (see Table 2).

Treatment

Invasive and disseminated infection
Antifungal chemotherapy. The optimal treatment strategy for patients who have severe fusarial infection remains unclear because of the lack of controlled trials and because the outcome is influenced largely by the immune status of the host. Hence, comparisons between different treatment reports are problematic. In a retrospective analysis of 84 patients who had hematologic diseases and invasive fusariosis, treatment consisted of deoxycholate amphotericin B (69 patients) or a lipid formulation of amphotericin B (13 patients), with 2 patients not receiving treatment. Twenty-seven patients (32%) responded to treatment, but only 18 patients (21%) were alive 90 days after diagnosis. The response rate to a lipid formulation of amphotericin B seemed superior to that of deoxycholate amphotericin B (46% versus 32%), but the difference was not statistically significant ($P = .36$) [29].

Among the 45 patients who underwent HSCT, deoxycholate amphotericin B was given to 30 patients, a lipid formulation of amphotericin B to 14 patients, and caspofungin to 1 patient. The outcome was poor, with only 13% of patients alive at 90 days after diagnosis [4].

In a retrospective study, amphotericin B lipid complex was given to 28 patients who had fusariosis (12 refractory to prior antifungal therapy) [77]. At a median daily dose of 4.5 mg/kg, the response rate (cure or improvement) in 26 evaluable patients was 46%. In another study, voriconazole was given to 11 patients who had fusariosis, all intolerant of or refractory to primary therapy [78]. The response rate (complete plus partial response) was 45%, with an actuarial survival at 90 days of 71%. These data contrast with the 21% 90-day survival of the previously reported 84 patients who had hematologic diseases [29] and the 13% 90-day survival in 61 HSCT recipients [4]. As mentioned before, however, it is difficult to draw any conclusion from these comparisons because of differences in patients' characteristics and because patients treated with salvage regimens may have a better prognosis because they have survived enough to receive a second treatment. Posaconazole has also been used in the treatment of fusariosis. Twenty-four patients (18 intolerant or refractory to prior antifungal therapy) were treated, with a 24% response rate [79].

If the organism is available, antifungal susceptibility testing should be performed, and the active agent should be applied at the highest tolerable doses.

Typically *Fusarium* spp are relatively resistant to most antifungal agents. In vitro susceptibility may vary among different species, however, with *Fusarium solani* exhibiting higher minimal inhibitory concentrations (MICs) than *Fusarium oxysporum* [80]. The MIC range for amphotericin B is usually 1 to 2 μg/mL, with MIC_{50} and MIC_{90} of 1 and 2 μg/mL, respectively. The same pattern is exhibited by other antifungal agents: itraconazole (MIC range, 1–16 μg/mL; $MIC_{50} > 8$ μg/mL; $MIC_{90} > 8$ μg/mL), voriconazole (MIC range, 0.25–16 μg/mL; $MIC_{50} = 8$ μg/mL; $MIC_{90} > 8$ μg/mL), posaconazole (MIC range, 0.5–8 μg/mL; $MIC_{50} > 8$ μg/mL; $MIC_{90} > 8$ μg/mL), and caspofungin (MIC range > 8 μg/mL; $MIC_{50} > 8$ μg/mL; $MIC_{90} > 8$ μg/mL) [81]. The echinocandins have no activity against *Fusarium* spp [82].

Adjunctive therapies

In addition to antifungal treatment, the optimal management of patients who have fusariosis includes surgical debulking of infected tissues [83] and removal of venous catheters in patients who have confirmed catheter-related fusariosis [17]. The roles of granulocyte colony-stimulating factor (G-CSF), granulocyte-macrophage colony-stimulating factor, and G-CSF–stimulated granulocyte transfusions in the adjuvant treatment of fusariosis are not established, but, because of the poor prognosis of fusariosis, especially in persistently neutropenic patients, they are frequently used. In support there are isolated case reports of the successful treatment of invasive fusariosis with a combination of medical treatment and some of these measures [56].

Localized infection

In the treatment of localized infection, débridement of infected tissue is even more critical. Keratitis usually is treated with topical antifungal agents; natamycin is the drug of choice, although limited data support its use [13]. Localized skin lesions in immunocompromised patients deserve special attention. Because the skin may be the source for disseminated and frequently life-threatening fusarial infections, local débridement should be performed, and topical antifungal agents (natamycin, amphotericin B) should be used before commencing immunosuppressive therapies.

Prevention

Because of the poor prognosis associated with fusariosis and the limited susceptibility of *Fusarium* spp to antifungal agents, prevention of infection remains the cornerstone of management. In severely immunosuppressed patients, especially leukemic patients who have prolonged neutropenia and HSCT recipients, every effort should be made to prevent patient exposure (eg, by avoiding contact with reservoirs of *Fusarium* spp, such as tap water [30] and cleaning showers before they are used by high-risk patients [84]).

Decreasing immunosuppression should be attempted in patients who have a prior history of *Fusarium* infection and can be achieved by a reduction in or discontinuation of immunosuppressive agents, shortening the duration of neutropenia (selection of nonmyeloablative as opposed to myeloablative preparative regimens for allogeneic HSCT and use of G-CSF or G-CSF and dexamethasone-elicited white blood cell transfusions) [85,86]. If the organism is available, antifungal susceptibility testing should be performed, and antifungal prophylaxis with an agent active against the fusarial strain should be considered. In addition, a thorough evaluation and treatment of skin lesions and breakdown (particularly onychomycoses that serve as a portal of entry for fusariosis) should be undertaken before HSCT [12].

Hyalohyphomycosis caused by other agents

Clinical spectrum

Scedosporium *spp*
S apiospermum. In normal hosts, *S apiospermum* causes localized infection after penetrating trauma and pneumonia or disseminated infection after near-drowning accidents. In North America, *S apiospermum* is the most frequent cause of eumycotic mycetoma, a chronic fistulous, suppurative infection of the subcutaneous tissue, fascia, and contiguous bones that arises after penetrating trauma.

In immunocompromised patients, *S apiospermum* causes deeply invasive infections such as pneumonia, sinusitis, and brain abscess [11,87]. The clinical presentation may be similar to aspergillosis. Neutropenia and organ transplantation are the most frequent underlying conditions. Pulmonary involvement is common in HSCT recipients: in a series of 10 cases, 9 had lung disease, frequently with sinusitis (6 cases). A recent publication described 23 cases of *S apiospermum* infection in recipients of solid-organ transplants from 1976 to 1999. There were 8 cases of disseminated disease, four cases of pneumonia, 3 cases of skin infection only, 2 cases each of brain abscess and fungus ball (1 in the lung and 1 in the sinuses), and 1 case each of endophthalmitis, meningitis, eye infection with brain abscess, and mycotic aneurysm [88].

S prolificans. *S prolificans* causes localized infections in immunocompetent patients, usually after surgery or trauma. Bones and soft tissues are the most frequent sites. Neutropenia is the predominant risk factor among immunocompromised patients [5]. Fifteen of 16 patients recently reported were neutropenic, and most developed disseminated infection with persistent fever, lung infiltrates, renal failure, and neurologic involvement. Skin lesions with central necrosis were present in four patients [89]. Like fusariosis, infection with *S prolificans* is associated with a high rate of bloodstream infection with 20 of 26 patients who had cancer presenting with positive blood cultures [90].

Paecilomyces *spp*

The clinical spectrum of infection caused by *Paecilomyces* spp in the immunocompetent host includes keratitis associated with corneal implants, endophthalmitis, endocarditis following valve replacement, sinusitis, cutaneous infections, and peritonitis in patients undergoing peritoneal dialysis. Disseminated infection, pneumonia, cellulitis, and pyelonephritis have been reported in immunosuppressed patients [90,91].

Acremonium *spp*

Acremonium spp may cause nail and corneal infection, mycetoma, peritonitis and dialysis fistulae infection, osteomyelitis, meningitis (following spinal anesthesia in an otherwise healthy individual), cerebritis in an intravenous drug abuser, endocarditis in a prosthetic valve operation, and a pulmonary infection in a child [91].

Prognosis and treatment

Like fusariosis, the optimal management of infection caused by the agents of hyalohyphomycoses is not established. In the immunocompetent host, surgery, local instillation of antifungal agents (intra-articular, intraocular, and at other sites), and systemic antifungal therapy are potentially curative. In the immunocompromised host, the outcome of disseminated infection remains poor [88,90]. In these patients, the critical factor is recovery from immunosuppression, with surgical resection of localized lesions and antifungal therapy playing an important adjunctive role. *S apiospermum* is susceptible to the antifungal triazoles. In a series of eight pediatric patients who had scedosporiosis, all six *S apiospermum* infections responded to voriconazole, but not the two *S prolificans* infections [92]. In another study, response to voriconazole was also observed in two of six patients who had *S apiospermum* infection and in one of four patients who had *S prolificans* infection [78].

Successful clinical outcomes of infection caused by *Acremonium* spp have been observed after treatment with amphotericin B, itraconazole, voriconazole, and posaconazole [63,93,94]. Infections caused by *Paecilomyces* have been treated successfully with amphotericin B, itraconazole, and voriconazole [95,96].

Summary

The hyalohyphomycetes (especially *Fusarium* spp) have emerged as significant pathogens in severely immunocompromised patients. Human infections by *Fusarium* spp can be superficial or limited to single organs in otherwise healthy patients. Such infections are rare and tend to respond well to therapy. By contrast, disseminated fusarial hyalohyphomycosis affects the immunocompromised host and frequently is fatal. Successful outcome is determined by the degree of immunosuppression and the extent of the infection. These infections may be suspected clinically on the basis of a constellation of clinical and laboratory findings, which should lead to prompt therapy.

References

[1] Pappas PG, Rex JH, Lee J, et al. A prospective observational study of candidemia: epidemiology, therapy, and influences on mortality in hospitalized adult and pediatric patients. Clin Infect Dis 2003;37(5):634–43.
[2] Marr KA, Carter RA, Crippa F, et al. Epidemiology and outcome of mould infections in hematopoietic stem cell transplant recipients. Clin Infect Dis 2002;34(7):909–17.
[3] Kauffman CA. Zygomycosis: reemergence of an old pathogen. Clin Infect Dis 2004;39(4): 588–90.
[4] Nucci M, Marr KA, Queiroz-Telles F, et al. Fusarium infection in hematopoietic stem cell transplant recipients. Clin Infect Dis 2004;38(9):1237–42.
[5] Revankar SG, Patterson JE, Sutton DA, et al. Disseminated phaeohyphomycosis: review of an emerging mycosis. Clin Infect Dis 2002;34(4):467–76.
[6] Procop GW, Roberts GD. Emerging fungal diseases: the importance of the host. Clin Lab Med 2004;24:691–719.
[7] Elvers KT, Leeming K, Moore CP, et al. Bacterial-fungal biofilms in flowing water photoprocessing tanks. J Appl Microbiol 1998;84(4):607–18.
[8] Nelson PE, Dignani MC, Anaissie EJ. Taxonomy, biology, and clinical aspects of Fusarium species. Clin Microbiol Rev 1994;7(4):479–504.
[9] Hayden RT, Isotalo PA, Parrett T, et al. In situ hybridization for the differentiation of Aspergillus, Fusarium, and Pseudallescheria species in tissue section. Diagn Mol Pathol 2003; 12(1):21–6.
[10] Issakainen J, Jalava J, Eerola E, et al. Relatedness of Pseudallescheria, Scedosporium and Graphium pro parte based on SSU rDNA sequences. J Med Vet Mycol 1997;35(6): 389–98.
[11] Walsh TJ, Groll A, Hiemenz J, et al. Infections due to emerging and uncommon medically important fungal pathogens. Clin Microbiol Infect 2004;10(Suppl 1):48–66.
[12] Nucci M, Anaissie E. Cutaneous infection by Fusarium species in healthy and immunocompromised hosts: implications for diagnosis and management. Clin Infect Dis 2002;35(8): 909–20.
[13] Doczi I, Gyetvai T, Kredics L, et al. Involvement of Fusarium spp. in fungal keratitis. Clin Microbiol Infect 2004;10(9):773–6.
[14] Rippon JW, Larson RA, Rosenthal DM, et al. Disseminated cutaneous and peritoneal hyalohyphomycosis caused by Fusarium species: three cases and review of the literature. Mycopathologia 1988;101(2):105–11.
[15] Kerr CM, Perfect JR, Craven PC, et al. Fungal peritonitis in patients on continuous ambulatory peritoneal dialysis. Ann Intern Med 1983;99(3):334–6.
[16] Flynn JT, Meislich D, Kaiser BA, et al. Fusarium peritonitis in a child on peritoneal dialysis: case report and review of the literature. Perit Dial Int 1996;16(1):52–7.
[17] Velasco E, Martins CA, Nucci M. Successful treatment of catheter-related fusarial infection in immunocompromised children. Eur J Clin Microbiol Infect Dis 1995;14(8):697–9.
[18] Raad I, Hachem R. Treatment of central venous catheter-related fungemia due to Fusarium oxysporum. Clin Infect Dis 1995;20(3):709–11.

[19] Ammari LK, Puck JM, McGowan KL. Catheter-related Fusarium solani fungemia and pulmonary infection in a patient with leukemia in remission. Clin Infect Dis 1993;16(1):148–50.

[20] Madhavan M, Ratnakar C, Veliath AJ, et al. Primary disseminated fusarial infection. Postgrad Med J 1992;68(796):143–4.

[21] Sander A, Beyer U, Amberg R. Systemic Fusarium oxysporum infection in an immunocompetent patient with an adult respiratory distress syndrome (ARDS) and extracorporeal membrane oxygenation (ECMO). Mycoses 1998;41(3–4):109–11.

[22] Jakle C, Leek JC, Olson DA, et al. Septic arthritis due to Fusarium solani. J Rheumatol 1983; 10(1):151–3.

[23] Kurien M, Anandi V, Raman R, et al. Maxillary sinus fusariosis in immunocompetent hosts. J Laryngol Otol 1992;106(8):733–6.

[24] Murray CK, Beckius ML, McAllister K. Fusarium proliferatum superficial suppurative thrombophlebitis. Mil Med 2003;168(5):426–7.

[25] Sturm AW, Grave W, Kwee WS. Disseminated Fusarium oxysporum infection in patient with heatstroke. Lancet 1989;1(8644):968.

[26] Pflugfelder SC, Flynn HW Jr, Zwickey TA, et al. Exogenous fungal endophthalmitis. Ophthalmology 1988;95(1):19–30.

[27] Gabriele P, Hutchins RK. Fusarium endophthalmitis in an intravenous drug abuser. Am J Ophthalmol 1996;122(1):119–21.

[28] Bourguignon RL, Walsh AF, Flynn JC, et al. Fusarium species osteomyelitis. Case report J Bone Joint Surg [Am] 1976;58(5):722–3.

[29] Nucci M, Anaissie EJ, Queiroz-Telles F, et al. Outcome predictors of 84 patients with hematologic malignancies and Fusarium infection. Cancer 2003;98(2):315–9.

[30] Anaissie EJ, Kuchar RT, Rex JH, et al. Fusariosis associated with pathogenic Fusarium species colonization of a hospital water system: a new paradigm for the epidemiology of opportunistic mold infections. Clin Infect Dis 2001;33(11):1871–8.

[31] Girmenia C, Arcese W, Micozzi A, et al. Onychomycosis as a possible origin of disseminated Fusarium solani infection in a patient with severe aplastic anemia. Clin Infect Dis 1992;14(5): 1167.

[32] Tanure MA, Cohen EJ, Sudesh S, et al. Spectrum of fungal keratitis at Wills Eye Hospital, Philadelphia, Pennsylvania. Cornea 2000;19(3):307–12.

[33] Rosa RH Jr, Miller D, Alfonso EC. The changing spectrum of fungal keratitis in south Florida. Ophthalmology 1994;101(6):1005–13.

[34] Dursun D, Fernandez V, Miller D, et al. Advanced Fusarium keratitis progressing to endophthalmitis. Cornea 2003;22(4):300–3.

[35] Ferrer C, Alio J, Rodriguez A, et al. Endophthalmitis caused by Fusarium proliferatum. J Clin Microbiol 2005;43(10):5372–5.

[36] Rezai KA, Eliott D, Plous O, et al. Disseminated Fusarium infection presenting as bilateral endogenous endophthalmitis in a patient with acute myeloid leukemia. Arch Ophthalmol 2005;123(5):702–3.

[37] Tiribelli M, Zaja F, Fili C, et al. Endogenous endophthalmitis following disseminated fungemia due to Fusarium solani in a patient with acute myeloid leukemia. Eur J Haematol 2002;68(5):314–7.

[38] Wickern GM. Fusarium allergic fungal sinusitis. J Allergy Clin Immunol 1993;92(4):624–5.

[39] Stammberger H. Endoscopic surgery for mycotic and chronic recurring sinusitis. Ann Otol Rhinol Laryngol Suppl 1985;119:1–11.

[40] Valenstein P, Schell WA. Primary intranasal Fusarium infection. Potential for confusion with rhinocerebral zygomycosis. Arch Pathol Lab Med 1986;110(8):751–4.

[41] Segal BH, Walsh TJ, Liu JM, et al. Invasive infection with Fusarium chlamydosporum in a patient with aplastic anemia. J Clin Microbiol 1998;36(6):1772–6.

[42] Lopes JO, de Mello ES, Klock C. Mixed intranasal infection caused by Fusarium solani and a zygomycete in a leukaemic patient. Mycoses 1995;38(7–8):281–4.

[43] Anaissie E, Kantarjian H, Ro J, et al. The emerging role of Fusarium infections in patients with cancer. Medicine (Baltimore) 1988;67(2):77–83.

[44] Nakar C, Livny G, Levy I, et al. Mycetoma of the renal pelvis caused by Fusarium species. Pediatr Infect Dis J 2001;20(12):1182–3.

[45] Pereiro M Jr, Abalde MT, Zulaica A, et al. Chronic infection due to Fusarium oxysporum mimicking lupus vulgaris: case report and review of cutaneous involvement in fusariosis. Acta Derm Venereol 2001;81(1):51–3.

[46] Sridhar H, Subramanyam JR, Appaji L, et al. Fusarium solani fungemia in a patient with acute lymphoblastic leukemia. Indian J Cancer 2001;38(1):19–21.

[47] Letscher-Bru V, Campos F, Waller J, et al. Successful outcome of treatment of a disseminated infection due to Fusarium dimerum in a leukemia patient. J Clin Microbiol 2002;40(3):1100–2.

[48] Pushker N, Chra M, Bajaj MS, et al. Necrotizing periorbital Fusarium infection–an emerging pathogen in immunocompetent individuals. J Infect 2002;44(4):236–9.

[49] Tomimori-Yamashita J, Ogawa MM, Hirata SH, et al. Mycetoma caused by Fusarium solani with osteolytic lesions on the hand: case report. Mycopathologia 2002;153(1):11–4.

[50] Apostolidis J, Bouzani M, Platsouka E, et al. Resolution of fungemia due to Fusarium species in a patient with acute leukemia treated with caspofungin. Clin Infect Dis 2003;36(10):1349–50.

[51] Bader M, Jafri AK, Krueger T, et al. Fusarium osteomyelitis of the foot in a patient with diabetes mellitus. Scand J Infect Dis 2003;35(11–12):895–6.

[52] Cocuroccia B, Gaido J, Gubinelli E, et al. Localized cutaneous hyalohyphomycosis caused by a Fusarium species infection in a renal transplant patient. J Clin Microbiol 2003;41(2):905–7.

[53] Consigny S, Dhedin N, Datry A, et al. Successful voriconazole treatment of disseminated Fusarium infection in an immunocompromised patient. Clin Infect Dis 2003;37(2):311–3.

[54] Durand-Joly I, Alfandari S, Benchikh Z, et al. Successful outcome of disseminated Fusarium infection with skin localization treated with voriconazole and amphotericin B-lipid complex in a patient with acute leukemia. J Clin Microbiol 2003;41(10):4898–900.

[55] Mansoory D, Roozbahany NA, Mazinany H, et al. Chronic Fusarium infection in an adult patient with undiagnosed chronic granulomatous disease. Clin Infect Dis 2003;37(7):e107–8.

[56] Rodriguez CA, Lujan-Zilbermann J, Woodard P, et al. Successful treatment of disseminated fusariosis. Bone Marrow Transplant 2003;31(5):411–2.

[57] Vincent AL, Cabrero JE, Greene JN, et al. Successful voriconazole therapy of disseminated Fusarium solani in the brain of a neutropenic cancer patient. Cancer Control 2003;10(5):414–9.

[58] Yera H, Bougnoux ME, Jeanrot C, et al. Mycetoma of the foot caused by Fusarium solani: identification of the etiologic agent by DNA sequencing. J Clin Microbiol 2003;41(4):1805–8.

[59] Bigley VH, Duarte RF, Gosling RD, et al. Fusarium dimerum infection in a stem cell transplant recipient treated successfully with voriconazole. Bone Marrow Transplant 2004;34(9):815–7.

[60] Guimera-Martin-Neda F, Garcia-Bustinduy M, Noda-Cabrera A, et al. Cutaneous infection by Fusarium: successful treatment with oral voriconazole. Br J Dermatol 2004;150(4):777–8.

[61] Guzman-Cottrill JA, Zheng X, Chadwick EG. Fusarium solani endocarditis successfully treated with liposomal amphotericin B and voriconazole. Pediatr Infect Dis J 2004;23(11):1059–61.

[62] Hamaki T, Kami M, Kishi A, et al. Vesicles as initial skin manifestation of disseminated fusariosis after non-myeloablative stem cell transplantation. Leuk Lymphoma 2004;45(3):631–3.

[63] Herbrecht R, Kessler R, Kravanja C, et al. Successful treatment of Fusarium proliferatum pneumonia with posaconazole in a lung transplant recipient. J Heart Lung Transplant 2004;23(12):1451–4.

[64] Kivivuori SM, Hovi L, Vettenranta K, et al. Invasive fusariosis in two transplanted children. Eur J Pediatr 2004;163(11):692–3.
[65] Moschovi M, Trimis G, Anastasopoulos J, et al. Subacute vertebral osteomyelitis in a child with diabetes mellitus associated with Fusarium. Pediatr Int 2004;46(6):740–2.
[66] Rothe A, Seibold M, Hoppe T, et al. Combination therapy of disseminated Fusarium oxysporum infection with terbinafine and amphotericin B. Ann Hematol 2004;83(6):394–7.
[67] Anandi V, Vishwanathan P, Sasikala S, et al. Fusarium solani breast abscess. Indian J Med Microbiol 2005;23(3):198–9.
[68] Dornbusch HJ, Buzina W, Summerbell RC, et al. Fusarium verticillioides abscess of the nasal septum in an immunosuppressed child: case report and identification of the morphologically atypical fungal strain. J Clin Microbiol 2005;43(4):1998–2001.
[69] Garbino J, Uckay I, Rohner P, et al. Fusarium peritonitis concomitant to kidney transplantation successfully managed with voriconazole: case report and review of the literature. Transpl Int 2005;18(5):613–8.
[70] Gardner JM, Nelson MM, Heffernan MP. Chronic cutaneous fusariosis. Arch Dermatol 2005;141(6):794–5.
[71] Sierra-Hoffman M, Paltiyevich-Gibson S, Carpenter JL, et al. Fusarium osteomyelitis: case report and review of the literature. Scand J Infect Dis 2005;37(3):237–40.
[72] Backman KS, Roberts M, Patterson R. Allergic bronchopulmonary mycosis caused by Fusarium vasinfectum. Am J Respir Crit Care Med 1995;152(4 Pt 1):1379–81.
[73] Castagnola E, Garaventa A, Conte M, et al. Survival after fungemia due to Fusarium moniliforme in a child with neuroblastoma. Eur J Clin Microbiol Infect Dis 1993;12(4):308–9.
[74] Eljaschewitsch J, Sandfort J, Tintelnot K, et al. Port-a-cath-related Fusarium oxysporum infection in an HIV-infected patient: treatment with liposomal amphotericin B. Mycoses 1996;39(3–4):115–9.
[75] Kiehn TE, Nelson PE, Bernard EM, et al. Catheter-associated fungemia caused by Fusarium chlamydosporum in a patient with lymphocytic lymphoma. J Clin Microbiol 1985;21(4):501–4.
[76] Musa MO, Al Eisa A, Halim M, et al. The spectrum of Fusarium infection in immunocompromised patients with haematological malignancies and in non-immunocompromised patients: a single institution experience over 10 years. Br J Haematol 2000;108(3):544–8.
[77] Perfect JR. Treatment of non-Aspergillus moulds in immunocompromised patients, with amphotericin B lipid complex. Clin Infect Dis 2005;40(Suppl 6):S401–8.
[78] Perfect JR, Marr KA, Walsh TJ, et al. Voriconazole treatment for less-common, emerging, or refractory fungal infections. Clin Infect Dis 2003;36(9):1122–31.
[79] Raad I, Chapman S, Bradsher R, et al. Posaconazole salvage therapy for invasive fungal infections [abstract M-669]. In: Programs and abstracts of the 40th Interscience Symposium on Antimicrobial Agents and Chemotherapy. Washington, DC: American Society for Microbiology; 2004.
[80] Cuenca-Estrella M, Gomez-Lopez A, Mellado E, et al. In vitro activity of ravuconazole against 923 clinical isolates of nondermatophyte filamentous fungi. Antimicrob Agents Chemother 2005;49(12):5136–8.
[81] Pfaller MA, Diekema DJ. Rare and emerging opportunistic fungal pathogens: concern for resistance beyond Candida albicans and Aspergillus fumigatus. J Clin Microbiol 2004;42(10):4419–31.
[82] Zaas AK, Alexander BD. Echinocandins: role in antifungal therapy, 2005. Expert Opin Pharmacother 2005;6(10):1657–68.
[83] Lupinetti FM, Giller RH, Trigg ME. Operative treatment of Fusarium fungal infection of the lung. Ann Thorac Surg 1990;49(6):991–2.
[84] Anaissie EJ, Stratton SL, Dignani MC, et al. Cleaning patient shower facilities: a novel approach to reducing patient exposure to aerosolized Aspergillus species and other opportunistic molds. Clin Infect Dis 2002;35(8):E86–8.

[85] Dignani MC, Anaissie EJ, Hester JP, et al. Treatment of neutropenia-related fungal infections with granulocyte colony-stimulating factor-elicited white blood cell transfusions: a pilot study. Leukemia 1997;11(10):1621–30.

[86] Hennequin C, Benkerrou M, Gaillard JL, et al. Role of granulocyte colony-stimulating factor in the management of infection with Fusarium oxysporum in a neutropenic child. Clin Infect Dis 1994;18(3):490–1.

[87] Bouza E, Munoz P. Invasive infections caused by Blastoschizomyces capitatus and Scedosporium spp. Clin Microbiol Infect 2004;10(Suppl 1):76–85.

[88] Castiglioni B, Sutton DA, Rinaldi MG, et al. Pseudallescheria boydii (Anamorph Scedosporium apiospermum). Infection in solid organ transplant recipients in a tertiary medical center and review of the literature. Medicine (Baltimore) 2002;81(5):333–48.

[89] Berenguer J, Rodriguez-Tudela JL, Richard C, et al. Deep infections caused by Scedosporium prolificans. A report on 16 cases in Spain and a review of the literature. Scedosporium Prolificans Spanish Study Group. Medicine (Baltimore) 1997;76(4):256–65.

[90] Maertens J, Lagrou K, Deweerdt H, et al. Disseminated infection by Scedosporium prolificans: an emerging fatality among haematology patients. Case report and review. Ann Hematol 2000;79(6):340–4.

[91] Fleming RV, Walsh TJ, Anaissie EJ. Emerging and less common fungal pathogens. Infect Dis Clin North Am 2002;16(4):915–33.

[92] Walsh TJ, Lutsar I, Driscoll T, et al. Voriconazole in the treatment of aspergillosis, scedosporiosis and other invasive fungal infections in children. Pediatr Infect Dis J 2002;21(3):240–8.

[93] Guarro J, Gams W, Pujol I, et al. Acremonium species: new emerging fungal opportunists—in vitro antifungal susceptibilities and review. Clin Infect Dis 1997;25(5):1222–9.

[94] Mattei D, Mordini N, Lo NC, et al. Successful treatment of Acremonium fungemia with voriconazole. Mycoses 2003;46(11–12):511–4.

[95] Gutierrez-Rodero F, Moragon M, Ortiz de IT, V, et al. Cutaneous hyalohyphomycosis caused by Paecilomyces lilacinus in an immunocompetent host successfully treated with itraconazole: case report and review. Eur J Clin Microbiol Infect Dis 1999;18(11):814–8.

[96] Garbino J, Ondrusova A, Baglivo E, et al. Successful treatment of Paecilomyces lilacinus endophthalmitis with voriconazole. Scand J Infect Dis 2002;34(9):701–3.

ELSEVIER
SAUNDERS

Infect Dis Clin N Am
20 (2006) 581–607

INFECTIOUS
DISEASE CLINICS
OF NORTH AMERICA

Invasive Zygomycosis: Update on Pathogenesis, Clinical Manifestations, and Management

Dimitrios P. Kontoyiannis, MD, ScD, FIDSA[a],*,
Russell E. Lewis, PharmD[b]

[a]Department of Infectious Diseases, Infection Control and Employee Health, Unit 402,
The University of Texas M. D. Anderson Cancer Center, 1515 Holcombe Boulevard,
Houston, TX 77030, USA
[b]Department of Clinical Sciences and Administration, University of Houston College
of Pharmacy, 1441 Moursund Street, Houston, TX 77030, USA

Zygomycosis encompasses a spectrum of infections caused by Zygomycetes, a class of fungi that produce predominantly aseptate or pauciseptate, wide, irregularly branching ribbon-like hyphae and reproduce sexually by the formation of zygospores [1]. Zygomycetes fungi are further classified into two orders, Mucorales and Entomophthorales, which produce distinct patterns of clinical infection (Fig. 1). Fungi belonging to the order Mucorales are angiotropic, cause tissue infarction, and are associated with disseminated and frequently fatal infections, especially in immunocompromised hosts [2]. In contrast, fungi of the order Entomophthorales are uncommon pathogens typically restricted to tropical areas that produce chronic cutaneous and subcutaneous infections that rarely disseminate to internal organs [2]. Because of the clinical and pathologic differences in disease patterns between these two orders, the term "mucormycosis" is frequently used for infections caused by molds of the order Mucorales, and the term "entomophthoromycosis" is often used for infections caused by molds of the order Entomophthorales. More recently, the geographic distribution and invasiveness of infections caused by Entomophthorales, along with the range of infected hosts, have broadened [3]. Therefore this article uses the unifying term "zygomycosis" to describe any invasive infection caused

This work was supported by a grant from the E. Cobb Endowment to D.P.K.
* Corresponding author.
E-mail address: dkontoyi@mdanderson.org (D.P. Kontoyiannis).

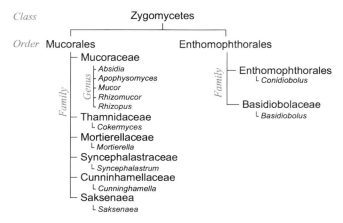

Fig. 1. Taxonomy of Zygomycetes fungi.

by Zygomycetes, because this term is more applicable to infections with positive histopathologic findings but negative cultures.

Etiology and epidemiology

Although a variety of Zygomycetes spp have been implicated in zygomycosis, those belonging to the family Mucoraceae are isolated more frequently than those of any other family (see Fig. 1). Mucorales fungi are thermotolerant molds that are ubiquitous in nature and widely found in organic substrates, including bread, fruits, vegetable matter, soil, compost piles, and animal excreta [4]. Mucorales fungi grow rapidly (in 2–5 days) and produce abundant spores when inoculated onto a carbohydrate-containing source [5]. Sporangiospores released by Mucorales fungi range from 3 to 11 μm in diameter, are easily aerosolized, and are the mechanism by which the fungi disperse throughout the environment and cause sinopulmonary infections in human hosts (Fig. 2) [5].

Although sporangiospores are the typical infective forms of zygomycetes, angioinvasive hyphal forms are responsible for tissue invasion and dissemination. Spore germination and unopposed hyphal proliferation occur primarily in immunocompromised patients, in whom migration of macrophages and neutrophils, phagocytosis, and killing of spores and hyphal elements are impaired [2].

Zygomycetes are unique among filamentous fungi in their greater ability to infect a broader, more heterogeneous population of human hosts than other opportunistic molds [5]. Although devastating infections caused by these fungi are rare, they have been reported in individuals who have no apparent underlying immunosuppressive condition [6]. For example, intravenous intake of illicit drugs contaminated with Zygomycetes

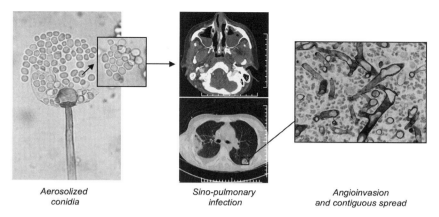

Aerosolized
conidia

Sino-pulmonary
infection

Angioinvasion
and contiguous spread

Fig. 2. Cellular morphology of zygomycosis during environmental and in vivo growth.

sporangiospores can produce disseminated and cerebral zygomycosis even in immunocompetent hosts [6]. Similarly, cutaneous and sinus disease has been reported in patients who have no underlying risk factors. Whereas most infections with zygomycetes are community acquired, nosocomial acquisition, sporadic cases, and pseudo-outbreaks have been linked with contaminated bandages [7], needles, and tongue depressors used to construct splints for intravenous and arterial cannulation sites in preterm infants [8]. The most common underlying risk factors for invasive zygomycosis are poorly controlled diabetes mellitus and metabolic acidosis, administration of high-dose systemic corticosteroids in solid-organ and hematopoietic stem cell transplantation, penetrating trauma or burns, persistent neutropenia, and use of deferoxamine-based therapy to chelate aluminum or iron in patients receiving dialysis or extensive blood transfusions [2,5,6]. The true incidence of invasive zygomycosis is not known, although a population-based survey in the United States estimated an incidence of 1.7 cases per 1 million people per year, that is, approximately 500 cases per year [9]. The incidence is probably underestimated because of difficulty in establishing an ante mortem diagnosis of this infection. In past autopsy series, the prevalence of zygomycosis ranged from one to five cases per 10,000 autopsies, making this infection 10- to 50-fold less common than infections with *Aspergillus spp* [10]. The incidence can be considerably higher in institutions that have larger populations of immunocompromised patients. In a recent review of autopsy data for patients who had hematologic malignancies from 1999 to 2003, there were eight reported cases of zygomycosis in 268 autopsy examinations, or roughly 30 cases per 1000 autopsies [11].

Historically, the majority of published cases of zygomycosis have been in diabetic patients and individuals who had no clear underlying risk factors (Fig. 3) [6]. During the past 20 years, however, there also has been an increase in the rates of zygomycosis in patient groups classically at risk for other

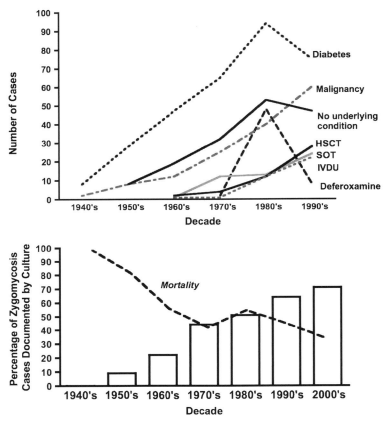

Fig. 3. Incidence, frequency, and mortality of invasive zygomycosis over a 60-year time span. HSCT, hematopoietic stem cell transplantation; IVDU, intravenous drug use, SOT, solid-organ transplantation. (*Data from* Roden MM, Zaoutis TE, Buchanan WL, et al. Epidemiology and outcome of zygomycosis: a review of 929 reported cases. Clin Infect Dis 2005;41(5):634–53.

opportunistic mold infections, such as those who have hematologic malignancies and recipients of hematopoietic stem cell or solid-organ transplants [6,9,12–15]. This rise in the number of reported cases may account for the sustained mortality rates of zygomycosis since the 1970s despite improvements in treatment options for this devastating infection. Surveillance data from The University of Texas M.D. Anderson Cancer Center confirm that zygomycosis has become an increasingly common mold infection in high-risk patients [9,12]. Specifically, among 109 cases of culture-proven invasive mold infections in patients who had hematologic malignancies and recipients of stem cell transplants, Zygomycetes were the second most common molds, after *Aspergillus,* representing 20% of all culture-confirmed cases [12]. Of concern is that an increasing number of zygomycosis cases since 2002 are presenting as breakthrough infections in patients receiving antifungal prophylaxis or treatment effective against *Aspergillus* but not Zygomycetes fungi (ie, vorico-nazole or echinocandins) [12,16–18] The authors' experience with patients who have high-risk leukemia and recipients of allogeneic hematopoietic stem cell transplants suggests that zygomycosis should be considered in these populations when fungal sinusitis develops in those receiving *Aspergillus*-ac-tive antifungal prophylaxis (ie, voriconazole), especially if the patient has been continuously and intensely immunosuppressed and has underlying dia-betes or malnutrition (albumin level < 3 g/dL) [12] On the other hand, zygo-mycosis is an uncommon opportunistic infection in patients who have advanced AIDS and typically is associated with intravenous drug abuse [6].

Several species of the order Mucorales predominate as causes of zygomy-cosis, suggesting potential differences in the virulence of different zygomy-cetes. In a published retrospective review of more than 900 reported cases of zygomycosis, *Rhizopus spp* (47%) were the most commonly isolated causes of culture-confirmed zygomycosis followed by *Mucor spp* (18%), *Cunninghamella bertholletiae* (7%), *Apophysomyces elegans* (5%), *Absidia spp* (5%), *Saksenaea spp* (5%), and *Rhizomucor pusillus* (4%), with other species representing less than 3% of cultured confirmed cases [6]. The rank order and frequency of zygomycetes are likely to differ by geographic location and climate. Significant weather events also have the potential to alter the environmental burden of relative Zygomycetes fungi. For example, over an 8-week period in September 2005 following the landfall of Hurri-cane Katrina in New Orleans, Louisiana, investigators identified four cases of lung or wound infections caused by fungi of the extremely rare genus *Syn-cephalastrum* of the order Mucorales in immunocompetent patients who lived in the New Orleans area [19]. Misidentification of zygomycetes in clin-ical laboratories also can affect the rank order of isolated species and their frequency. Comparison of molecular genotyping techniques with standard culture identification techniques in clinical laboratories has suggested that the divergence in species identification between the two methods may approach 20% [12]. Therefore, the exact frequency of distribution of zygo-mycetes causing human infections remains somewhat undefined.

Pathogenesis and host responses

Experimental animal data have been instrumental in clarifying the essential pathogenic features of zygomycosis. Because the infection develops following inhalation of sporangiospores, sinopulmonary disease is the most common initial presentation before dissemination outside the respiratory tract [2,20]. Most Zygomycetes spores are sufficiently small to avoid host upper airway defenses and reach the distal alveolar spaces. Larger sporan-giospores (> 10 μm) may lodge in the upper respiratory tract, however, pre-disposing patients to isolated sinusitis [1]. Inhalation of a large inoculum of Zygomycete sporangiospores, which can occur during excavation, construc-tion, and work in contaminated air ducts, can lead to slowly progressing pulmonary zygomycosis even in immunocompetent hosts [21,22]. Not surprisingly, cutaneous infection following traumatic inoculation of a high load of sporangiospores under the skin is the most common form of zygomycosis in normal hosts [2]. Cutaneous zygomycosis has even been described following insect bites and tattooing [23,24].

Intact mucosal and endothelial barriers serve as structural defenses against tissue invasion and angioinvasion by Zygomycetes (see Fig. 3) [2]. Relatively little is known about mechanisms of attachment to and invasion of mucosal surfaces used by Zygomycetes. One possibility, however, is that spores simply invade epithelium previously damaged by prior infection, cytotoxic chemotherapy, or direct trauma. Recent studies have suggested that Zygomycetes sporangiospores may have unique capability for tissue adherence and invasion of intact endothelial barriers [2]. For example, *Rhizopus* spores have the capacity to adhere tightly to subendothelial matrix proteins, including laminin and type IV collagen [25]. Once endothelialized, *Rhizopus* germlings are capable of damaging endothelial cells in vitro [26]. Surprisingly, viable spores are not essential for causing tissue damage, and injection of heat-killed *Rhizopus spp* can result in significant mortality in diabetic mice [2]. This observation suggests that some component of zygomycete sporangiospores, possibly a secreted toxin or protease, may be directly toxic to endothelial cells in the mucosal membranes. In plants, many Mucorales spp release polyketide metabolites that exhibit potent antimitotic effects, dramatically weakening plant responses to fungal invasion. Remarkably, biosynthesis of these mycotoxins in some zygomycetes may not be produced by the fungus itself but rather by endosymbiotic (free-living intracellular) bacteria of the genus *Burkholderia* [27]. This observation raises intriguing questions about whether reciprocal adaptation of toxin-producing endosymbiotic bacteria in response to antibacterial or environmental pressure may influence the epidemiology and pathogenesis of invasive zygomycosis.

Once spores are taken up in the endothelium, both mononuclear and polymorphonuclear phagocytes prevent germination of the conidia and kill the hyphal forms of the fungus [2,5,28–30]. Phagocytic defects because of cell-number deficiency (ie, neutropenia) and functional defects caused by corticosteroids, hyperglycemia, or acidosis allow proliferation of the fungus (Fig. 4). Corticosteroids are known to impair the migration, ingestion, and phagolysosome fusion of bronchoalveolar macrophages essential for clearing sporangiospores from the respiratory mucosa [31]. Similarly, hyperglycemia and decreased pH levels encountered in patients who have diabetic ketoacidosis, stress pseudodiabetes, severe burns, or corticosteroid-treated graft-versus-host disease impair neutrophil chemotaxis and oxidative and nonoxidative fungicidal mechanisms [32].

Prolonged neutropenia is one of the most important predisposing factors for invasive zygomycosis and is the sole identifying risk factor in approximately 15% of all reported cases [6,33]. Like aspergillosis, zygomycosis is increasingly reported as a late complication of hematopoietic stem cell

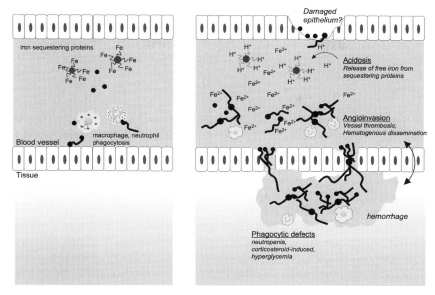

Fig. 4. Pathogenesis and host defense against invasive zygomycosis. Immunocompromised (*left panel*). Immunocompetent (*right panel*). (*Adapted from* Spellberg B, Edwards J Jr, Ibrahim A. Novel perspectives on mucormycosis: pathophysiology, presentation, and management. Clin Microbiol Rev 2005;18(3):556–69.)

transplantation after recovery from neutropenia (stem cell engraftment) [6]. In a previous study by the authors' group, the median onset of zygomycosis was significantly earlier (mean, 43 days) than that of aspergillosis (mean, 93 days), suggesting that delayed engraftment may be an important risk factor favoring zygomycosis, especially in patients receiving *Aspergillus*-active prophylaxis [12]. On the other hand, lymphopenia may not be as critical as neutropenia for protection against zygomycosis, as evidenced by the relative rarity of the infection in patients who have advanced AIDS [6].

Although iron is required for the growth and virulence of virtually all microbial pathogens [34], the ability to scavenge free iron from the host is clearly an essential component of the pathogenesis of zygomycetes, as suggested by the unique predisposition of patients who have iatrogenic or inherited conditions of iron overload [35,36] or diabetic ketoacidosis to develop zygomycosis [2]. In mammalian hosts very little serum iron is available to microorganisms because of its strong binding to serum proteins such as transferrin [2]. Fungi can acquire iron from the host using low-molecular-weight iron chelators (siderophores) or high-affinity iron permeases such as ferrirhizoferrin [4,37]. Of these two mechanisms, iron permeases are believed to play a more critical role for survival of fungi in human hosts.

More than a decade ago, Artis and colleagues [38,39] presented evidence supporting the central role of acidosis and free iron in the pathogenesis of zygomycosis when they compared the growth of *Rhizopus oryzae* in sera collected from patients who had diabetic acidosis with that in sera collected from healthy controls. The investigators found that normal human serum could not support the growth of *R oryzae* without the addition of free iron. Furthermore, exogenous iron supported the growth of *R oryzae* only under acidic conditions, not at an alkaline pH level (7.78–8.38) [38]. Similarly, sera collected from patients who had ketoacidosis supported exuberant growth of *R oryzae* even without exogenous iron, provided the pH level was maintained below 7.4. Simulated acidotic conditions also decreased the iron-binding capacity of sera obtained from healthy volunteers, suggesting that acidosis disrupts the capacity of iron transporter proteins such as transferrin to bind to iron [38,39].

Patients who have iron overload often receive treatment with iron chelators such as deferoxamine. Paradoxically, treatment with deferoxamine has been associated with a markedly increased incidence of *Rhizopus spp* infections, because these fungi can use this specific chelator as a siderophore to access iron previously unavailable to the fungus [40–43]. *Rhizopus spp* are thought to acquire iron from the iron–deferoxamine complex by binding to the complex and releasing the reduced iron, which is transported intracellularly by iron permeases [43]. This mechanism seems to be unique to *Rhizopus* spp, because in vitro studies of radiolabeled iron uptake in the presence of deferoxamine have demonstrated an 8- to 40-fold increase in iron uptake by *Rhizopus spp* when compared with *Candida* and *Aspergillus spp* [41]. Indeed, administration of deferoxamine worsens the survival in guinea pigs infected with *Rhizopus spp* but not in those infected with *Candida albicans* [41,42]. In contrast, the hydroxypyridinone iron chelator deferiprone does not seem to act as an iron siderophore in *Rhizopus spp* [42]. Hence, deferiprone could theoretically be used as an adjunct to antifungal therapy in the treatment of zygomycosis. Currently studies are underway to evaluate the therapeutic potential of novel chelators in animal models of zygomycosis. Furthermore, these novel chelators could help reverse dysregualtion of both innate and adaptive immune effector functions, which has been described in iron overload states [44].

The link between iron chelation and deferoxamine-based therapy is well established. It is unclear why this problem was not described earlier, because deferoxamine has been used extensively since the 1950s for treating iron overload in patients who have nonmalignant hematologic diseases (ie, thalassemia) [34]. Some have suggested that concomitant uremia plays a critical role in prolonging the half-life and serum retention of the siderophore–iron complex [45], thus improving iron availability for zygomycetes. The enhanced effect of deferoxamine in the setting of uremia may also explain why zygomycosis has been a more common complication of deferoxamine-based treatment in the setting of dialysis than in other nonmalignant states of iron overload (thalassemia, salicylate poisoning, methylmaloniciduria) [34]. Fortunately, the necessity of deferoxamine-based therapy to manage iron overload in patients who have end-stage renal disease has lessened with the replacement of aluminum salts with calcium salts as phosphate binders and the use of erythropoietin in lieu of blood transfusions for anemia [34]. Hence, deferoxamine-related zygomycosis cases are on the decline (see Fig. 3).

Clinical features of Zygomycetes infections

A hallmark of invasive zygomycosis is the rapid development of tissue necrosis resulting from invasion of blood vessels and subsequent thrombosis [4]. In most cases, the infection is relentlessly progressive and results in death unless underlying risk factors (ie, metabolic acidosis) are corrected and effective antifungal therapy combined with surgical excision is instituted. Based on clinical presentation and anatomic predilection, invasive zygomycosis can be classified as one of six forms: (1) rhinocerebral syndrome and (2) pulmonary, (3) cutaneous, (4) gastrointestinal, (5) disseminated, and (6) uncommon presentations.

Rhinocerebral syndromes

Rhinosinusitis, pansinusitis, rhino-orbital and rhinocerebral manifestations are characteristic manifestations of zygomycosis with significant clinical overlaps. The infection can progress rapidly to intracranial structures, notably, the cavernous sinuses, especially in patients who have diabetic ketoacidosis or profound cytopenia. There is host specificity in the presentation of this infection. Thus, the rhino-orbital form occurs more frequently in patients who have poorly controlled diabetes, whereas the sinopulmonary form is more common in patients who have malignant hematologic diseases (Table 1) [9]. In fact, rhino-orbital zygomycosis may be the first manifestation of undiagnosed diabetes mellitus [46].

Symptoms of zygomycosis are neither pathognomonic nor specific enough to distinguish pathogens from other causes of rhinosinusitis. Facial pressure, nasal obstruction or congestion, headache, mouth pain, otologic symptoms, and hyposmia/anosmia may be seen. Concomitant (dry) cough frequently reflects lung involvement. Also, necrosis or eschar in the nasal cavity and turbinates, necrotic facial lesions, and exophytic or necrotic lesions on the palate signify progressive and aggressive infections. Necrotic nasal or palate lesions may be seen in only 50% of patients within 3 days of the onset of infection [47]. Therefore, the absence of lesions or necrotic eschar should not decrease the index of suspicion for rhinocerebral infections. Rhinocerebral zygomycosis, if not aggressively treated, can result in intraorbital complications, intracranial complications, or both, with variable rates of progression. In intraorbital complications, the location and degree of penetration of the infection by contiguous extension to the orbit may lead

Table 1
Patterns of zygomycosis by host population

Predisposing condition	Predominant sites of infection (in order of frequency)
Diabetes	Rhinocerebral, pulmonary, sino-orbital, cutaneous
Malignancy (neutropenia)	Pulmonary, sinus, cutaneous, sino-orbital
Hematopoietic stem cell transplantation	Pulmonary, disseminated, rhinocerebral
Solid-organ transplantation	Sinus, cutaneous, pulmonary, rhinocerebral, disseminated
Intravenous drug use/abuse	Cerebral, endocarditis, cutaneous, disseminated
Malnutrition	Gastrointestinal, disseminated
Deferoxamine-based therapy	Disseminated, pulmonary, rhinocerebral, cerebral, cutaneous, gastrointestinal
No underlying condition	Cutaneous, pulmonary, sino-orbital, rhinocerebral, gastrointestinal

to preseptal cellulitis, orbital cellulitis, subperiosteal abscess, orbital abscess, or cavernous sinus thrombosis. Progressive eyelid edema (Fig. 5A), chemosis, ptosis, proptosis, or full-blown ophthalmoplegia and loss of vision could ensue rapidly. Trigeminal and facial cranial nerve palsy are common in patients who have extensive rhino-orbital or rhinocerebral zygomycosis [6]. In fact, perineural invasion is one of the most common histopathologic findings in patients who have rhinocerebral syndromes of zygomycosis [48]. Intracranial complications include epidural and subdural abscess and cavernous and, more rarely, sagittal sinus thrombosis. Frank meningitis is rarely observed.

Radiographic imaging often is suggestive of severe sinusitis but is in no way specific enough to diagnose rhinocerebral zygomycosis. CT scanning of the sinuses may reveal mucosal thickening, air-fluid levels, and bony

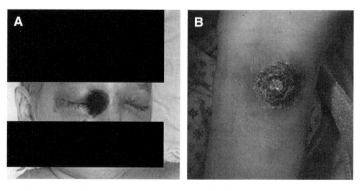

Fig. 5. (*A*) Rhino-orbital zygomycosis. (*B*) Cutaneous zygomycosis.

erosion. Orbital thickening may also be observed on CT scans but can be detected earlier by MRI [49]. MRI and CT images of the orbits also can be normal in the early stages of infection, highlighting the critical need for serial radiologic studies to monitor for possible progression [49]. Orbital infections often appear as thickening of the extraocular muscles on CT or MRI scans and mandate empiric antifungal therapy until surgical exploration or biopsy analysis of the sinuses and orbits is performed, which should be done as soon as possible. Obtaining biopsy samples of necrotic lesions and using frozen sections to make rapid histologic assessments are critical for early, definitive diagnosis of invasive zygomycosis. Impression smears from the wound edge may also reveal fungi characteristic of invasive zygomycosis [20].

A multidisciplinary approach involving consultants from the fields of infectious diseases, ophthalmology, otorhinolaryngology, or even neurosurgery is of paramount importance. Time is of the essence, because the infection could progress rapidly. Close monitoring with repeated daily otorhinolaryngologic evaluations and repeated imaging is required to detect early signs of progression after inadequate surgical or medical therapy. Isolated sinusitis without central nervous system or lung involvement is a curable infection provided prompt surgical intervention and systemic antifungal therapy follow an early diagnosis of zygomycosis [6].

Pulmonary infections

The clinical manifestations of pulmonary zygomycosis are similar to those of invasive pulmonary aspergillosis (IPA). In fact, these two entities are almost indistinguishable clinically [50]. Timely diagnosis of pulmonary zygomycosis is challenging because its symptoms are subtle and nonspecific even at the late stages of the infection, especially in patients given antiinflammatory agents that mask the immune response (eg, systemic corticosteroids, infliximab). Patients who have pulmonary zygomycosis present with fever refractory to broad-spectrum antibiotics, cough that is typically nonproductive, severe or subtle pleuritic chest pain, and rapidly progressive dyspnea. The absence of fever, however, does not rule out zygomycosis, especially in patients receiving corticosteroids. Zygomycetes are capable of producing infections that transverse tissue planes, such as chest wall cellulitis and pleural involvement. Also, a pleural friction rub may be heard upon auscultation. Angioinvasion results in necrosis of tissue parenchyma, which may lead ultimately to cavitation or hemoptysis. Fatal hemoptysis as a result of fungal invasion of a major blood vessel has been reported occasionally. In patients who have hematologic malignancies, clues for distinguishing pulmonary zygomycosis from IPA are the presence of concomitant pansinusitis, a history of antifungal prophylaxis with *Aspergillus*-active agents such as voriconazole and echinocandins, and possibly the repeated absence of detectable *Aspergillus* galactomannan antigen in serum [50]. Frequent coinfection with other molds and bacteria add to the difficulty of timely diagnosis of pulmonary zygomycosis [9,51].

A multitude of patterns may be present in a regular chest radiograph for a patient who has pulmonary zygomycosis, including, in descending order of frequency, lobar consolidation or nonspecific infiltrates, cavities, masses, and nodules [52,53]. Wedge-shaped infarcts of the lung also may be seen, particularly following thrombosis of the pulmonary vessels caused by fungal angioinvasion [52]. Furthermore, previous studies found that pulmonary lesions in patients who had zygomycosis had a predilection for the upper pulmonary lobes in 55% to 84% of all reported cases [52,53].

As with IPA, high-resolution chest CT is the best method of determining the extent of pulmonary zygomycosis and typically demonstrates evidence of infection before its appearance on standard chest radiographs. The halo and air-crescent signs are encountered in cases of zygomycosis at the same low frequency as in cases of IPA [50,52]. Importantly, the presence of the air-crescent sign has been associated with an increased risk of massive hemoptysis from centrally located lesions [20]. The authors recently found that the presence of multiple ($\geq$10) nodules and, to a lesser degree, pleural effusions on CT scans favors a diagnosis of pulmonary zygomycosis over IPA in high-risk patients who have cancer [50].

Pulmonary zygomycosis can spread to the contralateral lung and other organs when the infection is not treated promptly. Patients who have untreated pulmonary zygomycosis usually die from disseminated infection before respiratory failure occurs, and dissemination goes undetected ante mortem [9]. The overall mortality rate for pulmonary zygomycosis ranges from 50% to 70% but is higher than 95% when it is part of a disseminated infection [6,12].

Some atypical presentations of pulmonary zygomycosis include chronic infection with constitutional symptoms that last for several months in relatively immunocompetent hosts, multiple mycotic pulmonary artery aneurysms and pseudoaneurysms, bronchial obstruction, asymptomatic solitary nodules, and even normal chest radiographs. Of interest, patients who have diabetes mellitus have a predilection for the development of endobronchial lesions, accounting for more than 80% of cases reported in the literature [52]. Furthermore, pulmonary zygomycosis tends to present with a less fulminant, ($>$4 weeks) subacute clinical course in these patients. Occasionally, endobronchial lesions may lead to obstruction of major airways or erosion of major pulmonary blood vessels and fatal hemoptysis.

Similar to *Aspergillus spp*, Zygomycetes spp occasionally produce an asymptomatic mycetoma within a preexisting lung cavity [5]. Also, studies have reported allergic *Rhizomucor* sinusitis in immunocompetent individuals [54]. Hypersensitivity pneumonitis caused by *Rhizopus spp* has been described in farm workers as well as in Scandinavian sawmill workers (so-called "wood trimmer's disease") [55].

Skin and soft tissue infections

Primary cutaneous zygomycosis is seen in relation to disruption of skin integrity mainly in immunocompromised patients, patients who have burns or severe soft tissue trauma, and very premature neonates; it has been reported rarely in patients who have apparently normal skin. Recent cataclysmic events, such as the tsunami tragedy in southeast Asia, also have been associated with an increase in necrotizing soft tissue infections caused by Zygomycetes [56].

Cutaneous zygomycosis typically starts as erythema and induration of the skin at a puncture site and progresses to necrosis (Fig. 5B). Extension to the subcutaneous tissue or bone is common in patients who have delayed or ineffectively treated cutaneous zygomycosis [6]. Necrotizing fasciitis has been reported in cases of cutaneous zygomycosis and carries an extremely poor prognosis [57]. In neutropenic patients, the profound defect in local phagocytosis allows fungal sporangiospores to produce local necrosis, tissue infarction, vessel invasion, and, if immunosuppression persists, dissemination. Unlike infections caused by other opportunistic molds, the skin seems to be a much less common site of secondary involvement in disseminated zygomycosis [6]. Nevertheless, a skin lesion caused by Zygomycetes should prompt careful, expeditious clinical and laboratory examinations to rule out disseminated infection.

Because necrotic skin lesions in immunocompromised patients have a very broad differential diagnosis, skin biopsy analysis is required. The biopsy specimen should be taken from the center of the lesion and include subcutaneous fat, because molds frequently invade blood vessels of the dermis and subcutis, resulting in an ischemic cone at the skin surface. Wide débridement that resects all the necrotic or semiviable lesion coupled with systemic antifungal therapy and possibly hyperbaric oxygen (HBO) therapy can further reduce mortality rates. The timing of surgical excision, need for repeated surgery, and duration of antifungal therapy are highly individualized.

Gastrointestinal zygomycosis

Only 25% of cases of gastrointestinal zygomycosis are diagnosed ante mortem, although gastrointestinal involvement in the setting of dissemination is not as uncommon as previously thought [6]. Extreme malnutrition, persistent ingestion of non-nutritional substances (pica), severe systemic illness, age extremes, and systemic immunosuppression are the typical predisposing conditions for gastrointestinal zygomycosis, and this infection is thought to be acquired by ingestion of sporangiospores [4]. In cases of liver abscess caused by zygomycetes, ingestion of herbal medications contaminated with *Mucor indicus* has been described [58–59]. In premature neonates, gastrointestinal zygomycosis presents as necrotizing enterocolitis, whereas in neutropenic patients, a masslike appendiceal or ileal lesion is observed [5,60]. Neutropenic fever, typhlitis, and hematochezia also have been described in neutropenic patients. Diagnosis of gastrointestinal zygomycosis usually is delayed, because the nonspecific presentation requires a high degree of suspicion leading to early endoscopic biopsy. Although any component of the gastrointestinal tract can be involved with this infection, the stomach is a common site of involvement, with frequent presentation of peptic ulceration [6,60].

Disseminated zygomycosis

Disseminated zygomycosis is often clinically unapparent ante mortem. Its symptoms vary widely, reflecting the location and degree of vascular invasion and tissue infarction of the affected organs. Pneumonia is common in patients who have disseminated zygomycosis and is assumed to be the source of dissemination. Patients who have iron overload states (especially those who receive deferoxamine), patients who have profound immunosuppression (eg, recipients of allogeneic bone marrow transplants who have graft-versus-host disease treated with corticosteroids), and neutropenic patients who have active leukemia are the classic groups at risk for disseminated zygomycosis [6]. Because of the low yield of blood cultures and suboptimal recovery of the fungus from respiratory secretions, biopsy of the affected site or sites is the mainstay of diagnosis of this infection. The elusive presentation of disseminated zygomycosis requires a high index of suspicion for early diagnosis. For example, an acute abdomen in a patient with known pulmonary zygomycosis should alert the clinician to check for bowel ischemia because of dissemination of zygomycetes in the gastrointestinal tract.

Less common clinical presentations of zygomycosis

Peritonitis has been rarely described in patients undergoing continuous ambulatory peritoneal dialysis who have central venous catheter–related zygomycosis [61,62]. Prior bacterial peritonitis is common in patients undergoing continuous ambulatory peritoneal dialysis, and the infection tends to have a slowly progressive course, although the attributable mortality rate in patients who receive delayed or inappropriate treatment has been as high as 60% [61,63]. In all cases of catheter-related zygomycosis, prompt removal of the catheter and use of systemic antifungal therapy for several weeks are essential.

Reports describing isolated zygomycosis of the trachea [64], mediastinum [65,66], kidney [67], or bone [68] are rare. Intravenous drug abuse is the typical risk factor for both native and prosthetic valve Zygomycetes endocarditis [69–72] and brain abscess (typically involving the basal ganglia) in the absence of concomitant pneumonia [6]. Zygomycosis has protean manifestations and can affect any organ. Unusual manifestations such as otitis externa, corneal infection, and superior vena cava syndrome have been reported [73,74].

Diagnosis

Definitive diagnosis of zygomycosis almost always requires histopathologic evidence of fungal invasion of tissue. Not surprisingly, the site of infection has a major impact on the likelihood of histopathologic diagnosis, with the sinuses being the most common site of definite infection [9]. In tissue, Zygomycetes hyphae can be distinguished from more common opportunistic molds such as *Aspergillus spp* by their broad (3–25 μm in diameter), thin-walled, mostly aseptate hyphae [75]. Frequently, these hyphae have focal bulbous dilation and nondichotomous, irregular branching that occasionally occurs at right angles (see Fig. 2) [75]. Histopathologic sections occasionally show folded, twisted, and compressed hyphae, which may be mistaken for septated hyphae or, if transected, large empty yeast cells or spherules of *Coccidioides immitis* [75]. Sporangia, the reproductive hyphal structures that contain spores, are seen rarely in tissue in patients infected with zygomycetes [75].

Zygomycetes do not stain as deeply as other filamentous fungi with specialized fungus stains (eg, Gomori's methenamine silver stain, periodic acid-Schiff stain), but they often can be detected in tissue sections stained with hematoxylin and eosin [75]. Costaining with hematoxylin and eosin uniquely intensifies Gomori's methenamine silver staining of Zygomycetes hyphae, potentially providing a unique clue for identification of the fungus [75]. In hematoxylin and eosin–stained tissue sections, Entomophthorales organisms demonstrate hyphal encasement by eosinophilic Splendore-Hoeppli material. This material may be the first indication that a patient has an infection with either a *Basidiobolus* or *Conidiobolus spp* instead of one of the Mucorales organisms, which rarely demonstrate this phenomenon in tissues [5]. Distinguishing zygomycetes from hyphal forms of *Aspergillus* can be challenging, however, and the mere observation of septations does not rule out the possibility of zygomycetes [75].

Identification of zygomycetes at the genus and species levels requires culture studies, because all members of this group are morphologically similar in tissue. The level of development of the rhizoids, the shape of the sporangium, and the location of the sporangiospores are the morphologic features used to distinguish different genera of Zygomycetes. The positive predictive value of a Zygomycetes-positive culture is directly linked to the degree of the host immunosuppression [9]. Poor recovery of Zygomycetes organisms may reflect limited septation of the hyphae, making the fungi more liable to damage as a result of tissue manipulation. Culture techniques that attempt to simulate physiologic conditions of zygomycete growth in vivo (ie, relative anaerobic conditions, incubation at 35°C–37°C) may enhance recovery of zygomycetes from tissue. Zygomycetes are rarely isolated from cultures of

blood, cerebrospinal fluid, sputum, urine or feces, or swabs of infected areas
[20]. Early differentiation of zygomycosis from other opportunistic molds is
critical to the management of suspected infections, especially in patients who
have cancer and transplant recipients, in whom the clinical presentation of
zygomycosis is frequently indistinguishable from that of more common
mold infections such as aspergillosis [12,50]. Hence, there is considerable interest in the detection and differentiation of zygomycosis using nonhistopa-
thologic and non–culture-based methods, such as early detection of
Zygomycetes-specific antigens or nucleic acid in clinical samples. Importantly, there are no reliable serologic or skin tests for zygomycosis. Unfortunately, the recently introduced antigen tests for *Aspergillus*
(galactomannan) and other fungal species (β-D-glucan) do not detect zygomycosis because of the limited amount of galactomannan and glucan in
their cell walls [19]. Recently, some have attempted to improve the diagnosis
of zygomycosis by detecting Zygomycetes nucleic acid in serum using polymerase chain reaction (PCR) or in situ hybridization techniques. Researchers have examined diagnostic methods relying on the detection of
nucleic acid as an adjunctive diagnostic tool, which have proven to be the
most useful for confirming the presence of presumptive organisms when histopathology is positive and cultures are negative. Hence, at the present time,
PCR testing is unlikely to replace tissue-based diagnosis. In one recent series, use of a semi-nested PCR assay suggested the presence of a causative
organism in six patients who had histopathologic evidence of an angioinvasive mold but mold-negative cultures and detected a mixed mold infection in
two patients [76–78]. Sequencing of PCR products provided a presumptive
identification of the Zygomycetes organisms at the genus level, which provided some guidance in selecting antifungal therapy that would not have
been available using histopathology alone.

Some methods of molecular typing of zygomycetes, such as repetitive-
sequence–based PCR, have been shown to be effective for the molecular
typing of isolates [12], although much more work is needed in this area.
Molecular typing is most useful for characterizing zygomycete epidemiology
in the setting of a cluster of nosocomial cases, outbreaks, or pseudo-outbreaks (ie, to rule out clonal spread or a common infecting source).

Antifungal susceptibility testing

Once zygomycetes are grown in culture, antifungal susceptibility testing
can be performed using broth microdilution or an agar-based method
such as the Epsilometer test (AB Biodisk, Solna, Sweden) (Fig. 6). The Clinical and Laboratory Standards Institute has proposed a standardized broth
microdilution method for testing of *Rhizopus spp* (M38-A); however, inter-
pretative breakpoints have yet to be established, and the relationship between clinical response and the mean inhibitory concentration (MIC) as
determined in vitro remains uncertain [31,79]. Therefore, antifungal

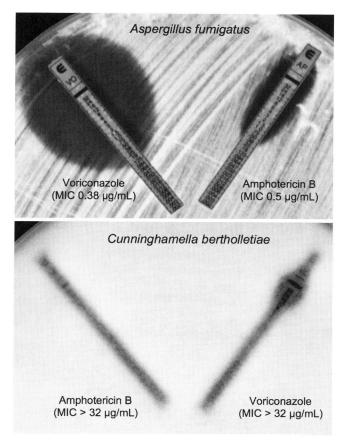

Fig. 6. Comparative amphotericin B and voriconazole susceptibility of *Cunninghamella berthol-letiae* and *Aspergillus fumigatus* following 18 hours of incubation as determined using the Ep-silometer test. Hyphal overgrowth covering the epsilometer strip is evident in the bottom panel.

susceptibility testing to guide routine clinical decisions, including selection of antifungal therapy, is not recommended at this time.

Antifungal susceptibility testing performed in research laboratories has clearly revealed that zygomycetes are relatively resistant to many antifungal drugs, including flucytosine, ketoconazole, fluconazole, voriconazole, and the echinocandins. Studies in this area are often limited by a relatively small number of tested isolates. In general, *Rhizopus* and *Cunninghamella* isolates seem to be significantly less susceptible to amphotericin B (AMB) and tria-zoles than are zygomycetes of the order Mucorales [80]. Itraconazole and terbinafine have variable activity against Mucorales isolates, but these agents have limited clinical utility in the treatment of serious infections. Most Mucorales isolates seem to be susceptible to AMB when tested using broth microdilution methods, with an MIC_{90} less than 0.5 µg/mL [80].

Agar-based testing methods have revealed substantially higher MICs (2 to > 32 μg/mL), however (see Fig. 5) [12]. Posaconazole, an investigational triazole, has been shown to possess enhanced activity against Zygomycetes (MIC_{90}, ≤ 1 μg/mL) that falls within the range of serum concentrations in high-risk patients who received oral posaconazole in phase II-III clinical studies [81–83]. In preclinical studies, combinations of antifungal agents occasionally seem to be more effective than single agents, including combinations of drugs that have minimal activity alone against zygomycetes [84,85]. For example, caspofungin inhibited 1,3-β-D-glucan synthase in R oryzae [86] and enhanced the activity of AMB in an experimental model of invasive zygomycosis [84].

Management

Successful treatment of zygomycosis largely depends on timely diagnosis, reversal of the underlying predisposing factors, early and ideally broad surgical débridement of infected tissue, and rapid initiation of effective systemic antifungal therapy. Early diagnosis, in particular, is critical to the outcome of zygomycosis because small focal lesions often can be excised surgically before the infection progresses to involve critical structures or disseminates to other organs. Time is of the essence in the treatment of zygomycosis because the infection has the ability to rapidly spread and disseminate even in relatively asymptomatic patients. For example, studies have shown that making therapeutic decisions based on examination of frozen tissue sections instead of waiting for fixed and stained histopathology is correlated with improved outcome in patients who have zygomycosis [87]. In addition, rapid correction of underlying conditions, such as appropriate control of hyperglycemia or correction of diabetic ketoacidosis, immediate tapering of corticosteroids and immunosuppressive drugs, and discontinuation of deferoxamine-based treatment, is critical to outcome [6]. Notably, there have been rare cases in which a patient who had cavitary pulmonary zygomycosis recovered from the infection without undergoing antifungal treatment after correction of diabetic ketoacidosis [6].

Antifungal treatment

There have been no prospective studies of primary treatment of zygomycosis. Most of the evidence of the activity of existing antifungal agents has come from small case series, anecdotal case reports, and in vivo studies of animal models of zygomycosis. Therefore, the optimal therapy is uncertain. Currently, the recommended antifungal therapy for zygomycosis includes AMB deoxycholate administered at the highest tolerated dosage, usually 1.0 to 1.5 mg/kg/d [4]. The nephrotoxic and acute infusional toxic effects of high-dose conventional AMB frequently preclude long-term, high-dose therapy. As a result, the liposomal preparations of AMB present an attractive alternative for treating zygomycosis. Lipid formulations have been used to treat zygomycosis, although no comparative studies have been performed thus far [88]. Outcomes of the use of lipid formulations of AMB seem to be similar to those historically reported for conventional AMB-based therapy, albeit with fewer adverse effects [88]. In the largest reported case series of zygomycosis, 64 patients, most of whom had diabetes as the underlying risk factor for zygomycosis, received a lipid complex of AMB for refractory disease or intolerance of conventional AMB. The overall response rate (improvement in or cure of infection) was 50%, and there were no significant toxic effects, even in patients who had preexisting renal disease [88]. Several case reports of liposomal AMB used for zygomycosis have also indicated favorable responses, including the use of particularly high doses of liposomal AMB (10 mg/kg/d) or prolonged therapy to achieve a cure in some cases [89]. The necessity of administering high dosages of liposomal formulations of AMB for zygomycosis may be questionable, considering the biopharmaceutical properties of AMB (high protein binding, limited solubility) [90] and the recently reported results of the AmBiLoad trial, which demonstrated no benefit and enhanced toxicity of a 2-week loading regimen of liposomal AMB (AmBisome) at 10 mg/kg/d versus 3 mg/kg/d in the treatment of invasive aspergillosis [91]. Researchers have also reported that drainage of abscesses and instillation of AMB into pulmonary cavitary lesions was successful in a limited number of patients [20]. Successful treatment of pulmonary zygomycosis with an aerosolized lipid complex of AMB (50 mg/d administered using a Respiguard II nebulizer) and combination antifungal treatment with terbinafine or rifampicin and AMB has been described in single case reports [89,92].

Most azoles, including fluconazole and voriconazole, have no meaningful activity against Zygomycetes fungi. Posaconazole, an orally available broad-spectrum investigational triazole (800 mg/d given in divided doses), seems to possess potent activity against these fungi, however [93]. In a recently reported open-label salvage trial, the overall success rate of posaconazole (800 mg) was 70% in 24 patients [82]. The drug was well tolerated with only minimal gastrointestinal side effects. Similarly, a recent retrospective review of posaconazole-based salvage therapy in 91 patients who had refractory zygomycosis indicated an overall success rate of 61%, including a success rate of 65% in patients who had pulmonary zygomycosis [87]. Furthermore, an additional 21% of subjects had stable disease after 12 weeks of treatment. These encouraging preliminary data suggest that the use of posaconazole fills an unmet need in the treatment of zygomycosis. Determining whether posaconazole alone or in combination with a lipid formulation of AMB is preferable will require further studies. Finally, secondary prophylaxis often is desired for patients requiring further immunosuppression after treatment of zygomycosis. Posaconazole seems to be a favorable option for patients who need continuous long-term antifungal therapy because they remain at high risk for relapse of infection.

Caspofungin lacks significant activity against zygomycetes in vitro, and clinical experience with caspofungin in the treatment of zygomycosis is extremely limited. Nevertheless, in case reports and a study of a model of disseminated zygomycosis in diabetic mice, echinocandins seemed to have some activity especially in combination with a polyene [84]. Because several cases of breakthrough zygomycosis have occurred in patients receiving echinocandin-based therapy [12], further studies of the role of echinocandins in the treatment of zygomycosis are needed.

Finally, the optimal duration of therapy for zygomycosis remains poorly defined. Treatment decisions are highly individualized. Near normalization of radiographic imaging, negative biopsy specimens and cultures from the affected site, and recovery from immunosuppression are important indicators that a patient is a candidate for stopping antifungal therapy.

Surgical management

Because zygomycosis is a highly angioinvasive infection with resulting extensive thrombosis and tissue necrosis, antifungal agents often display poor penetration at the site of infection. Even if the causative strain of an angioinvasive mold infection is susceptible to an antifungal agent in vitro, the agent may be ineffective in vivo [94]. Surgical débridement of infected tissue should be performed on an urgent basis. In patients who have pulmonary zygomycosis, surgical treatment in conjunction with antifungal therapy has been shown to improve survival significantly when compared with antifungal therapy alone [6,51]. In one of these studies, a comprehensive review of cases of pulmonary zygomycosis, the mortality rate was 55% in patients who received antifungal agents alone versus 27% in patients who received antifungal agents and underwent surgery [51]. The reported improved outcomes may partly reflect a bias toward offering surgery to less severely ill patients, however. Removal of as much of the infected or devitalized tissue as possible while the infection is localized has the greatest benefit. Lobectomy often is required, and pneumonectomy may be necessary for proximal or extensive involvement. Also, repeated procedures may be needed. The benefit of pulmonary resection diminishes as dissemination of zygomycosis occurs.

A recent review of 28 cases of zygomycosis suggested that treatment with HBO may be a beneficial adjunct to standard surgical and antifungal therapy for zygomycosis, particularly in diabetic patients who have rhinocerebral disease [95–100]. The increased oxygen pressure achieved with HBO treatment seems to improve the ability of neutrophils to kill organisms. Furthermore, by correcting lactic acidosis, treatment with HBO promotes the oxidative action of AMB. Additionally, high oxygen pressure inhibits fungal growth in vitro and improves the rate of wound healing by elevating tissue oxygen levels and releasing growth factors [100]. Data on treatment of zygomycosis with HBO are scarce, however, and its role in this setting remains uncertain.

The role of adjunctive cytokine therapy for zygomycosis has not been studied in detail. Cytokines that enhance phagocytic activity, such as interferon-γ and granulocyte-macrophage colony-stimulating factor, increase the killing efficacy of phagocytic cells against Zygomycetes fungi in vitro [101]. Case reports have indicated a favorable outcome in patients who had rhinocerebral zygomycosis after the addition of interferon-γ and granulocyte-macrophage colony-stimulating factor to the treatment regimen [101,102]. Further studies of cytokines that activate host phagocyte function are warranted for this infection. Occasional case reports have suggested a benefit of granulocyte transfusions [103], but prospective trials are needed.

The central role of iron metabolism in the pathogenesis of zygomycosis supports the use of effective iron chelators such as deferiprone and deferasirox as adjunctive antifungal therapy. Unlike deferoxamine, these newer iron chelators do not allow the fungus to take up iron, thereby inhibiting its growth in vitro in the presence of iron. Novel iron chelators could be effective adjunctive agents in suppressing the growth of zygomycetes in the absence of intact mononuclear and polymorphonuclear cell responses [2].

Prognosis

The disease site and host factors are key determinants of prognosis for zygomycosis. Hence, active hematologic malignancy, allogeneic bone marrow transplantation, and disseminated infection are associated with poor outcome. In a series of 391 patients who had hematologic malignancies and invasive fungal infections, Pagano and colleagues [14] found that the infections caused by Mucorales organisms had significantly poorer prognoses than did aspergillosis. In the authors' experience, most patients who have cancer and zygomycosis infection die within 12 weeks of diagnosis [9,12]. Correction of underlying immunodeficiency (eg, rapid tapering of steroids) and early diagnosis coupled with an aggressive multimodality treatment approach offer the best chance for survival in these patients.

Future needs

A number of important questions remain concerning the epidemiology, pathobiology, and management of invasive zygomycosis. The epidemiology of this infection requires careful study, particularly with the increasing appearance of zygomycetes as breakthrough pathogens in patients receiving *Aspergillus*-active antifungal therapy and the increasing incidence of this infection in the transplant setting. An improved understanding of whether zygomycetes are acquired in the community or nosocomially could help identify potentially important unrecognized risk factors that may explain the emerging epidemiology of this infection. Clearly, the greatest need for epidemiologic and clinical investigations of zygomycosis is an early, accurate, non–culture-based diagnostic test using a novel antigen or nucleic acid detection technology (ie, ELISA PCR). Such tests would be essential for early differentiation of zygomycosis from aspergillosis in high-risk patients in whom the two opportunistic molds infections frequently overlap and would allow the development of preemptive treatment protocols in lieu of the largely empiric treatment approaches that are currently required.

Prospective studies are urgently needed to address fundamental questions in the management of invasive zygomycosis:

1. What is the most effective primary antifungal therapy: lipid AMB formulations, posaconazole, or combination therapy?
2. What are the benefits and risks of antifungal prophylaxis in high-risk patients to prevent infections by both *Aspergillus* and Zygomycetes organisms (eg, posaconazole) versus *Aspergillus spp* alone (eg, voriconazole)?
3. What is the optimal timing and degree of surgical resection required to improve survival?
4. What is the potential for improving outcomes through the use of adjunctive immune-enhancement strategies such as cytokine administration, granulocyte transfusions, and possibly adoptive cellular immunotherapy for zygomycosis?
5. Can current antifungal and immune therapies be improved using novel approaches such as iron chelation therapy and HBO therapy?

References

[1] Larone DH. Medically important fungi–a guide to identification. 3rd edition. Washington (DC): American Society for Microbiology Press; 1995.
[2] Spellberg B, Edwards J Jr, Ibrahim A. Novel perspectives on mucormycosis: pathophysiology, presentation, and management. Clin Microbiol Rev 2005;18(3):556–69.
[3] Chayakulkeeree M, Ghannoum MA, Perfect JR. Zygomycosis: the re-emerging fungal infection. Eur J Clin Microbiol Infect Dis 2006;25:28.
[4] Ibrahim A, Edwards JE Jr, Filler SG. Zygomycosis. Philadelphia: Harcourt Brace; 2004.
[5] Ribes JA, Vanover-Sams CL, Baker DJ. Zygomycetes in human disease. Clin Microbiol Rev 2000;13(2):236–301.
[6] Roden MM, Zaoutis TE, Buchanan WL, et al. Epidemiology and outcome of zygomycosis: a review of 929 reported cases. Clin Infect Dis 2005;41(5):634–53.
[7] Mead JH, Lupton GP, Dillavou CL, et al. Cutaneous Rhizopus infection. Occurrence as a postoperative complication associated with an elasticized adhesive dressing. JAMA 1979;242(3):272–4.
[8] Mitchell SJ, Gray J, Morgan ME, et al. Nosocomial infection with *Rhizopus microsporus* in preterm infants: association with wooden tongue depressors. Lancet 1996;348(9025):441–3.
[9] Kontoyiannis DP, Wessel VC, Bodey GP, et al. Zygomycosis in the 1990s in a tertiary-care cancer center. Clin Infect Dis 2000;30(6):851–6.
[10] Rees JR, Pinner RW, Hajjeh RA, et al. The epidemiological features of invasive mycotic infections in the San Francisco Bay area, 1992–1993: results of population-based laboratory active surveillance. Clin Infect Dis 1998;27(5):1138–47.
[11] Chamilos G, Luna M, Lewis RE, et al. Invasive fungal infections in patients with hematological malignancies in a tertiary care cancer center: an autopsy study over a 15-year period (1989–2003). Hematologica 2006;91:988–91.

[12] Kontoyiannis DP, Lionakis MS, Lewis RE, et al. Zygomycosis in a tertiary-care cancer center in the era of *Aspergillus-active* antifungal therapy: a case-control observational study of 27 recent cases. J Infect Dis 2005;191(8):1350–60.

[13] Marr KA, Carter RA, Crippa F, et al. Epidemiology and outcome of mould infections in hematopoietic stem cell transplant recipients. Clin Infect Dis 2002;34(7):909–17.

[14] Pagano L, Girmenia C, Mele L, et al. Infections caused by filamentous fungi in patients with hematologic malignancies. A report of 391 cases by GIMEMA Infection Program. Haematologica 2001;86(8):862–70.

[15] Pagano L, Ricci P, Tonso A, et al. Mucormycosis in patients with haematological malignancies: a retrospective clinical study of 37 cases. GIMEMA Infection Program (Gruppo Italiano Malattie Ematologiche Maligne dell'Adulto). Br J Haematol 1997;99(2):331–6.

[16] Imhof A, Balajee SA, Fredricks DN, et al. Breakthrough fungal infections in stem cell transplant recipients receiving voriconazole. Clin Infect Dis 2004;39(5):743–6.

[17] Park B, Kontoyiannis D, Pappas P, et al. Comparison of zygomycosis and fusariosis to invasive aspergillosis (IA) among transplant recipients reporting TRANSNET. Presented at the 44th Interscience Conference on Antimicerobial Agents and Chemotherapy [*M-666]. Washington, DC, October 30–November 2.

[18] Siwek GT, Dodgson KJ, de Magalhaes-Silverman M, et al. Invasive zygomycosis in hematopoietic stem cell transplant recipients receiving voriconazole prophylaxis. Clin Infect Dis 2004;39(4):584–7.

[19] Kurukularatne C, Garcia-Diaz J, Kemmerly S, Reed D, et al. Beyond *Rhizopus* and *Mucor*: Hurricane Katrina stirs up *Synephalastrum* in New Orleans. Presented at Focus on Fungal Infections 16. Las Vegas, March 8–10, 2006.

[20] Greenberg RN, Scott LJ, Vaughn HH, et al. Zygomycosis (mucormycosis): emerging clinical importance and new treatments. Curr Opin Infect Dis 2004;17(6):517–25.

[21] Abzug MJ, Gardner S, Glode MP, et al. Heliport-associated nosocomial mucormycoses. Infect Control Hosp Epidemiol 1992;13(6):325–6.

[22] Weems JJ Jr, Davis BJ, Tablan OC, et al. Construction activity: an independent risk factor for invasive aspergillosis and zygomycosis in patients with hematologic malignancy. Infect Control 1987;8(2):71–5.

[23] Parker C, Kaminski G, Hill D. Zygomycosis in a tattoo, caused by *Saksenaea vasiformis*. Australas J Dermatol 1986;27(3):107–11.

[24] Prevoo RL, Starink TM, de Haan P. Primary cutaneous mucormycosis in a healthy young girl. Report of a case caused by *Mucor hiemalis Wehmer*. J Am Acad Dermatol 1991;24 (5 Pt 2):882–5.

[25] Bouchara JP, Oumeziane NA, Lissitzky JC, et al. Attachment of spores of the human pathogenic fungus *Rhizopus oryzae* to extracellular matrix components. Eur J Cell Biol 1996;70(1):76–83.

[26] Ibrahim AS, Spellberg B, Avanessian V, et al. *Rhizopus oryzae* adheres to, is phagocytosed by, and damages endothelial cells in vitro. Infect Immun 2005;73(2):778–83.

[27] Partida-Martinez LP, Hertweck C. Pathogenic fungus harbours endosymbiotic bacteria for toxin production. Nature 2005;437(7060):884–8.

[28] Waldorf AR, Diamond RD. Neutrophil chemotactic responses induced by fresh and swollen *Rhizopus oryzae* spores and *Aspergillus fumigatus conidia*. Infect Immun 1985; 48(2):458–63.

[29] Waldorf AR, Levitz SM, Diamond RD. In vivo bronchoalveolar macrophage defense against *Rhizopus oryzae* and *Aspergillus fumigatus*. J Infect Dis 1984;150(5):752–60.

[30] Waldorf AR, Ruderman N, Diamond RD. Specific susceptibility to mucormycosis in murine diabetes and bronchoalveolar macrophage defense against *Rhizopus*. J Clin Invest 1984;74(1):150–60.

[31] Lionakis MS, Kontoyiannis DP. Glucocorticoids and invasive fungal infections. Lancet 2003;362(9398):1828–38.

[32] Chinn RY, Diamond RD. Generation of chemotactic factors by *Rhizopus oryzae* in the presence and absence of serum: relationship to hyphal damage mediated by human neutrophils and effects of hyperglycemia and ketoacidosis. Infect Immun 1982;38(3):1123–9.

[33] Richardson M, Warnock D. Mucormycosis. Oxford (UK): Blackwell; 2003.

[34] Crichton R. Iron and infection. 2nd edition. London: Wiley and Sons; 2001.

[35] Gaziev D, Baronciani D, Galimberti M, et al. Mucormycosis after bone marrow transplantation: report of four cases in thalassemia and review of the literature. Bone Marrow Transplant 1996;17(3):409–14.

[36] Sands JM, Macher AM, Ley TJ, et al. Disseminated infection caused by *Cunninghamella bertholletiae* in a patient with beta-thalassemia. Case report and review of the literature. Ann Intern Med 1985;102(1):59–63.

[37] Howard DH. Acquisition, transport, and storage of iron by pathogenic fungi. Clin Microbiol Rev 1999;12(3):394–404.

[38] Artis WM, Fountain JA, Delcher HK, et al. A mechanism of susceptibility to mucormycosis in diabetic ketoacidosis: transferrin and iron availability. Diabetes 1982;31(12): 1109–14.

[39] Artis WM, Patrusky E, Rastinejad F, et al. Fungistatic mechanism of human transferrin for *Rhizopus oryzae* and *Trichophyton mentagrophytes*: alternative to simple iron deprivation. Infect Immun 1983;41(3):1269–78.

[40] Boelaert JR, de Locht M, Schneider YJ. The effect of deferoxamine on different zygomycetes. J Infect Dis 1994;169(1):231–2.

[41] Boelaert JR, de Locht M, Van Cutsem J, et al. Mucormycosis during deferoxamine therapy is a siderophore-mediated infection. In vitro and in vivo animal studies. J Clin Invest 1993; 91(5):1979–86.

[42] Boelaert JR, Van Cutsem J, de Locht M, et al. Deferoxamine augments growth and pathogenicity of *Rhizopus*, while hydroxypyridinone chelators have no effect. Kidney Int 1994; 45(3):667–71.

[43] de Locht M, Boelaert JR, Schneider YJ. Iron uptake from ferrioxamine and from ferrirhizoferrin by germinating spores of *Rhizopus microsporus*. Biochem Pharmacol 1994;47(10): 1843–50.

[44] Mencacci A, Cenci E, Boelaert JR, et al. Iron overload alters innate and T helper cell responses to *Candida albicans* in mice. J Infect Dis 1997;175(6):1467–76.

[45] Verpooten GA, D'Haese PC, Boelaert JR, et al. Pharmacokinetics of aluminoxamine and ferrioxamine and dose finding of desferrioxamine in haemodialysis patients. Nephrol Dial Transplant 1992;7(9):931–8.

[46] Bhansali A, Bhadada S, Sharma A, et al. Presentation and outcome of rhino-orbital-cerebral mucormycosis in patients with diabetes. Postgrad Med J 2004;80(949):670–4.

[47] Yohai RA, Bullock JD, Aziz AA, et al. Survival factors in rhino-orbital-cerebral mucormycosis. Surv Ophthalmol 1994;39(1):3–22.

[48] Frater JL, Hall GS, Procop GW. Histologic features of zygomycosis: emphasis on perineural invasion and fungal morphology. Arch Pathol Lab Med 2001;125(3):375–8.

[49] Fatterpekar G, Mukherji S, Arbealez A, et al. Fungal diseases of the paranasal sinuses. Semin Ultrasound CT MR 1999;20(6):391–401.

[50] Chamilos G, Marom EM, Lewis RE, et al. Predictors of pulmonary zygomycosis versus invasive pulmonary aspergillosis in patients with cancer. Clin Infect Dis 2005;41(1):60–6.

[51] Lee FY, Mossad SB, Adal KA. Pulmonary mucormycosis: the last 30 years. Arch Intern Med 1999;159(12):1301–9.

[52] McAdams HP, Rosado de Christenson M, Strollo DC, et al. Pulmonary mucormycosis: radiologic findings in 32 cases. AJR Am J Roentgenol 1997;168(6):1541–8.

[53] Tedder M, Spratt JA, Anstadt MP, et al. Pulmonary mucormycosis: results of medical and surgical therapy. Ann Thorac Surg 1994;57(4):1044–50.

[54] Goldstein MF, Dvorin DJ, Dunsky EH, et al. Allergic Rhizomucor sinusitis. J Allergy Clin Immunol 1992;90(3 Pt 1):394–404.

[55] Dykewicz MS, Laufer P, Patterson R, et al. Woodman's disease: hypersensitivity pneumonitis from cutting live trees. J Allergy Clin Immunol 1988;81(2):455–60.

[56] Andresen D, Donaldson A, Choo L, et al. Multifocal cutaneous mucormycosis complicating polymicrobial wound infections in a tsunami survivor from Sri Lanka. Lancet 2005; 365(9462):876–8.

[57] Patino JF, Castro D, Valencia A, et al. Necrotizing soft tissue lesions after a volcanic cataclysm. World J Surg 1991;15(2):240–7.

[58] Bittencourt AL, Ayala MA, Ramos EA. A new form of abdominal zygomycosis different from mucormycosis: report of two cases and review of the literature. Am J Trop Med Hyg 1979;28(3):564–9.

[59] Oliver MR, Van Voorhis WC, Boeckh M, et al. Hepatic mucormycosis in a bone marrow transplant recipient who ingested naturopathic medicine. Clin Infect Dis 1996;22(3):521–4.

[60] Park YS, Lee JD, Kim TH, et al. Gastric mucormycosis. Gastrointest Endosc 2002;56(6): 904–5.

[61] Branton MH, Johnson SC, Brooke JD, et al. Peritonitis due to *Rhizopus* in a patient undergoing continuous ambulatory peritoneal dialysis. Rev Infect Dis 1991;13(1):19–21.

[62] Polo JR, Luno J, Menarguez C, et al. Peritoneal mucormycosis in a patient receiving continuous ambulatory peritoneal dialysis. Am J Kidney Dis 1989;13(3):237–9.

[63] Nakamura M, Weil WB Jr, Kaufman DB. Fatal fungal peritonitis in an adolescent on continuous ambulatory peritoneal dialysis: association with deferoxamine. Pediatr Nephrol 1989;3(1):80–2.

[64] Schwartz JR, Nagle MG, Elkins RC, et al. Mucormycosis of the trachea: an unusual cause of acute upper airway obstruction. Chest 1982;81(5):653–4.

[65] Connor BA, Anderson RJ, Smith JW. *Mucor* mediastinitis. Chest 1979;75(4):525–6.

[66] Marwaha RK, Banerjee AK, Thapa BR, et al. Mediastinal zygomycosis. Postgrad Med J 1985;61(718):733–5.

[67] Lussier N, Laverdiere M, Weiss K, et al. Primary renal mucormycosis. Urology 1998;52(5): 900–3.

[68] Echols RM, Selinger DS, Hallowell C, et al. *Rhizopus* osteomyelitis. A case report and review. Am J Med 1979;66(1):141–5.

[69] Mishra B, Mandal A, Kumar N. Mycotic prosthetic-valve endocarditis. J Hosp Infect 1992; 20(2):122–5.

[70] Roy TM, Anderson KC, Farrow JR. Cardiac mucormycosis complicating diabetes mellitus. J Diabetes Complications 1990;4(3):132–5.

[71] Sanchez-Recalde A, Merino JL, Dominguez F, et al. Successful treatment of prosthetic aortic valve mucormycosis. Chest 1999;116(6):1818–20.

[72] Zhang R, Zhang JW, Szerlip HM. Endocarditis and hemorrhagic stroke caused by *Cunninghamella bertholletiae* infection after kidney transplantation. Am J Kidney Dis 2002;40(4):842–6.

[73] Bosken CH, Szporn AH, Kleinerman J. Superior vena cava syndrome due to mucormycosis in a patient with lymphoma. Mt Sinai J Med 1987;54(6):508–11.

[74] Tierney MR, Baker AS. Infections of the head and neck in diabetes mellitus. Infect Dis Clin North Am 1995;9(1):195–216.

[75] Chandler F, Kaplan W, Ajello L. A colour atlas and textbook of the histopathology of mycotic diseases. London: Wofle Medical Publications, Ltd.; 1980.

[76] Bialek R, Konrad F, Kern J, et al. PCR based identification and discrimination of agents of mucormycosis and aspergillosis in paraffin wax embedded tissue. J Clin Pathol 2005;58(11): 1180–4.

[77] Kobayashi M, Togitani K, Machida H, et al. Molecular polymerase chain reaction diagnosis of pulmonary mucormycosis caused by *Cunninghamella bertholletiae*. Respirology 2004; 9(3):397–401.

[78] Rickerts V, Just-Nubling G, Konrad F, et al. Diagnosis of invasive aspergillosis and mucormycosis in immunocompromised patients by seminested PCR assay of tissue samples. Eur J Clin Microbiol Infect Dis 2006;25(1):8–13.

[79] National Committee for Clinical Laboratory Standards. Reference method for broth dilution antifungal susceptibility testing of filamentous fungi; approved standard NCCLS document M38-A. Wayne, PA: National Committee for Clinical Laboratory Standards; 2002.

[80] Dannaoui E, Meletiadis J, Mouton JW, et al. In vitro susceptibilities of zygomycetes to conventional and new antifungals. J Antimicrob Chemother 2003;51(1):45–52.

[81] Ullmann AJ, Cornely OA, Burchardt A, et al. Pharmacokinetics, safety, and efficacy of posaconazole in patients with persistent febrile neutropenia or refractory invasive fungal infection. Antimicrob Agents Chemother 2006;50(2):658–66.

[82] Greenberg RN, Mullane K, van Burik JA, et al. Posaconazole as salvage therapy for zygomycosis. Antimicrob Agents Chemother 2006;50(1):126–33.

[83] Courtney R, Pai S, Laughlin M, Lim J, et al. Pharmacokinetics, safety, and tolerability of oral posaconazole administered in single and multiple doses in healthy adults. Antimicrob Agents Chemother 2003;47(9):2788–95.

[84] Spellberg B, Fu Y, Edwards JE Jr, et al. Combination therapy with amphotericin B lipid complex and caspofungin acetate of disseminated zygomycosis in diabetic ketoacidotic mice. Antimicrob Agents Chemother 2005;49(2):830–2.

[85] Dannaoui E, Afeltra J, Meis JF, et al. In vitro susceptibilities of zygomycetes to combinations of antimicrobial agents. Antimicrob Agents Chemother 2002;46(8):2708–11.

[86] Ibrahim AS, Bowman JC, Avanessian V, et al. Caspofungin inhibits *Rhizopus oryzae* 1,3-beta-D-glucan synthase, lowers burden in brain measured by quantitative PCR, and improves survival at a low but not a high dose during murine disseminated zygomycosis. Antimicrob Agents Chemother 2005;49(2):721–7.

[87] van Burik JA, Hare RS, Solomon HF, et al. Posaconazole is effective as salvage therapy in zygomycosis: a retrospective summary of 91 cases. Clin Infect Dis 2006;42(7):e61–5.

[88] Perfect JR. Treatment of non-*Aspergillus* moulds in immunocompromised patients, with amphotericin B lipid complex. Clin Infect Dis 2005;40(Suppl 6):S401–8.

[89] Gleissner B, Schilling A, Anagnostopolous I, et al. Improved outcome of zygomycosis in patients with hematological diseases? Leuk Lymphoma 2004;45(7):1351–60.

[90] Lewis RE, Wiederhold NP. The solubility ceiling: a rationale for continuous infusion amphotericin B therapy? Clin Infect Dis 2003;37(6):871–2.

[91] Cornely OA, Maertens J, Bresnik M, et al. Liposomal amphotericin B (L-AMB) as initial therapy for invasive filamentous fungal infections (IFFI): a randomized, prospective trial of a high loading regimen vs. standard dosing (AmBiLoad Trial). Presented at the 47th annual meeting of the American Society for Hematology. Atlanta, December 10–13 2005.

[92] Dannaoui E, Mouton JW, Meis JF, et al. Efficacy of antifungal therapy in a nonneutropenic murine model of zygomycosis. Antimicrob Agents Chemother 2002;46(6):1953–9.

[93] Torres HA, Hachem RY, Chemaly RF, et al. Posaconazole: a broad-spectrum triazole antifungal. Lancet Infect Dis 2005;5(12):775–85.

[94] Paterson PJ, Seaton S, Prentice HG, et al. Treatment failure in invasive aspergillosis: susceptibility of deep tissue isolates following treatment with amphotericin B. J Antimicrob Chemother 2003;52(5):873–6.

[95] Shafer MR. Use of hyperbaric oxygen as adjunct therapy to surgical debridement of complicated wounds. Semin Perioper Nurs 1993;2(4):256–62.

[96] Price JC, Stevens DL. Hyperbaric oxygen in the treatment of rhinocerebral mucormycosis. Laryngoscope 1980;90(5 Pt 1):737–47.

[97] Kajs-Wyllie M. Hyperbaric oxygen therapy for rhinocerebral fungal infection. J Neurosci Nurs 1995;27(3):174–81.

[98] Ferguson BJ, Mitchell TG, Moon R, et al. Adjunctive hyperbaric oxygen for treatment of rhinocerebral mucormycosis. Rev Infect Dis 1988;10(3):551–9.

[99] Couch L, Theilen F, Mader JT. Rhinocerebral mucormycosis with cerebral extension successfully treated with adjunctive hyperbaric oxygen therapy. Arch Otolaryngol Head Neck Surg 1988;114(7):791–4.

[100] Barratt DM, Van Meter K, Asmar P, et al. Hyperbaric oxygen as an adjunct in zygomycosis: randomized controlled trial in a murine model. Antimicrob Agents Chemother 2001; 45(12):3601–2.

[101] Gil-Lamaignere C, Simitsopoulou M, Roilides E, et al. Interferon-gamma and granulocyte-macrophage colony-stimulating factor augment the activity of polymorphonuclear leukocytes against medically important zygomycetes. J Infect Dis 2005;191(7):1180–7.

[102] Abzug MJ, Walsh TJ. Interferon-gamma and colony-stimulating factors as adjuvant therapy for refractory fungal infections in children. Pediatr Infect Dis J 2004;23(8):769–73.

[103] Slavin MA, Kannan K, Buchanan MR, et al. Successful allogeneic stem cell transplant after invasive pulmonary zygomycosis. Leuk Lymphoma 2002;43(2):437–9.

ELSEVIER
SAUNDERS

Infect Dis Clin N Am
20 (2006) 609–620

INFECTIOUS
DISEASE CLINICS
OF NORTH AMERICA

Phaeohyphomycosis

Sanjay G. Revankar, MD

Division of Infectious Diseases, Wayne State University, Harper University Hospital,
3990 John R., 5 Hudson, Detroit, MI 48201, USA

Phaeohyphomycosis is the general term used to describe infections caused by dematiaceous, or darkly pigmented, fungi. These are uncommon causes of human disease, but they can be responsible for life-threatening infections in immunocompromised and immunocompetent individuals. They are commonly found in the soil and are generally distributed worldwide. This suggests that most if not all individuals are exposed to them, presumably from inhalation. Phaeohyphomycosis, however, should be distinguished from other specific pathologic conditions associated with dematiaceous fungi, which include chromoblastomycosis and mycetoma. Chromoblastomycosis, which is caused by a small group of fungi that produce characteristic sclerotic bodies in tissue, is usually seen in tropical areas [1]. Mycetoma is a deep-tissue infection usually of the lower extremities characterized by the presence of mycotic granules [1]. These pathologic conditions are discussed in detail in other reviews [1–3].

In recent years, agents of phaeohyphomycosis have been increasingly recognized as important pathogens. The spectrum of disease they are associated with has also broadened. For the purposes of this article, these are divided into superficial infections, allergic disease, pneumonia, brain abscess, and disseminated disease. These are not necessarily mutually exclusive, and other groupings could be devised also. For some infections in immunocompetent individuals, such as allergic fungal sinusitis and brain abscess, they are among the most common etiologic fungi.

The fungi

More than 100 species and 60 genera of dematiaceous fungi have been implicated in human disease [3]. As the number of patients immunocompromised from diseases and medical therapy increases, additional species are

E-mail address: srevankar@med.wayne.edu

id.theclinics.com

being reported as causes of human disease, expanding an already long list of potential pathogens. Common genera associated with specific clinical syndromes are listed in Table 1. The distinguishing characteristic common to all these various species is the presence of melanin in their cell walls, which imparts the dark color to their conidia or spores and hyphae. The colonies are typically brown to black also. In tissue, they stain strongly with the Fontana-Masson stain, which is specific for melanin [2]. This can be helpful in distinguishing these fungi from other species, particularly *Aspergillus*. In addition, hyphae typically appear more fragmented in tissue than is seen with *Aspergillus*, with irregular septate hyphae and yeast-like forms [2].

Guidelines are available regarding the handling of potentially infectious fungi in the laboratory setting. Cultures of certain well-known fungi, such as *Coccidioides immitis* and *Histoplasma capsulatum*, are suggested to be worked with in a Biosafety Level 3 facility, which requires a separate negative pressure room. Recently agents of phaeohyphomycosis, in particular *Cladophialophora bantiana*, have been included in the list of fungi that should be kept under Biosafety Level 2 containment [4]. This seems reasonable given their propensity, albeit rarely, for causing life-threatening infection in normal individuals.

Table 1
Clinical syndromes associated with phaeohyphomycosis

Clinical syndrome	Commonly associated fungal genera[a]	Suggested therapy
Onychomycosis	*Onychocola*	Itra or Terb +/− topical agents
	Alternaria	
Subcutaneous nodules	*Exophiala*	Surgery +/− Itra
	Alternaria	
	Phialophora	
Keratitis	*Curvularia*	Topical natamycin +/− Itra
	Bipolaris	
	Exserohilum	
	Lasiodiplodia	
Allergic disease	*Bipolaris*	Steroids +/− Itra
	Curvularia	
Pneumonia	*Ochroconis*	Itra (AmB if severe)
	Exophiala	
	Chaetomium	
Brain abscess	*Cladophialophora* (*C bantiana*)	High-dose azole + lipid
	Ramichloridium (*R mackenzei*)	AmB +/− 5-FC
	Ochroconis	
Disseminated disease	*Scedosporium* (*S prolificans*)	Lipid AmB + azole +/−
	Bipolaris	echinocandin
	Wangiella	

Abbreviations: AmB, amphotericin B; azole, itraconazole or voriconazole; 5-FC, flucytosine; Itra, itraconazole; Terb, terbinafine

[a] Taxonomy notes: *Bipolaris* = *Dreschlera* and *Helminthosporium* (older terms); *Ochroconis* = *Dactylaria* (older term); *Cladophialophora* = *Xylohypha* and *Cladosporium* (older terms).

Diagnosis

The diagnosis of phaeohyphomycosis currently rests on pathologic examination of clinical specimens and careful gross and microscopic examination of cultures, occasionally requiring the expertise of a mycology reference laboratory. Because many of these are rarely seen in practice, a high degree of clinical suspicion is required when interpreting culture results. Unlike other common mycoses that cause human disease, there are no simple serologic or antigen tests available to detect these fungi in blood or tissue. Polymerase chain reaction is being studied as an aid to the diagnosis of fungal infections, but as yet it does not reliably distinguish between dematiaceous fungi and other more common mycoses, and it is not widely available.

Pathogenesis

Little is known regarding the pathogenic mechanisms by which these fungi cause disease, particularly in immunocompetent individuals. One of the likely candidate virulence factors is the presence of melanin in the cell wall, which is common to all dematiaceous fungi. There are several mechanisms proposed by which melanin may act as a virulence factor [5–7]. It is believed to confer a protective advantage by scavenging free radicals and hypochlorite that are produced by phagocytic cells in their oxidative burst and that would normally kill most organisms [5]. In addition, melanin may bind to hydrolytic enzymes, thereby preventing their action on the plasma membrane [5]. These multiple functions may help explain the pathogenic potential of some dematiaceous fungi, even in immunocompetent hosts. Considerable work has been done in several fungi that contain melanin. Specifically, in the yeasts *Cryptococcus neoformans* and *Wangiella dermatitidis*, disruption of melanin production leads to markedly reduced virulence in animal models [8,9]. Melanin has also been shown to reduce the susceptibility of *C neoformans* and *H capsulatum* to amphotericin B and caspofungin, possibly by binding these drugs [10,11]. This effect is not apparent with azole drugs [10].

Almost all allergic disease and eosinophilia caused by agents of phaeohyphomycosis is caused by two genera, *Bipolaris* and *Curvularia*. These organisms are common in the environment, so exposure is practically universal. The virulence factors in these fungi that are responsible for eliciting allergic reactions are unclear at present.

In vitro susceptibility

Although in vitro antifungal testing has come a long way in the past several years, with the development of standardized methods for testing yeasts and molds [12,13], the available in vitro data for dematiaceous fungi are sparse and often rely on small numbers of isolates per species. Recent years have seen an increased interest in dematiaceous fungi and reports of in vitro testing.

Azoles were the first oral, broad spectrum antifungal agents available and are widely used. Itraconazole and voriconazole have the most consistent activity against dematiaceous fungi. Almost all the recent in vitro data with dematiaceous fungi include itraconazole. Apart from the species *Scedosporium prolificans* and *Scopulariopsis brumptii*, itraconazole and voriconazole demonstrate good activity against the vast majority of dematiaceous fungi tested [14–18]. MICs generally are ≤0.125 μg/mL for this group of fungi. Minimum inhibitory concentrations (MICs), however, are usually slightly higher for voriconazole, though the clinical significance of this is unclear. In vitro data with posaconazole are more limited. Fluconazole has negligible activity against dematiaceous molds, and use of ketoconazole is limited by several side effects.

Amphotericin B is usually rapidly fungicidal against susceptible species in vitro and generally has good activity against most clinically important dematiaceous fungi [16]. Some species have been consistently resistant (MIC ≥2 μg/mL) in vitro, however, including *S prolificans* and *S brumptii* [14].

Limited data are available for other agents. Terbinafine is the only oral allylamine available for systemic use. Its extensive binding to serum proteins and distribution into skin and adipose tissue, however, have diminished enthusiasm for its use in treating serious systemic fungal infections [19,20]. In vitro studies against dematiaceous fungi are emerging, and fairly broad spectrum activity is seen. The echinocandins are the latest group of antifungal agents to be developed, and they have a unique mechanism of action, inhibiting β-1,3 glucan synthesis and thereby disrupting the fungal cell wall [21]. Caspofungin, micafungin, and anidulafungin are available for clinical use, though in vitro studies with dematiaceous fungi are limited. In general, MICs for dematiaceous fungi are higher than for *Aspergillus* spp [22]. 5-FC is unique in its mechanism of action, inhibiting DNA and RNA synthesis. It has a limited role in therapy of these fungi, though some species are susceptible [23].

Use of antifungal combinations is a potentially useful strategy for refractory infections, though it has not been studied extensively in phaeohyphomycosis. The combination of itraconazole and terbinafine has been studied against *S prolificans*, which is otherwise generally resistant to all agents. In vitro, synergistic activity was found against most isolates of this species, and no antagonism was noted [24]. Voriconazole and terbinafine also display similar synergy in vitro [25]. The mechanism is presumably potent inhibition of ergosterol synthesis at two different steps of the pathway by these agents. This should be interpreted with caution, however, because terbinafine is not generally used for systemic infections. Another report suggested synergy for *S prolificans* with voriconazole and caspofungin [26].

Clinical syndromes and therapy

There are no standard therapies for infections caused by dematiaceous fungi with regard to choice of agent or duration of therapy. Far more experience has accumulated with itraconazole than for any other single drug, though newer agents may have specific advantages. Length of therapy is generally based on clinical response and ranges from several weeks to several months or longer. A summary of suggested therapies is presented in Table 1.

Superficial infections

Superficial infections are the most common form of infection caused by dematiaceous fungi. These cases are generally associated with minor trauma or other environmental exposure. Although many pathogens have been reported, a few are responsible for most infections. Although they rarely lead to life-threatening disease, significant morbidity can occur depending on the site of infection and response to therapy.

Onychomycosis

Dematiaceous fungi are rare causes of onychomycosis. Clinical features may include a history of trauma, involvement of only one or two toenails, and lack of response to standard systemic therapy [27]. *Onychocola* and *Alternaria* have been reported, with the former being highly resistant to therapy [27,28]. Itraconazole and terbinafine are the most commonly used systemic agents and may be combined with topical therapy for refractory cases [28]. No published data are available for the newer azole agents.

Subcutaneous lesions

There are numerous case reports of subcutaneous infection caused by a wide variety of species [29–31]. *Exophiala*, *Alternaria*, *Phialophora*, and *Bipolaris* are among the more common etiologic agents [32]. Minor trauma is the usual inciting factor, though it may be unrecognized by the patient. Lesions typically occur on exposed areas of the body and often appear as isolated cystic or papular lesions. Immunocompromised patients are at increased risk for subsequent dissemination, though rare cases have been described in apparently immunocompetent patients also. Occasionally infection may involve joints or bone, requiring more extensive surgery or prolonged antifungal therapy.

As for many of the infectious syndromes associated with dematiaceous fungi, therapy is not standardized. Surgical excision alone has been successful in several cases [33]. Oral systemic therapy with an azole antifungal agent in conjunction with surgery is frequently used and has been successful. Two cases of refractory bone and joint infection caused by *S prolificans* were treated effectively with voriconazole and the combination of voriconazole and caspofungin [26,34].

Keratitis

Fungal keratitis is an important ophthalmologic problem, particularly in tropical areas of the world. In one large series, 40% of all infectious keratitis was caused by fungi, almost exclusively molds [35]. The most common fungi are *Fusarium* and *Aspergillus*, followed by dematiaceous fungi (up to 8%–17% of cases) [36]. Approximately half the cases are associated with trauma; prior eye surgery, diabetes and contact lens use have also been noted as important risk factors [35,36]. Diagnosis rests on potassium hydroxide (KOH) smear and culture.

Some of the largest case series with dematiaceous fungi have come from India [37,38]. In a large experience of keratitis caused by dematiaceous fungi, 88 cases were examined [37]. The most common dematiaceous genus causing keratitis was *Curvularia*, followed by *Bipolaris*, *Exserohilum*, and *Lasiodiplodia*. Almost half the cases were associated with trauma. Most patients received topical agents only (5% natamycin ± azole), though more severe cases also received oral ketoconazole. Overall response was 72% in those available for follow-up. Surgery was needed in 13 patients, with an additional 6 requiring enucleation because of poor response.

In a study from the United States of 43 cases of *Curvularia* keratitis, almost all were associated with trauma [39]. Plants were the most common source, though several cases of metal injury were seen also. Topical natamycin was used almost exclusively, with only a few severe cases requiring adjunctive therapy, usually with an azole. Of the oral agents, itraconazole had the best in vitro activity. Surgery, including penetrating keratoplasty, was required in 19% of patients. At the end of therapy, only 78% had a visual acuity of 20/40 or better.

Topical polyenes, such as amphotericin B and natamycin, are commonly used, but oral and topical itraconazole has been found to be useful also [35,40]. Voriconazole is a potentially useful agent, but published clinical experience is primarily limited to cases caused by *Scedosporium apiospermum* (teleomorph: *Pseudallescheria boydii*) [41]. Many patients are left with residual visual deficits at the end of therapy, however, suggesting that further advances in therapy are needed for this debilitating disease.

Allergic disease

Fungal sinusitis

Patients who have this condition usually present with chronic sinus symptoms that are not responsive to antibiotics. Previously *Aspergillus* was believed to be the most common fungus responsible for allergic sinusitis, but it is now appreciated that disease caused by dematiaceous fungi actually comprises most cases [42,43]. The most common species isolated are *Bipolaris* and *Curvularia*. Criteria have been suggested for this disease, and include (1) nasal polyps, (2) presence of allergic mucin containing Charcot–Leyden crystals and eosinophils, (3) hyphal elements in the mucosa without evidence of tissue invasion, (4) positive skin test to fungal allergens, and (5) on computed tomography (CT) scans, characteristic areas of central hyperattenuation within the sinus cavity [44]. Diagnosis generally depends on demonstration of allergic mucin, with or without actual culture of the organism. Therapy consists of surgery to remove the mucin, which is often tenacious, and systemic steroids. Antifungal therapy, usually in the form of itraconazole, may play a role in reducing the requirement for steroids, but this is not routinely recommended [45]. Other azoles have only rarely been used for this disease.

Allergic bronchopulmonary mycosis

Allergic bronchopulmonary mycosis (ABPM) is similar in presentation to allergic bronchopulmonary aspergillosis (ABPA), which is typically seen in patients who have asthma or cystic fibrosis [46]. There is a suggestion that allergic fungal sinusitis and ABPM may actually be a continuum of disease and should be referred to as sinobronchial allergic mycosis (SAM) [47]. Criteria for the diagnosis of ABPA in patients who have asthma include: (1) asthma, (2) positive skin test for fungal allergens, (3) elevated IgE levels, (4) *Aspergillus*-specific IgE, and (5) proximal bronchiectasis [46]. Similar criteria for ABPM are not established, but may include elevated IgE levels, positive skin tests, and response to systemic steroids.

In reviewing cases of ABPM caused by dematiaceous fungi, essentially all cases are caused by *Bipolaris* or *Curvularia* [48] These two genera are commonly found in the environment, and their spores are large (20–30 μm × 8–12 μm) compared with *Aspergillus* (2–3 μm). Asthma was common in these cases, but bronchiectasis was often not present, perhaps reflecting somewhat different pathogenic mechanisms. All cases had either eosinophilia or elevated IgE levels. Therapy was primarily systemic steroids, usually prednisone at 0.5 mg/kg/day for 2 weeks, followed by a slow taper over 2–3 months or longer, if necessary. Itraconazole has been used as a steroid-sparing agent, but its efficacy is not clear and routine use of itraconazole is not generally recommended [46,49].

Pneumonia

Nonallergic pulmonary disease is usually seen in immunocompromised patients and may be caused by a wide variety of species, in contrast to allergic disease [50–53]. Clinical manifestations include pneumonia, asymptomatic solitary pulmonary nodules, and endobronchial lesions that may cause hemoptysis. Therapy consists of systemic antifungal agents, usually amphotericin B or itraconazole initially, followed by itraconazole for a more prolonged period. Mortality rates are high in immunocompromised patients. Experience with the newer azoles is anecdotal.

Brain abscess

This is a rare but frequently fatal manifestation of phaeohyphomycosis, often in immunocompetent individuals [54]. In a review of 101 cases of central nervous system infection caused by dematiaceous fungi, 87 were found to be brain abscess [55]. More than half of the cases were in patients who had no risk factor or immunodeficiency. The most common species was *C bantiana*, accounting for half of the cases. Other species included *Ramichloridium mackenzei*, *Ochroconus gallopavum*, and *W dermatitidis*. Symptoms include headache, neurologic deficits, and seizures. The pathogenesis may be hematogenous spread from an initial, presumably subclinical pulmonary focus. It remains unclear why these fungi preferentially cause CNS disease in immunocompetent individuals.

Therapy varied depending on the case report. A retrospective analysis of reported cases suggested that the combination of amphotericin B, flucytosine, and itraconazole may be associated with improved survival, though it was not frequently used. Complete excision of brain abscesses seemed to have better outcomes than aspiration or partial excision. Outcomes were poor, with an overall mortality exceeding 70%.

The newer azoles (voriconazole and the investigational posaconazole) were not used in the case series mentioned. More recent reports, however, have used both agents. Voriconazole was unsuccessful in treating three cases of *C bantiana* brain abscess, though two of these patients were immunocompromised [56–58]. Clinical improvement, however, was seen in one of the severely immunosuppressed patients while receiving voriconazole, despite later succumbing to the infection [58]. In a more recent report, voriconazole alone was successful in a case of *C bantiana* brain abscess in an immunocompetent patient [59]. Posaconazole has been reported effective in a case of *R mackenzei* brain abscess, which represents the first reported survival of infection caused by this species [60]. In addition, use of lipid formulations of amphotericin B may allow for better efficacy by administration of much higher doses than possible with standard amphotericin B, though this has not been systematically studied for these infections [61].

Disseminated infection

This is the most uncommon manifestation of infection seen with dematiaceous fungi. In a recent review, most patients were immunocompromised, though occasional patients who had no known immunodeficiency or risk factors developed disseminated disease also [62]. In contrast to most invasive mold infections, blood cultures were positive in more than half of the cases. The most common isolate was *S prolificans*, accounting for more than a third of the cases. This species should be distinguished from *Scedosporium apiospermum* (teleomorph: *Pseudallescheria boydii*), which some experts do not consider truly dematiaceous and which has different antifungal susceptibilities.

The mortality rate was greater than 70% despite aggressive antifungal therapy. There were no antifungal regimens associated with improved survival in disseminated infection. Infection with *S prolificans* was associated with nearly 100% mortality in the absence of recovery from neutropenia, because it is generally resistant to all available antifungal agents. Recent case reports have suggested, however, that the combination of itraconazole or voriconazole with terbinafine may be synergistic against this species and may improve outcomes [24,63].

Other combinations or therapies have not been shown to be effective, though clinical experience is limited and is likely confined to anecdotal reports, given the rarity of this infection. More recently a case of disseminated *Exophiala spinifera* infection was treated successfully with posaconazole after failing itraconazole and amphotericin B [64].

Summary

Phaeohyphomycosis is an uncommon infection, but has become increasingly recognized in a wide variety of clinical syndromes. Many species are associated with human infection, though a few are responsible for most cases. Because these are typically soil organisms and common laboratory contaminants, they are often disregarded from clinical specimens as non-pathogenic. The clinical setting in which they are isolated, however, should always be carefully considered before making decisions regarding therapy. *Bipolaris* and *Curvularia* are often associated with allergic disease. Diagnosis depends on a high degree of clinical suspicion and appropriate pathologic and mycologic examination of clinical specimens. Therapy is evolving for many of the clinical syndromes described, and randomized clinical trials are unlikely given the sporadic nature of cases. Case reporting of successful and unsuccessful clinical experiences is important in attempting to better define optimal therapy for the more refractory infections. Itraconazole and voriconazole demonstrate the most consistent in vitro activity against this group of fungi. Itraconazole should be considered the drug of choice for most situations, given the greater clinical experience associated with its use for these infections. Given the lack of comparative clinical data, however, decisions over which azole to use in a particular setting are largely empiric. Much additional work is needed to better understand the pathogenic mechanisms underlying phaeohyphomycosis and to optimize therapy for these often refractory infections.

References

[1] McGinnis MR. Chromoblastomycosis and phaeohyphomycosis: new concepts, diagnosis, and mycology. J Am Acad Dermatol 1983;8:1–16.
[2] Rinaldi MG. Phaeohyphomycosis. Dermatol Clin 1996;14:147–53.
[3] Matsumoto T, Ajello L, Matsuda T, et al. Developments in hyalohyphomycosis and phaeohyphomycosis. J Med Vet Mycol 1994;32(Suppl 1):329–49.
[4] Padhye AA, Bennett JE, McGinnis MR, et al. Biosafety considerations in handling medically important fungi. Med Mycol 1998;36(Suppl 1):258–65.
[5] Jacobson ES. Pathogenic roles for fungal melanins. Clin Microbiol Rev 2000;13:708–17.
[6] Butler MJ, Day AW. Fungal melanins: a review. Can J Microbiol 1998;44:1115–36.

[7] Hamilton AJ, Gomez BL. Melanins in fungal pathogens. J Med Microbiol 2002;51:
    189–91.
[8] Dixon DM, Polak A, Szaniszlo PJ. Pathogenicity and virulence of wild-type and melanin-
    deficient Wangiella dermatitidis. J Med Vet Mycol 1987;25:97–106.
[9] Kwon-Chung KJ, Polacheck I, Popkin TJ. Melanin-lacking mutants of *Cryptococcus neofor-*
    mans and their virulence for mice. J Bacteriol 1982;150:1414–21.
[10] van Duin D, Casadevall A, Nosanchuk JD. Melanization of *Cryptococcus neoformans* and
     Histoplasma capsulatum reduces their susceptibilities to amphotericin B and caspofungin.
     Antimicrob Agents Chemother 2002;46:3394–400.
[11] Ikeda R, Sugita T, Jacobson ES, et al. Effects of melanin upon susceptibility of *Cryptococcus*
     to antifungals. Microbiol Immunol 2003;47:271–7.
[12] National Committee for Clinical Laboratory Standards. Reference method for broth
     dilution antifungal susceptibility testing of yeasts. Approved standard M27–A2. 2nd edition.
     Villanova, PA: National Committee for Clinical Laboratory Standards; 2002.
[13] National Committee for Clinical Laboratory Standards. Reference method for broth dilu-
     tion antifungal susceptibility testing of conidium-forming filamentous fungi. Approved
     M38-A. Wayne, PA: National Committee for Clinical Laboratory Standards; 2002.
[14] McGinnis MR, Pasarell L. In vitro testing of susceptibilities of filamentous ascomycetes to
     voriconazole, itraconazole, and amphotericin B, with consideration of phylogenetic implica-
     tions. J Clin Microbiol 1998;36:2353–5.
[15] Meletiadis J, Meis JF, Mouton JW, et al. In vitro activities of new and conventional antifun-
     gal agents against clinical *Scedosporium* isolates. Antimicrob Agents Chemother 2002;46:
     62–8.
[16] Espinel-Ingroff A, Boyle K, Sheehan DJ. In vitro antifungal activities of voriconazole and
     reference agents as determined by NCCLS methods: review of the literature. Mycopatholo-
     gia 2001;150:101–15.
[17] McGinnis MR, Pasarell L. In vitro evaluation of terbinafine and itraconazole against dema-
     tiaceous fungi. Med Mycol 1998;36:243–6.
[18] Espinel-Ingroff A. In vitro fungicidal activities of voriconazole, itraconazole, and amphoter-
     icin B against opportunistic moniliaceous and dematiaceous fungi. J Clin Microbiol 2001;39:
     954–8.
[19] Hosseini-Yeganeh M, McLachlan AJ. Physiologically based pharmacokinetic model for ter-
     binafine in rats and humans. Antimicrob Agents Chemother 2002;46:2219–28.
[20] Ryder NS, Frank I. Interaction of terbinafine with human serum and serum proteins. J Med
     Vet Mycol 1992;30:451–60.
[21] Deresinski SC, Stevens DA. Caspofungin. Clin Infect Dis 2003;36:1445–57.
[22] Espinel-Ingroff A. In vitro antifungal activities of anidulafungin and micafungin, licensed
     agents and the investigational triazole posaconazole as determined by NCCLS methods
     for 12,052 fungal isolates: review of the literature. Rev Iberoam Micol 2003;20:121–36.
[23] Vermes A, Guchelaar HJ, Dankert J. Flucytosine: a review of its pharmacology, clinical in-
     dications, pharmacokinetics, toxicity and drug interactions. J Antimicrob Chemother 2000;
     46:171–9.
[24] Meletiadis J, Mouton JW, Rodriguez-Tudela JL, et al. In vitro interaction of terbinafine with
     itraconazole against clinical isolates of *Scedosporium prolificans*. Antimicrob Agents Chemo-
     ther 2000;44:470–2.
[25] Meletiadis J, Mouton JW, Meis JF, et al. In vitro drug interaction modeling of combinations
     of azoles with terbinafine against clinical *Scedosporium prolificans* isolates. Antimicrob
     Agents Chemother 2003;47:106–17.
[26] Steinbach WJ, Schell WA, Miller JL, et al. *Scedosporium prolificans* osteomyelitis in an im-
     munocompetent child treated with voriconazole and caspofungin, as well as locally applied
     polyhexamethylene biguanide. J Clin Microbiol 2003;41:3981–5.
[27] Gupta AK, Ryder JE, Baran R, et al. Non-dermatophyte onychomycosis. Dermatol Clin
     2003;21:257–68.

[28] Tosti A, Piraccini BM, Lorenzi S, et al. Treatment of nondermatophyte mold and *Candida* onychomycosis. Dermatol Clin 2003;21:491–7.

[29] Kimura M, Goto A, Furuta T, et al. Multifocal subcutaneous phaeohyphomycosis caused by *Phialophora verrucosa*. Arch Pathol Lab Med 2003;127:91–3.

[30] Agarwal A, Singh SM. A case of cutaneous phaeohyphomycosis caused by *Exserohilum rostratum*, its in vitro sensitivity and review of literature. Mycopathologia 1995;131:9–12.

[31] Chuan MT, Wu MC. Subcutaneous phaeohyphomycosis caused by *Exophiala jeanselmei*: successful treatment with itraconazole. Int J Dermatol 1995;34:563–6.

[32] Koga T, Matsuda T, Matsumoto T, et al. Therapeutic approaches to subcutaneous mycoses. Am J Clin Dermatol 2003;4:537–43.

[33] Summerbell RC, Krajden S, Levine R, et al. Subcutaneous phaeohyphomycosis caused by Lasiodiplodia theobromae and successfully treated surgically. Med Mycol 2004;42:543–7.

[34] Studahl M, Backteman T, Stalhammar F, et al. Bone and joint infection after traumatic implantation of *Scedosporium prolificans* treated with voriconazole and surgery. Acta Paediatr 2003;92:980–2.

[35] Gopinathan U, Garg P, Fernandes M, et al. The epidemiological features and laboratory results of fungal keratitis: a 10-year review at a referral eye care center in South India. Cornea 2002;21:555–9.

[36] Srinivasan M. Fungal keratitis. Curr Opin Ophthalmol 2004;15:321–7.

[37] Garg P, Gopinathan U, Choudhary K, et al. Keratomycosis: clinical and microbiologic experience with dematiaceous fungi. Ophthalmology 2000;107:574–80.

[38] Chowdhary A, Singh K. Spectrum of fungal keratitis in North India. Cornea 2005;24:8–15.

[39] Wilhelmus KR, Jones DB. Curvularia keratitis. Trans Am Ophthalmol Soc 2001;99:111–30.

[40] Thomas PA. Fungal infections of the cornea. Eye 2003;17:852–62.

[41] Hernandez PC, Llinares TF, Burgos SJ, et al. Voriconazole in fungal keratitis caused by *Scedosporium apiospermum*. Ann Pharmacother 2004;38:414–7.

[42] Ferguson BJ. Definitions of fungal rhinosinusitis. Otolaryngol Clin N Am 2000;33:227–35.

[43] Schubert MS. Allergic fungal sinusitis: pathogenesis and management strategies. Drugs 2004;64:363–74.

[44] Houser SM, Corey JP. Allergic fungal rhinosinusitis: pathophysiology, epidemiology, and diagnosis. Otolaryngol Clin N Am 2000;33:399–409.

[45] Kuhn FA, Javer AR. Allergic fungal rhinosinusitis: perioperative management, prevention of recurrence, and role of steroids and antifungal agents. Otolaryngol Clin N Am 2000;33: 419–33.

[46] Greenberger PA. Allergic bronchopulmonary aspergillosis. J Allergy Clin Immunol 2002; 110:685–92.

[47] Venarske DL, deShazo RD. Sinobronchial allergic mycosis: the SAM syndrome. Chest 2002; 121:1670–6.

[48] Lake FR, Froudist JH, McAleer R, et al. Allergic bronchopulmonary fungal disease caused by Bipolaris and Curvularia. Aust N Z J Med 1991;21:871–4.

[49] Wark PAB, Gibson PG. Allergic bronchopulmonary aspergillosis: new concepts of pathogenesis and treatment. Respirology 2001;6:1–7.

[50] Burns KE, Ohori NP, Iacono AT. *Dactylaria gallopava* infection presenting as a pulmonary nodule in a single-lung transplant recipient. J Heart Lung Transplant 2000;19:900–2.

[51] Odell JA, Alvarez S, Cvitkovich DG, et al. Multiple lung abscesses due to *Ochroconis gallopavum*, a dematiaceous fungus, in a nonimmunocompromised wood pulp worker. Chest 2000;118:1503–5.

[52] Tamm M, Malouf M, Glanville A. Pulmonary *Scedosporium* infection following lung transplantation. Transpl Infect Dis 2001;3:189–94.

[53] Mazur JE, Judson MA. A case report of a *Dactylaria* fungal infection in a lung transplant patient. Chest 2001;119:651–3.

[54] Carter E, Boudreaux C. Fatal cerebral phaeohyphomycosis due to *Curvularia lunata* in an immunocompetent patient. J Clin Microbiol 2004;42:5419–23.

[55] Revankar SG, Sutton DA, Rinaldi MG. Primary central nervous system phaeohyphomycosis: a review of 101 cases. Clin Infect Dis 2004;38:206–16.

[56] Levin TP, Baty DE, Fekete T, et al. *Cladophialophora bantiana* brain abscess in a solid-organ transplant recipient: case report and review of the literature. J Clin Microbiol 2004;42: 4374–8.

[57] Fica A, Diaz MC, Luppi M, et al. Unsuccessful treatment with voriconazole of a brain abscess due to *Cladophialophora bantiana*. Scand J Infect Dis 2003;35:892–3.

[58] Trinh JV, Steinbach WJ, Schell WA, et al. Cerebral phaeohyphomycosis in an immunodeficient child treated medically with combination antifungal therapy. Med Mycol 2003;41: 339–45.

[59] Lyons MK, Blair JE, Leslie KO. Successful treatment with voriconazole of fungal cerebral abscess due to *Cladophialophora bantiana*. Clin Neurol Neurosurg 2005;107:53–4.

[60] Al Abdely HM, Alkhunaizi AM, Al Tawfiq JA, et al. Successful therapy of cerebral phaeohyphomycosis due to *Ramichloridium mackenzei* with the new triazole posaconazole. Med Mycol 2005;43:91–5.

[61] Walsh TJ, Goodman JL, Pappas P, et al. Safety, tolerance, and pharmacokinetics of high-dose liposomal amphotericin B (AmBisome) in patients infected with *Aspergillus* species and other filamentous fungi: maximum tolerated dose study. Antimicrob Agents Chemother 2001;45(12):3487–96.

[62] Revankar SG, Patterson JE, Sutton DA, et al. Disseminated phaeohyphomycosis: review of an emerging mycosis. Clin Infect Dis 2002;34:467–76.

[63] Howden BP, Slavin MA, Schwarer AP, et al. Successful control of disseminated *Scedosporium prolificans* infection with a combination of voriconazole and terbinafine. Eur J Clin Microbiol Infect Dis 2003;22:111–3.

[64] Negroni R, Helou SH, Petri N, et al. Case study: posaconazole treatment of disseminated phaeohyphomycosis due to *Exophiala spinifera*. Clin Infect Dis 2004;38:e15–20.

INFECTIOUS DISEASE CLINICS OF NORTH AMERICA

Infect Dis Clin N Am
20 (2006) 621–643

Coccidioidomycosis

Gregory M. Anstead, MD, PhD[a,b,*],
John R. Graybill, MD[a]

[a]*Department of Medicine, Division of Infectious Diseases, University of Texas Health Science
Center at San Antonio, 7703 Floyd Curl Drive, San Antonio, TX 78229, USA*
[b]*Research Service, South Texas Veterans Healthcare System, 7400 Merton Minter Boulevard,
San Antonio, TX 78229, USA*

Coccidioidomycosis is an infection caused by inhalation of arthroconidia of dimorphic fungi of the genus *Coccidioides*. This genus has recently been divided on the basis of genomic analyses into two species, *C immitis* (isolates from California) and *C posadasii* (isolates from outside California). There is no obvious difference in the disease states produced by these two species [1]. These soil-dwelling fungi have an endemic range that encompasses semiarid to arid life zones, principally in the southwestern United States and northern Mexico [2]. *Coccidioides* also is found in parts of Argentina, Brazil Columbia, Guatemala, Honduras, Nicaragua, Paraguay, and Venezuela [3]. Hyperendemic areas include Kern, Tulare, and Fresno counties in the San Joaquin Valley of California and Pima, Pinal, and Maricopa counties in Arizona. Major cities within these hyperendemic areas include Bakersfield, California, and Phoenix and Tucson, Arizona [4]. There are approximately 150,00 infections per year in the United States [5].

The ecology of *Coccidioides*

There is a relationship between climatic conditions and the incidence of coccidioidomycosis. A period of moisture is required for the hyphae to grow in the soil. During a subsequent dry period the hyphae die, leaving viable arthroconidia (spores). The arthroconidia may be dispersed by natural forces (wind, earthquakes) or by anthropogenic disturbance of the soil [6].

* Corresponding author. Department of Medicine, Division of Infectious Diseases, University of Texas Health Science Center at San Antonio, 7703 Floyd Curl Drive, San Antonio, TX 78229.
E-mail address: anstead@uthscsa.edu (G.M. Anstead).

0891-5520/06/$ - see front matter © 2006 Elsevier Inc. All rights reserved.
doi:10.1016/j.idc.2006.06.005   *id.theclinics.com*

Persons at risk

Residence in or travel to these endemic areas is a risk factor for becoming infected with this fungus and provides an important clue to the diagnosis [7]. Persons with occupations that have soil exposure, such as agricultural workers, excavators, military personnel, and archeologists, are at the greatest risk of acquiring coccidioidomycosis [3,8]. Immunocompromised persons are also at high risk, including patients who have AIDS [9], transplant recipients (especially those who received *Coccidioides*-infected organs) [10], patients treated with tumor necrosis factor-α antagonists [11]; pregnant women (especially in the third trimester) [12], and patients who have cancer [13]. Certain ethnic groups are also at high risk of suffering disseminated disease. Persons of Filipino or African American descent have a 10- to 175-fold higher risk for dissemination [3]. Persons with blood group B are also at risk for more severe disease [14].

Epidemics

Outbreaks of coccidioidomycosis may follow natural events that result in atmospheric soil dispersion, such as dust storms, earthquakes, and droughts [15–17]. Notable events include a dust storm in the San Joaquin Valley in 1977 and the Northridge, California, earthquake in 1994 [16,17]. A large epidemic occurred in California between 1991 and 1993, during which the incidence of coccidioidomycosis increased to as much as 10 times the usual rate. Factors responsible for the epidemic were (1) a drought, which was followed by abundant rainfall; (2) new building construction, which resulted in soil disruption; and (3) an influx of susceptible individuals into the area [18]. An epidemic in Arizona from 1998 to 2001 involved 7599 persons; the disease was most common during periods of hot, dry weather [4].

Common-source outbreaks can occur among persons who participate in an activity that disrupts the soil, such as an archaeological dig. Often those affected are not from the endemic area and thus have no prior immunity. Also, these patients may have extensive pulmonary infiltrates because of the intense exposure to the fungus in a confined area [19].

Pathogenesis

Arthroconidia are inhaled, ingested by pulmonary macrophages, and convert to a round cell that enlarges over 3 or more days to become a spherule. The spherule (8–30 μm in diameter) has thick outer walls and contains hundreds of asexual endospores. This spherule ruptures, dispersing the endospores, thereby initiating the endospore-spherule cycle. The endospores may disseminate hematogenously to meninges, bones, skin, or other soft tissues. Host control of coccidioidomycosis depends on competent cell-mediated immunity [20].

Diagnosis

Culture

The diagnosis of coccidioidomycosis is based on clinical suspicion supported by microbiologic, histopathologic, or serologic evidence. Culture is the most definitive method for making a diagnosis [21]. In nature *Coccidioides* forms fragile mycelia that are very liable to disruption and dispersion by air currents. It grows readily (in about 5–7 days) on many culture media. The mycelia are formed by barrel-shaped arthroconidia (1–4 × 5–6 μm) with intercalated "ghost" cells. This morphology is characteristic of *Coccidioides* but is not unique. A single arthroconidium may be sufficient to cause disease if inhaled, so this organism should be given great respect in the laboratory. All mycelial organisms should be handled only in a laminar flow hood. Confirmation of identify can be made in vitro by conversion into the spherule form using Converse medium at 39°C. Spherules, in vitro or in tissue, are 20 to 150 μm in diameter, have double walls, and are filled with endospores.

Histopathologic findings

Coccidioides in the host forms a large spherule, readily seen on hematoxylin-eosin, periodic acid-Schiff, or Gomori's methenamine silver staining (Fig. 1). The main distinguishing feature of *Coccidioides* spherules is the presence of endospores. There are a few fungi or funguslike organisms that may superficially resemble spherules. These include *Rhinosporidium seeberi*, *Prototheca wickerham*, and *Chrysosporium parvum*. Should there be any ambiguity in the histopathologic appearance, specific antibody staining is available at the Centers for Disease Control and Prevention. Histopathologic findings of lesions may vary, from abscesses with many spherules, endospores, and neutrophils (in immunocompromised patients and in uncontrolled disease) to

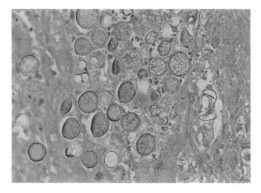

Fig. 1. Spherules of *Coccidioides posadasii* showing internal endospores in tissue specimen (Gomori's methenamine silver-hematoxylin-eosin, ×100).

well-formed granulomas with very few organisms seen within the lesion (in patients who have competent cell-mediated immunity).

Immunologic methods

Coccidioidin and spherulin skin tests are no longer available. Traditional immunologic methods have involved complement fixation and immunodiffusion using the complement-fixing antigen (IDCF) [22,23]. Tests for precipitin antibody (IgM) become positive within the first few weeks of infection and clear within a month or two. Tests for IgG require several months to convert to positive but remain positive for years. The tests can be run more simply using immunodiffusion with the tube precipitin (IgM) or complement-fixing (IgG) antigens. With these tests a distinct pattern of antibody responses has been documented (Table 1). Traditionally, a serum complement fixation titer of 1:16 or higher was associated with worsening or disseminated disease [24]. Serologic titers tend to be higher in osteoarticular than in soft tissue or chronic pulmonary disease [25]. Most patients who have active coccidioidomycosis will have a positive antibody titer. Although older literature suggests that antibody titers wane with clinical resolution of disease, treatment trials done by the Mycoses Study Group have found serum titers to be insensitive to the course of disease, even when followed over several years [25]. Indeed, some consideration has been given to removing the serologic titer from the scoring system, because it changes so little during therapy. Any positive titer in the cerebrospinal fluid (CSF) confirms a diagnosis of coccidioidal meningitis, except when the approach of the lumbar puncture is through infected paraspinous tissue or a lumbar puncture is contaminated by CSF containing peripheral blood [26,27]. In coccidioidal meningitis, the CSF IgG titer is positive (in titers of 1:2 or more) more than 75% of the time, whereas cultures of CSF are positive in less than 50% of patients [28]. The CSF serologic titer declines more slowly than the severity of symptoms and the CSF leukocyte count but ultimately became undetectable in most patients receiving chronic fluconazole therapy [29].

More recently, the ELISA for coccidioidal IgG and IgM antibodies has been used increasingly [30]. The optical density by ELISA correlates reasonably well with the titer of the IDCF test [31]. The correlation is looser at higher titers, however. Recently, Crum and coworkers [3] evaluated the

Table 1
Serologic methods for detecting *Coccidioides* infection

Method	IgM	IgG	Utilization in 2006
Tube precipitin	Yes	No	No
Immunodiffusion tube precipitin	Yes	No	Yes
Complement fixation	No	Yes	Rarely
Immunodiffusion complement fixation	No	Yes	Yes
ELISA	Yes	Yes	Yes

characteristics of an ELISA for the diagnosis of coccidioidomycosis. The overall characteristics of the ELISA were 100% sensitivity, 99% specificity, a positive predictive value of 82%, and a negative predictive value of 100%. Early in the course of the disease, however, the ELISA can be falsely negative; false positives can occur also.

Serologic testing for coccidioidomycosis is hampered by serologic cross-reactivity with *Histoplasma capsulatum* and *Paracoccidioides braziliensis* [32]. Antigen testing, which is so useful for the diagnosis of histoplasmosis and cryptococcosis, is not currently available for coccidioidomycosis. An assay based on the polymerase chain reaction is in development and may have future application [33].

Clinical presentation and recommended treatment

In vitro susceptibility testing

Coccidioides exists in nature as a mycelial form with arthroconidia and in humans as the spherule form. Although spherules can be generated in vitro using Converse medium at 39°C, this is not commonly done, and the arthroconidia are used for in vitro susceptibility testing. The Clinical Laboratory Sciences Institute methods for testing mycelial fungi have been used [34]. In vitro, *Coccidioides* is susceptible to most antifungal agents, including amphotericin B, azoles, and the echinocandins [35]. In no other mycosis, however, is the discordance between in vitro susceptibility and clinical response as dramatic as with coccidioidomycosis. Therefore, although one may assume that *Coccidioides* is susceptible to most antifungal drugs in vitro, it is only through clinical experience that one gains an understanding of the strengths and limitations of the available drugs against this formidable fungal pathogen.

Clinical presentation and treatment

Evidence-based guidelines for the treatment of coccidioidomycosis are more limited than for other endemic mycoses; in fact, there has been only one single controlled, prospective trial, of fluconazole versus itraconazole [36]. In the 2005 Infectious Disease Society of America (IDSA) guidelines, treatment decisions are often the strongly recommended "A" level but are based on relatively weak evidence, at the "II or III" level (ie, few randomized, prospective trials) [5]. Recently, an expert review of coccidioidal meningitis was, by necessity, largely focused on clinical experience, because of the paucity of clinical trial data [37].

Primary infection

Primary coccidioidomycosis is a pulmonary infection in which as many as 60% of subjects are asymptomatic [38,39]. Persons who received heavy exposure to arthroconidia have a higher incidence of clinically apparent primary disease. In one example, 103 nonresidents of an endemic zone were heavily exposed at an archeological site [40]. Of the 94 persons who completed a survey, 61 developed an illness compatible with primary coccidioidomycosis. Of these, 27 were confirmed with positive serology or skin tests. No patients received treatment, and all resolved their disease spontaneously. Symptomatic primary pulmonary infection typically resembles community-acquired pneumonia or influenza. The illness begins 1 to 3 weeks after inhalation of arthroconidia and presents with fever, cough, and pulmonary infiltrates [38]. The usual course is resolution over several weeks. More than 95% of patients who have symptomatic primary coccidioidomycosis recover spontaneously without further sequelae [2,5]. Several aspects of primary coccidioidomycosis merit special consideration, however:

1. Rheumatologic syndromes: Rheumatologic syndromes are manifestations of hypersensitivity and include erythema nodosum, erythema multiforme, polyarthralgia, and polyarthritis; antifungal therapy is not required [39].
2. Pleural effusions: In one series of 28 patients published in the pre-azole era (1976), cultures were positive in all of 18 pleural biopsies [41]. Most patients recovered without receiving antifungal therapy, but two suffered disseminated disease and succumbed within 3 days. Three others received amphotericin B. The authors concluded that uncomplicated pleural effusion did not warrant antifungal therapy, but this study was published before azoles were available. At present, azole therapy would seem appropriate, given that fungi are recoverable from pleural biopsies, and a few patients had life-threatening disease.
3. Immunosuppression: Primary coccidioidomycosis may develop into progressive disease and dissemination in persons who have mild or severe immunosuppression. These conditions include pregnancy and the immunosuppression associated with solid-organ transplantation, diabetes, end-stage liver disease, receipt of systemic steroids, or HIV infection [2,9,12,42–52]. These patients warrant aggressive antifungal therapy. Initial reports of coccidioidomycosis in the setting of AIDS were associated with poor responses to antifungal therapy [48]. More recently, with the widespread use of highly active antiretroviral therapy, coccidioidomycosis has been easier to tame, although it still can be a formidable adversary. When AIDS patients' CD4 cell count is brought above 250 cells/μL by highly active antiretroviral therapy, and the fungal disease is quiescent, antifungal therapy may be discontinued, as recommended for histoplasmosis and cryptococcosis [47].
4. Pregnancy: The third trimester of pregnancy has been associated with severe coccidioidomycosis, premature delivery, and spontaneous abortion [12,53–55].
5. Race. For unclear reasons, Filipinos and African Americans are much more likely than whites to develop persistent, progressive, and disseminated disease [56,57]. At present, there is no recommendation to treat all

African Americans who have primary coccidioidomycosis, but they should be followed carefully.

There has been interest in whether the course of primary coccidioidomycosis, which accounts for substantial loss of work time as well as a risk of progression, can be shortened by antifungal therapy. To date, there has not been a prospective, randomized, placebo-controlled trial in primary coccidioidomycosis. In the absence of clinical trial data, some physicians may elect to observe patients who have relatively mild disease, but others may initiate a course of fluconazole. Patients who have diffuse pneumonia are more likely to progress to chronic disease or death and should be treated. High-dose fluconazole or amphotericin B has been recommended in the 2005 IDSA guidelines [5]. The dose and duration of therapy are undefined.

Outcomes of primary infection

The outcomes of primary coccidioidomycosis include uneventful healing, coccidioma, progressive or persistent pneumonia, chronic pulmonary coccidioidomycosis, disseminated coccidioidomycosis, osteoarticular disease, and central nervous system involvement.

Uneventful healing

Uneventful healing with resolution of pulmonary infiltrates is the usual outcome, and many of these infections are not diagnosed during the course of illness.

Coccidioima

Coccidioima follows the contraction of pulmonary infiltrates into a mass that is asymptomatic and may persist for years. It is usually diagnosed inadvertently at surgery directed at potential lung cancer. In the immunocompetent patient there is no need for antifungal therapy [5].

Progressive or persistent pneumonia

In its most acute form, progressive pneumonia manifests as diffuse pulmonary disease or military disease [58]. Acute respiratory failure may occur in immunosuppressed persons or persons with heavy inoculum exposures (Fig. 2) [59]. In this situation, amphotericin B would be recommended. Recently, two patients who had fulminant coccidioidomycosis with septic shock were treated successfully with drotrecogin alfa in addition to antifungal therapy [60]. Persistent pneumonia is defined as lasting more than 2 months and manifests as extensive infiltrates, sometimes with cavitation (Fig. 3) [61]. Amphotericin B may be the initial choice if the patient is severely ill. Recent IDSA guidelines suggest 3 to 6 months for the duration of antifungal therapy [5], but the authors favor treatment for more than 6 months after resolution of symptoms and for more than a year for diffuse miliary disease. Conversion to an oral azole is appropriate when the patient is improving.

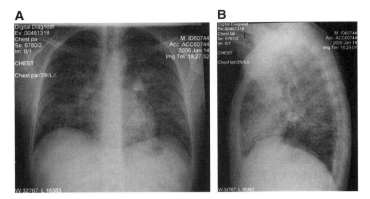

Fig. 2. Chest radiographs. (*A*) Posteroanterior and (*B*) lateral views showing diffuse bilateral pulmonary infiltrates in a patient who has coccidioidomycosis. This patient was a 42-year-old undocumented Mexican immigrant who had AIDS and a CD4 cell count of 25 cells/μL. The patient had stopped taking fluconazole and highly active antiretroviral therapy. He died of respiratory failure 1 week after this radiograph was obtained.

Termination of therapy should be followed by years of close observation, given the unpleasant propensity of coccidioidomycosis to relapse [25,62,63]. Oldfield and colleagues [64] have suggested that relapse can be anticipated in patients who have complement fixation antibody titers of 1:256 or higher (relative risk 4.7) [64].

Chronic pulmonary coccidioidomycosis

Chronic pulmonary coccidioidomycosis occurs in about 5% of patients who have symptomatic primary coccidioidomycosis and often is a smoldering process, waxing and waning over years. Nodular lesions may cavitate, with surrounding infiltrates and fibrosis. Cavitary disease may be asymptomatic or be associated with rupture and pneumothorax, hemorrhage, or

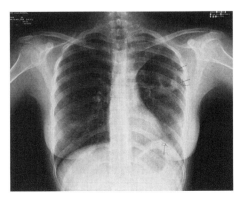

Fig. 3. Chest radiograph (posteroanterior view) showing cavitary lesions in a patient who has pulmonary coccidioidomycosis.

secondary infection. Cavities smaller than 2.5 cm in diameter tend to resolve spontaneously over a year, but cavities larger than 5 cm persist. A study from 1958 recommended surgical resection of these large cavities and of secondarily infected cavities, empyema, ruptured cavities, and bronchopleural fistula [41]. This series is remarkable in that it summarized 400 patients before the era of antifungal therapy. These cases had a postoperative complication rate of 13%, with a mortality rate of 1.7% over a variable time of follow-up. Complications included persistent cavities, recurrent cavities, and empyema, with and without bronchopleurocutaneous fistula. In a report from the early years of amphotericin B, Grant and Melick [65] noted that the postoperative complication rate fell from 20% of 44 cases without amphotericin B to 4% of 48 cases with perioperative amphotericin B.

Cavities may remain stable for years, may become secondarily infected with *Aspergillus* with subsequent fungus ball formation, or may wax and wane with intermittent infiltrates and fibrocavitary disease. Hemorrhage may occur from secondarily infected cavities. Chronic pulmonary coccidioidomycosis may destroy the lungs progressively and should be treated medically. The duration of therapy is unclear, but in general for coccidioidomycosis "longer is better," which may be more than a year [5]. Fluconazole and itraconazole are the standard drugs [25,63], but posaconazole or voriconazole probably will be more effective. There have been recommendations to follow the serologic titers of the IDCF test, because these decline during successful therapy. In the Mycoses Study Group azole trials, however, there was little change of the titer during years of therapy, and thus it is not a key parameter for assessing response [25]. If there is structural damage to the lung, surgical resection may be required [66]. After a period of observation over years, large asymptomatic cavities may be resected. Cavities that persist for more than 6 months rarely close and should be resected [67]. Rarely, coccidioidal mycetoma may occur in preexisting cavities and is treated by resection [68].

Disseminated coccidioidomycosis

Disseminated coccidioidomycosis may occur locally or hematogenously. Local dissemination may produce pleural and pericardial invasion [69–71]. Hematogenous dissemination occurs within a few months after infection and manifests as a single chronic remote focus or widespread multiorgan involvement [49]. In its disseminated form, coccidioidomycosis may involve nearly any organ of the body; the most common sites of involvement are the lungs, skin and soft tissue, bones, joints, and meninges. Other reported sites include the liver and spleen, peritoneum, pericardium, prostate, epididymus, urethra, and female genital tract. In contrast to histoplasmosis and tuberculosis, in coccidioidomycosis the gastrointestinal tract is usually spared. Ocular disease is also rare. Pregnancy, particularly the third trimester, is also risk factor for disseminated disease. Some patients who have uncommon manifestations of coccidioidomycosis, such as acute coccidioidal pericarditis, may be misdiagnosed as having tuberculosis and treated with corticosteroids [72]. The authors have had similar experiences with patients misdiagnosed as having "aseptic" meningitis and treated with corticosteroids [73]. This distinction is important because the level of the host immune response is critical in determining the outcome of coccidioidomycosis. Chronic involvement is seen commonly with isolated skin, bone, or joint lesions, although almost any tissue can be involved. Skin lesions may take the form of papules, nodules, abscesses, verrucous plaques, or ulcers (Fig. 4) [3]. Biopsies often show variable levels of granuloma formation, with occasional organisms usually well contained within the granuloma. These lesions may worsen spontaneously, improve over months to years, or remain stable for long periods of time. Widespread dissemination is associated with poor granuloma formation and with purulent abscesses packed with neutrophils and abundant spherules and endospores. Cutaneous abscesses, paraspinous abscesses, necrotic lymph nodes, diffuse vertebral osteomyelitis, and often-draining sinus tracts may be present (Fig. 5). Soft tissue involvement may also include the omentum and peritoneum [74–76]. Medical therapy often is combined with surgical therapy to debulk lesions.

In chronic forms of coccidioidomycosis, azoles are the first line of therapy. Fluconazole at 400 or 800 mg/d or itraconazole at 200 mg two times per day may be used [25,63]. The treatment of the unfortunate patients who have chronic coccidioidomycosis can be most challenging, and death may ensue despite heroic efforts at medical and surgical intervention.

Osteoarticular disease

Although any bone and joint may be targeted, the weight-bearing joints and bones are more vulnerable. Vertebral disease is of particular concern because the process can destroy the vertebral body, with collapse and joint instability. Treatment for vertebral disease should include debulking paraspinous abscesses and, if the spine is unstable, surgery to stabilize the

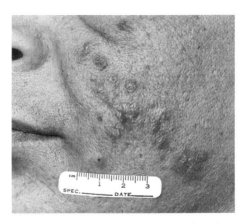

Fig. 4. Papular skin lesions in a patient who has disseminated coccidioidomycosis.

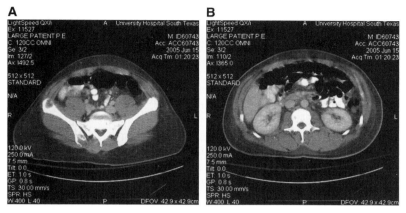

Fig. 5. CT of abdomen in a patient who has disseminated coccidioidomycosis. (*A*) Multiple lytic lesions are visible in lumbar spine. (*B*) Lytic lesions of right iliac bone with extension into adjacent paraspinous tissue. This patient is a 31 year-old African American man who presented with severe back pain and in respiratory distress. He had diffuse bilateral pulmonary infiltrates and extensive bony and paraspinous soft tissue involvement. He had innumerable lytic lesions throughout the lumbar spine and pelvis, left eleventh rib involvement, and fluid collections in the right paraspinous, right psoas, and left piriformis muscles. This patient went into respiratory failure, requiring mechanical ventilation for 3 weeks. He did not respond to amphotericin B therapy and improved on posaconazole. At the time of this writing, he has remained on posaconazole maintenance therapy for 8 months without relapse.

involved joints [77,78]. Medical therapy alone is considered inadequate for vertebral disease with unstable articulations.

Central nervous system involvement

Disseminated coccidioidomycosis in the central nervous system manifests as meningitis with granuloma formation or coccidioima. In general, basilar meningeal reaction causes chronic inflammation and progressive resistance to resorption of CSF that manifests as either obstructive or communicating hydrocephalus [79]. With current azole-based regimens, lifetime medical treatment is indicated for coccidioidal meningitis [73]. Fluconazole has received the greatest attention in the treatment of coccidioidal meningitis [29,80]. At present, most clinicians are using doses of 800 mg/d or higher [37]. There have been a few reports of success with voriconazole [81,82]. Itraconazole, despite some early successes, was not pursued, because of irregular oral absorption [83]. Obstructive hydrocephalus requires ventriculoperitoneal shunting.

Selection of antifungal agents

Amphotericin B

For primary disease amphotericin B has been administered to a total dose of 500 to 1000 mg over 2 to 4 weeks [84]. Clinical responses vary from complete resolution to undetectable change, and later relapse is common. Total courses of 2 to 4 g have been used, with dose ranges of more than 35 mg/kg [84]. Overall, it is likely that 50% to 70% of patients who have nonmeningeal disease respond well to amphotericin B.

Coccidioidal meningitis is lethal if untreated, with virtually all patients dead within 2 years [85]. Coccidioidal meningitis may produce vasculitis and infarction or communicating or obstructive hydrocephalus [86,87]. One method for treatment of coccidioidal meningitis before the advent of fluconazole was intrathecal amphotericin B, in which the drug was instilled into the CSF, directly or through an Ommaya reservoir [88]. The outlet of the reservoir typically was placed in the lateral ventricle or, occasionally, in the fourth ventricle. Lateral cervical punctures have also used to deliver amphotericin B. Finally, amphotericin B has been mixed with hyperbaric glucose and administered by the lumbar route, with the patient placed in a head-down position to facilitate delivery of the solution to the basilar meninges [89]. The regimen typically was initiated at 0.05 mg three times weekly and was gradually increased to 5 mg/dose [90]. As CSF pleocytosis and serologic titers wane, the dose is decreased gradually, to terminate over 2 to 8 years. Intrathecal amphotericin B may cause arachnoiditis, vasculitis, and infarctions. Dexamethasone is used for the treatment of vasculitis or infarction [37]. Accordingly, intrathecal amphotericin B is commonly administered with 20 mg methylprednisolone [26,88].

The use of Ommaya reservoirs may be complicated by bacterial shunt infections [91]. With this difficult regimen, 50% to 60% of patients could be weaned eventually from amphotericin B [26,88]. In authors' opinion, the place of amphotericin B therapy today in the treatment of coccidioidomycosis is largely as a salvage drug and as the drug of choice for pregnant patients because of the potential teratogenicity of azoles.

Azole antifungal drugs

Azoles are currently the preferred agents for the treatment of most forms of coccidioidomycosis [5,92]. Clinical experience has been acquired with each of these drugs, with responses documented for each. There are vast differences in tolerance, efficacy, and amount of clinical experience with each agent. Coccidioidomycosis may present as a multifocal disease, involving multiple skin, bone, soft tissue, and pulmonary sites; some of these lesions, but not necessarily all, may respond to amphotericin B. In the era of amphotericin B, quantifying the patient response often was a problematic task. This problem in total patient assessment led members of the Mycoses Study Group to propose a multicomponent scoring system for patients who have nonmeningeal coccidioidomycosis (Box 1) [63]. Using this system, patients initially were scored according to culture-confirmed sites of disease (soft tissue, osteoarticular, or pulmonary), serologic titer, and extent of lesions. Later revisions allowed for scoring symptoms and signs and lesion size or

---

Box 1. Recent version of the coccidioidomycosis clinical scoring system

Determination of baseline score: baseline cumulative point count = 100%

1. Symptoms: 1 point each, no limit of points
2. Lesions: 2 points for each lesion at each site of disease (soft tissue, osteoarticular, pulmonary), no limit of points
3. Serology: 0 points for immunodiffusion complement fixation ≤ 1:2; 1 point for titer 1:4 or 1:8; 2 points if 1:16 or 1:32; 3 points if ≥ 1:64.
4. Cultures: 4 points for each site positive to a maximum of 12 points; if follow-up culture is not done, points carry over to next visit or end of therapy

Serial scoring: cumulative point score at each visit/baseline cumulative points = % response

A patient is a responder if

1. There is any reduction in score at 4 months
2. There is a 51% to 100% response at 8 months

Recrudescence is defined by a score under 50% that reverts back to higher than 50%.

More recently, authors have eliminated the culture scoring, because many invasive cultures were not done. Also, because serologic titers often did not change even with chronic therapy, and because the evaluation method changed to ELISA, some authors have eliminated the serology as well, retaining the score based on symptoms and signs [93].

Data from Catanzaro A, Galgiani JN, Levine BE, et al. Fluconazole in the treatment of chronic pulmonary and nonmeningeal disseminated coccidioidomycosis. Am J Med 1995;98:249–56.

---

severity. The sum of points pretreatment was the baseline score. A successful response was considered a reduction of the baseline score by 50% or more within a set period of time. Because coccidioidomycosis tends to improve relatively slowly, scoring was done at 3-month intervals. The scoring system, although far from ideal, allows physicians to estimate a total body burden of disease and follow that index.

Ketoconazole

Ketoconazole was the first azole studied against coccidioidomycosis. Because so many physicians wished to try anything other than amphotericin B, it was not possible to enroll patients in any comparative trial with an azole versus amphotericin B. Unfortunately, to this day, there are no systematic trials comparing azoles with amphotericin B. Ketoconazole absorption is maximized when taken with fatty food and an acidic beverage [94,95]. The initial trial with ketoconazole was a complicated dose-finding study that used a scoring system; only 20% to 30% of patients had a clinical response to 200–400 mg/d, and the regimen was continued 9 months after the patient was scored as a success (Table 2). Unfortunately, even with this extended period of treatment, 45% of patients relapsed. Higher doses of ketoconazole, up to 1200 mg/d, were explored in follow-up studies [98,100]. Gastrointestinal intolerance, testosterone and cortisol suppression, and frequent liver function abnormalities limit the highest tolerable dose of ketoconazole [101–103]. Thus, ketoconazole never became a clear drug of choice for the treatment of coccidioidomycosis.

Itraconazole

Itraconazole in the capsular form is best absorbed after a high-fat meal and when administered with an acidic beverage [104]. Itraconazole clearly was tolerated better than ketoconazole [103]. Initial trials found higher response rates and fewer relapses than with ketoconazole. Itraconazole, initially in capsules, 200 mg twice daily, and then in cyclodextrin solution, 100 to 200 mg twice daily, became the drug of choice for coccidioidomycosis [105]. Relapse rates after successful treatment courses were 15%, markedly less than with ketoconazole. Because responses were not 100%, there were several studies directed at raising the dose to 800 mg/d or more. At this dose, however, one encounters a syndrome of hypertension, hypokalemia, and edema [106]. The itraconazole solution has increased oral bioavailability (160% over the capsules), and the drug is maximally absorbed in the fasting state; however, it is somewhat unpalatable, and higher doses are not well

Table 2
Comparison of results in treatment studies of coccidioidomycosis, by dose of drugs

Drug	Dose	N	% response	Dose	N	% response	Dose	N	% response	% relapse as % successes off drug
Ketoconazole [96]	200	16	66	400	38	48	>400	20	50	58
Ketoconazole [97]	200	26	28	400	22	75	>400	4	Unknown	Unknown
Ketoconazole [98]	200	20	20	400	15	74	>400	2	50	Unknown
Ketoconazole [99]				400	21	57	>400	3	33	Unknown
Ketoconazole [100]				400	56	23	800	56	32	18
Itraconazole [25]	100	6	0	200	6	14	400	44	56	9
Itraconazole [36]							400	97	72[a]	18
Fluconazole [36]							400	94	57	28
Fluconazole [63]	200	73	60	400	41	64				37

[a] Itraconazole superior to fluconazole at 12 months of therapy ($P = .04$).

tolerated. Itraconazole was not detectable in the CSF after oral or intravenous administration. In a small series of 10 patients treated with itraconazole for coccidioidal meningitis, however, the response rate was 80% [83]. The results from this small series does not constitute a recommendation for using itraconazole to treat coccidioidal meningitis, but it does indicate that high penetration of itraconazole into the CSF is not necessarily required for successful therapy of coccidioidal meningitis.

Fluconazole

Fluconazole has different properties from itraconazole: it is easily administered intravenously, has high oral bioavailability, few drug interactions, and penetrates readily into most tissues. These characteristics quickly made fluconazole the drug of choice for coccidioidal meningitis [29]. Initial reports of 70% responses with doses of 400 mg/d were encouraging, but failures led to doses to as high as 2 g/d [37]. At present, most patients begin therapy for coccidioidal meningitis with 800 mg/d. This dosage may be decreased gradually over months, but fluconazole therapy for coccidioidal meningitis is lifelong. One small series found that as many as two thirds of patients treated for as long as 8 years had prompt relapses after discontinuation of therapy [73]. Fluconazole is also effective for nonmeningeal coccidioidomycosis. In a randomized trial comparing fluconazole with itraconazole, response rates were similar, 50% to 60% for both drugs. Patients who had osteoarticular diseases fared significantly better with itraconazole than with fluconazole, but the number of patients was limited (Table 3) [36]. At present, both fluconazole and itraconazole have been used for primary therapy of coccidioidomycosis. Treatment is often done with 400 mg/d of either drug, given for a year or longer after the patient achieves clinical success.

Voriconazole

Voriconazole has been used to treat coccidioidomycosis, but at present there have been very few reports. The authors have treated two patients with voriconazole, neither of whom had responded to multiple prior regimens. One patient had no clinical response to as much as 7 mg/kg twice

Table 3
Results after 12 months of therapy, itraconazole versus fluconazole

Drug	Pulmonary (N)	Pulmonary response (%)	Soft tissue (N)	Soft tissue response (%)	Osteoarticular (N)	Osteoarticular response (%)
Itraconazole	22/35	57	31/39	79	16/23	70
Fluconazole	22/35	63	22/32	69	10/27	37
P	NS		NS		0.03	

Data from Galgiani JN, Catanzaro A, Cloud GA, et al. Comparison of oral fluconazole and itraconazole for progressive, nonmeningeal coccidioidomycosis—a randomized, double-blind trial. Ann Intern Med 2000;133:676–86.

daily and ultimately succumbed to the inexorable progression of her disease [93]. The other patient, having not responded to amphotericin B, itraconazole, interferon gamma with itraconazole, and fluconazole, and with extensive involvement of her right lung and mediastinum, responded very well to voriconazole and became asymptomatic for more than a year. Unfortunately, more than a year after discontinuing voriconazole, she relapsed with a coccidioidal soft tissue abscess. She died from complications unrelated to coccidioidomycosis.

Posaconazole

Posaconazole is licensed in Europe for salvage therapy of coccidioidomycosis. Experience with posaconazole has been obtained for a larger number of patients than with voriconazole but is still very limited. In one unpublished early trial, 20 patients were treated with posaconazole, 400 mg/d for up to 6 months [107]. Unfortunately, the trial was terminated prematurely because of (later) unsubstantiated questions of drug toxicity. Nevertheless, 15 of 20 patients who completed more than 23 weeks of therapy responded, and none died from coccidioidomycosis. By 16 weeks of therapy the median score had been reduced to 40% of baseline; by 24 weeks, the median score was 22% of baseline. Of 10 patients who stopped therapy, 3 relapsed, and 7 had inactive disease. In another study, six patients, all of whom had severe refractory disease, were treated with posaconazole, 200 mg four times per day; all these patients initially responded, and five maintained a response [93].

Echinocandins

Caspofungin is the only echinocandin that has been evaluated in coccidioidomycosis. In vitro, the mycelial form is highly resistant to caspofungin at the traditional minimal inhibitory concentration, but C immitis is quite susceptible to caspofungin at the minimum effective concentration (the lowest concentration needed to produce abnormal hyphal growth). There is not a broad range of susceptibility among isolates. Mice infected with C immitis respond well to caspofungin, suggesting that it has clinical potential [35]. There has been almost no published experience with patients treated with caspofungin [108]. Caspofungin is a costly intravenous drug, and coccidioidomycosis is a disease that requires treatment for many months. The authors' experience has been with very few patients treated for periods of weeks, not months. Thus, they are unable to assess the contribution of caspofungin to patient outcome.

Interferon gamma

There are only two reports on the use of interferon gamma as an adjunct in the treatment of coccidioidomycosis [109]. In one report, a patient who had persistent ventilator dependency despite treatment with amphotericin B lipid complex recovered when given interferon gamma at 50 $\mu g/m^2$ three times per week for 9 weeks. The authors have treated two patients with interferon gamma for refractory coccidioidomycosis. One unsuccessful use of interferon gamma was reported by Anstead and colleagues [93]. Another patient who had not responded to itraconazole, amphotericin B, lipid amphotericin B formulations, and fluconazole was stable for some months on a regimen of interferon gamma added to itraconazole. When the interferon gamma was discontinued, her disease again slowly progressed. She ultimately responded to voriconazole, and it was not clear whether interferon gamma had an impact on her outcome. There is a tremendous selection bias, because failures are unlikely to be reported, and thus it is difficult to know whether interferon gamma has a role in the treatment of refractory coccidioidomycosis.

Considerations in pregnancy

The course of coccidioidomycosis in the first two trimesters of pregnancy is thought to follow the same path as in nonpregnant women. The third trimester of pregnancy, however, is a time of high risk for dissemination and, rarely, placental transmission to the fetus. If a woman presents with a history of prior coccidioidomycosis or an inactive lesion, such as a pulmonary coccidioima, one need not embark on therapy. For primary coccidioidomycosis and for extrapulmonary disease treatment should be prompt, aggressive, and sustained through pregnancy and for some months thereafter. Because of issues of azole teratogenicity, amphotericin B is the drug of choice. If there are problems with nephrotoxicity or progression of disease, the patient may be transferred to azole therapy. There is no clear indication of which azole to use, because both fluconazole and itraconazole have risk of teratogenicity. Presumably, the later in pregnancy the switch to an azole is made, the lower will be the risk of teratogenesis [110].

Discontinuation of therapy for coccidioidomycosis

Finally, when should therapy be stopped? In coccidioidal meningitis, azole therapy should be life-long. For other patients, 6, 9, or 12 months after "success" (as evaluated by the Mycoses Study Group criteria) were the durations of therapy used in various clinical trials. Success was defined as a weighted score of less than 50% of the baseline disease severity score and was defined as response, not cure. Because the disease can relapse in more than a third of the cases of nonmeningeal disease after azole therapy, it is recommended that observation be continued for years, and that "remission" rather than "cure" be the operative term for response [36,62,111–113].

Coccidioides as a potential bioterrorism weapon

Coccidioides recently has been declared a potential organism of bioterrorism. A variety of laboratory modifications are required for any laboratory to work with this organism, both to assure the safety of laboratory personnel and to prevent access by unauthorized persons.

Specific approval by the Centers for Disease Control/Federal Bureau of Investigation is required to conduct investigations with this organism, and strict regulations govern its laboratory use. *Coccidiodes* seems an unattractive agent for bioterrorism, however, because incubation requires weeks to months, there is virtually no human-to-human transmission, most patients remain asymptomatic, the disease is chronic, good therapy exists, and the mortality rates, overall, are low. These considerations suggest that designation of coccidioidomycosis as a potential bioterrorism agent is based more on anxiety than on substantive evidence.

Summary

The difficulties in managing this potentially horrific disease, with its myriad manifestations, are immense, because host factors dramatically impact outcome. Coccidioidomycosis should warrant great respect among clinicians, because, even with dramatic improvements in therapies, outcomes remain poor. Although there have been outstanding successes with these new therapies, tragic losses after years of immense patient suffering still occur. Coccidioidomycosis is a geographically restricted fungus but is one that inflicts tremendous suffering on affected patients. In addition, because of travel and the influx of susceptible hosts, dramatic increases in patients at risk for infection are seen throughout the southwest United States. The extended-spectrum azoles, such as posaconazole and voriconazole, may prove to be more efficacious in the treatment of coccidioidomycosis than prior agents, including amphotericin B, fluconazole, and itraconazole. Additional resources are needed to conduct randomized, controlled clinical trials for the treatment of this disease.

References

[1] Bailek R, Kern J, Herrmann T, et al. PCR assays for the identification of *Coccidioides posadasii* based on the nucleotide sequence of antigen 2/proline-rich antigen. J Clin Microbiol 2004;42:778–83.
[2] Stevens DA. Current concepts: coccidioidomycosis. N Engl J Med 1995;332:1077–82.
[3] Crum NF, Lederman ER, Stafford CM, et al. Coccidioidomycosis: a descriptive survey of a reemerging disease. Clinical characteristics and emerging controversies. Medicine (Baltimore) 2004;83:149–75.
[4] Park BJ, Sigel K, Vaz V, et al. An epidemic of coccidioidomycosis in Arizona associated with climatic changes, 1998–2001. J Infect Dis 2005;191:1981–7.
[5] Galgiani JN, Ampel NM, Blair JE, et al. Coccidioidomycosis. Clin Infect Dis 2005;41: 1217–23.

[6] Kolivras KN, Comrie AC. Modeling valley fever (coccidioidomycosis) incidence on the basis of climatic conditions. Int J Biometeorol 2003;47:87–101.
[7] Galgiani JN. Coccidioidomycosis: a regional disease of national importance. Rethinking approaches to control. Ann Intern Med 1999;130:293–300.
[8] Petersen LR, Marshall SL, Barton-Dickson C, et al. Coccidioidomycosis among workers at an archaeological site, northeastern Utah. Emerg Infect Dis 2004;10: 637–42.
[9] Ampel NM. Coccidioidomycosis in persons infected with HIV type 1. Clin Infect Dis 2005; 41:1174–8.
[10] Wright PW, Pappagiannis D, Wilson M, et al. Donor-related coccidioidomycosis in organ transplant recipients. Clin Infect Dis 2003;37:1265–9.
[11] Bergstrom L, Yocum DE, Ampel NM, et al. Increased risk of coccidioidomycosis in patients treated with tumor necrosis factor alpha antagonists. Arthritis Rheum 2004;50: 1959–66.
[12] Peterson CM, Schuppert K, Kelly PC, et al. Coccidioidomycosis and pregnancy. Obstet Gynecol Surv 1993;48:149–56.
[13] Blair JE, Smilack JD, Caples SM. Coccidioidomycosis in patients with hematologic malignancies. Arch Intern Med 2005;165:113–7.
[14] Deresinski SC, Pappagianis D, Stevens D. Association of ABO blood group and outcome of coccidioidal infections. Sabouraudia 1979;17:261–4.
[15] Flynn N, Hoeprich P, Kawachi M, et al. An unusual outbreak of windborne coccidioidomycosis. N Engl J Med 1979;301:358–61.
[16] Schneider E, Hajjeh R, Spiegel R, et al. A coccidioidomycosis outbreak following Northridge, Calif, earthquake. JAMA 1997;277:904–8.
[17] Williams PL, Sable DL, Mendez P, et al. Symptomatic coccidioidomycosis following a severe natural dust storm. An outbreak at the Naval Air Station, Lemoore, Calif. Chest 1979;76:566–70.
[18] Pappagianis D. Marked increases in cases of coccidioidomycosis in California: 1991, 1992, and 1993. Clin Infect Dis 1994;19(Suppl 1):S14–8.
[19] Ampel NM. Coccidioidomycosis. In: Dismukes W, Pappas P, Sobel J, editors. Clinical mycology. New York: Oxford University Press; 2003. p. 311–27.
[20] Galgiani J. *Coccidioides* species. In: Mandel GL, Bennett JE, Dolin R, editors. Principles and practice of infectious diseases. 6th edition. New York: Churchill Livingstone; 2005. p. 3040–50.
[21] Pappagianis D. Coccidioidomycosis. In: Merz W, Hay RJ, editors. Topley and Wilson's medical mycology. 10th edition. Washington (DC): ASM Press; 2005. p. 502–18.
[22] Pappagianis D, Zimmer BL. Serology of coccidioidomycosis. Clin Microbiol Rev 1990;3: 247–68.
[23] Pappagianis D. Serologic studies in coccidioidomycosis. Semin Respir Infect 2001;16: 242–50.
[24] Smith CE, Saito MT, Simons SA. Pattern of 39,500 serologic tests in coccidioidomycosis. JAMA 1956;160:546–52.
[25] Graybill JR, Stevens DA, Galgiani JN, et al, for the NIAID Mycoses Study Group. Itraconazole treatment of coccidioidomycosis. Am J Med 1990;89:292–300.
[26] Kelly PC. Coccidioidal meningitis. In: Stevens DA, editor. Coccidioidomycosis: a text. New York: Plenum; 1980. p. 163–93.
[27] Pappagianis D, Saito M, Van Hoosear KH. Antibody in cerebrospinal fluid in non-meningitis coccidioidomycosis. Sabouraudia 1972;10:173–9.
[28] Kelly PC, Sievers ML, Thompson R, et al. Coccidioidal meningitis: results of treatment in 22 patients. In: Ajello L, editor. Coccidioidomycosis, current clinical and diagnostic studies. Miami (FL): Symposia Specialists; 1977. p. 239–51.
[29] Galgiani JN, Catanzaro A, Cloud GA, et al. Fluconazole therapy for coccidioidal meningitis. Ann Intern Med 1993;119:28–35.

[30] Kaufman L, Sekhon AS, Molidina N, et al. Comparative evaluation of commercial premier EIA and microimmunodiffusion and complement fixation tests for *Coccidioides immitis* antibodies. J Clin Microbiol 1995;33:618–9.
[31] Martins TB, Jaskowski TD, Mouritsen CL, et al. Comparison of commercially available enzyme immunoassay with traditional serological tests for detection of antibodies to *Coccidioides immitis*. J Clin Microbiol 1995;33:940–3.
[32] Wheat LJ, Wheat H, Connolly P, et al. Cross-reactivity in *Histoplasma capsulatum* variety *capsulatum* antigen assays of urine samples from patients with endemic mycoses. Clin Infect Dis 1997;24:1169–71.
[33] Bialek R, Johnson SM, Pappagianis KA. Amplification of coccidioidal DNA in clinical specimens by PCR. J Clin Microbiol 2005;43:1492–3.
[34] National Committee for Clinical Laboratory Standards. Reference method for broth dilution antifungal susceptibility testing of conidium forming filamentous fungi: proposed standard. NCCLS document M38-P. Wayne (PA): National Committee for Clinical Laboratory Standards; 1998.
[35] Gonzalez GM, Tijerna R, Najvar LK, et al. Correlation between antifungal susceptibilities of *Coccidioides immitis* (CI) in vitro and antifungal treatment with caspofungin in a mouse model. Antimicrob Agents Chemother 2001;45:1854–9.
[36] Galgiani JN, Catanzaro A, Cloud GA, et al. Comparison of oral fluconazole and itraconazole for progressive, nonmeningeal coccidioidomycosis—a randomized, double-blind trial. Ann Intern Med 2000;133:676–86.
[37] Johnson RH, Einstein HE. Coccidioidal meningitis. Clin Infect Dis 2006;42:103–6.
[38] Drutz D. Coccidioidal pneumonia. In: Pennington J, editor. Respiratory infections: diagnosis and management. New York: Raven Press; 1983. p. 353–73.
[39] Fiese MJ. Coccidioidomycosis. Springfield (IL): Charles C. Thomas; 1958.
[40] Werner SB, Pappagianis D, Heindl I, et al. An epidemic of coccidioidomycosis among archeology students in northern California. N Engl J Med 1972;286:507–12.
[41] Lonky SA, Catanzaro A, Moser K, et al. Acute coccidioidal pleural effusion. Am Rev Respir Dis 1976;114:681–8.
[42] Blair JE, Douglas DD. Coccidioidomycosis in liver transplant recipients relocating to an endemic area. Dig Dis Sci 2004;49:1981–5.
[43] Wright PW, Pappagianis D, Wilson M, et al. Donor-related coccidioidomycosis in organ transplant recipients. Clin Infect Dis 2003;37:1265–9.
[44] Hart PD, Russell E Jr, Remington JS. The compromised host and infection. II. Deep fungal infection. J Infect Dis 1969;120:169–91.
[45] Blair JE, Logan JL. Coccidioidomycosis in solid organ transplantation. Clin Infect Dis 2001;33:1536–44.
[46] Cohen IM, Galgiani JN, Potter D, et al. Coccidioidomycosis in renal replacement therapy. Arch Intern Med 1982;142:489–94.
[47] Ampel NM. Coccidioidomycosis among persons with human immunodeficiency virus infection in the era of highly active antiretroviral therapy (HAART). Semin Respir Infect 2001;16:257–62.
[48] Fish DG, Ampel NM, Galgiani JN, et al. Coccidioidomycosis during human immunodeficiency virus infection. Medicine (Baltimore) 1990;69:394–8.
[49] Deresinski SC, Stevens DA. Coccidioidomycosis in compromised hosts. Medicine (Baltimore) 1974;54:377–95.
[50] Holt CD, Winston DJ, Kubak BM, et al. Coccidioidomycosis in liver transplant patients. Clin Infect Dis 1997;24:216–21.
[51] Rosenstein N, Emery K, Werner S, et al. Risk factors for severe pulmonary and disseminated coccidioidomycosis: Kern County, California, 1995–1996. Clin Infect Dis 2001;32:708–15.
[52] Woods CW, McRill C, Plikaytis BD, et al. Coccidioidomycosis in human immunodeficiency virus-infected persons in Arizona, 1994–1997: incidence, risk factors, and prevention. J Infect Dis 2000;181:1428–34.

[53] Harris RE. Coccidioidomycosis complicating pregnancy. Obstet Gynecol 1966;28:401–5.

[54] Wack EE, Ampel NM, Galgiani JN, et al. Coccidioidomycosis during pregnancy. Chest 1988;94:376–9.

[55] Caldwell JW, Arsura EL, Kilgore WB, et al. Coccidioidomycosis in pregnancy during an epidemic in California. Obstet Gynecol 2000;95:236–9.

[56] Louie L, Ng S, Hajjeh R. Influence of host genetics on the severity of coccidioidomycosis. Emerg Infect Dis 1999;5:672–80.

[57] Pappagianis D, Lindsay S, Beall S, et al. Ethnic background and the clinical course of coccidioidomycosis. Am Rev Respir Dis 1979;120:959–61.

[58] Lopez AM, Williams PL, Ampel NM. Acute pulmonary coccidioidomycosis mimicking bacterial pneumonia and septic shock: a report of two cases. Am J Med 1993;95:236–9.

[59] Larsen RA, Jacobson JA, Morris AH, et al. Acute respiratory failure caused by primary pulmonary coccidioidomycosis. Am Rev Respir Dis 1985;131:797–9.

[60] Crum NF, Groff HL, Parrish JS, et al. A novel use for drotrecogin alfa (activated): successful treatment of septic shock associated with coccidioidomycosis. Clin Infect Dis 2004;39:E122–3.

[61] Drutz DJ, Catanzaro A. Coccidioidomycosis: state of the art. Part I. Am Rev Respir Dis 1978;117:559–85.

[62] Graybill JR, Galgiani JN, Stevens DA, et al, for the NIAID Mycoses Study Group. Progress in treatment of systemic mycoses: recent trials of the mycoses study group. In: In vitro and in vivo evaluation of antifungal agents. Amsterdam: Elsevier; 1986.

[63] Catanzaro A, Galgiani JN, Levine BE, et al. Fluconazole in the treatment of chronic pulmonary and nonmeningeal disseminated coccidioidomycosis. Am J Med 1995;98:249–56.

[64] Oldfield ECI, Bone WD, Martin CR, et al. Prediction of relapse after treatment of coccidioidomycosis. Clin Infect Dis 1997;25:1205–10.

[65] Grant AR, Melick DW. The surgical treatment of cavitary pulmonary coccidioidomycosis. Arch Surg 1967;94:559–65.

[66] Bayer AS. Fungal pneumonias: pulmonary coccidioidal syndromes (part 2). Chest 1981;79: 686–91.

[67] Cotton BH, Paulsen GA. Surgical considerations in pulmonary coccidioidomycosis. Am J Surg 1955;90:101–6.

[68] Thadepalli H, Salem FA, Mandal AK, et al. Pulmonary mycetoma due to *Coccidioides immitis*. Chest 1977;71:429–30.

[69] Amundson DE. Perplexing pericarditis caused by coccidioidomycosis. South Med J 1993; 86:694–6.

[70] Schwartz EL, Waldmann EB, Payne RM, et al. Coccidioidal pericarditis. Chest 1976;70: 670–2.

[71] Chowdhury JK, Habibzadeh MA. Disseminated coccidioidomycosis with pericarditis. Chest 1977;71:533–5.

[72] Bayer AS, Yoshikawa TT, Galpin JE, et al. Unusual syndromes of coccidioidomycosis: diagnostic and therapeutic considerations. Medicine (Baltimore) 1976;55:131–52.

[73] Dewsnup DH, Galgiani JN, Graybill JR, et al. Is it ever safe to stop azole therapy for *Coccidioides immitis* meningitis? Ann Intern Med 1996;124:305–10.

[74] Weisman IM, Moreno AJ, Parker AL, et al. Gastrointestinal dissemination of coccidioidomycosis. Am J Gastroenterol 1986;81:589–93.

[75] Dooley DP, Reddy RK, Smith CE. Coccidioidomycosis presenting as an omental mass. Clin Infect Dis 1994;19:802–3.

[76] Phillips P, Ford B. Peritoneal coccidioidomycosis: case report and review. Clin Infect Dis 2000;30:971–6.

[77] Deresinski SC. Coccidioidomycosis of bones and joints. In: Stevens DA, editor. Coccidioidomycosis: a text. New York: Plenum; 1980. p. 195–211.

[78] Lewicky YM, Roberto RF, Curtin SL. The unique complications of coccidioidomycosis of the spine. A detailed time line of disease progression and suppression. Spine 2004;29:E435–41.

[79] Kelly PC. Coccidioidal meningitis. In: Stevens DA, editor. Coccidioidomycosis: a text. New York: Plenum; 1980. p. 163–93.

[80] Tucker RM, Galgiani JN, Denning DW, et al. Treatment of coccidioidal meningitis with fluconazole. Rev Infect Dis 1990;12(Suppl 3):S380–9.

[81] Proia LA, Tenorio AR. Successful use of voriconazole for treatment of *Coccidioides* meningitis. Antimicrob Agents Chemother 2004;48:2341.

[82] Cortez SAE, Walsh TJ, Bennett JE. Successful treatment of coccidioidal meningitis with voriconazole. Clin Infect Dis 2003;36:1619–22.

[83] Tucker RM, Denning DW, DuPont B, et al. Itraconazole therapy for chronic coccidioidal meningitis. Ann Intern Med 1990;112:108–12.

[84] Drutz DJ. Amphotericin B in the treatment of coccidioidomycosis. Drugs 1983;26: 337–46.

[85] Vincent T, Galgiani JN, Huppert M, et al. The natural history of coccidioidal meningitis: VA-Armed Forces cooperative studies, 1955–1958. Clin Infect Dis 1993;16:247–54.

[86] Kleinschmidt-DeMasters BK, Mazowiecki M, Bonds LA, et al. Coccidioidomycosis meningitis with massive dural and cerebral venous thrombosis and tissue arthroconidia. Arch Pathol Lab Med 2000;124:310–4.

[87] Williams PL, Johnson R, Pappagianis D, et al. Vasculitic and encephalitic complications associated with *Coccidioides immitis* infection of the central nervous system in humans: report of 10 cases and review. Clin Infect Dis 1992;14:673–82.

[88] Johnson RH, Brown JF Jr, Holeman CW, et al. Coccidioidal meningitis: a 25-year experience with 194 patients. In: Einstein HE, Catanzaro A, editors. Coccidioidomycosis: proceedings of the 4th International Conference. Washington (DC): National Foundation for Infectious Diseases; 1985. p. 411–21.

[89] Alazracki NP, Fierer J, Halpern SE, et al. Use of a hyperbaric solution for administration of intrathecal amphotericin B. N Engl J Med 1974;290:641–6.

[90] Stevens D, Shatsky S. Intrathecal amphotericin B in the management of coccidioidal meningitis. Semin Respir Infect 2001;16:263–9.

[91] Graybill JR, Ellenbogen C. Complications with the Ommaya reservoirs in patients with granulomatous meningitis. J Neurosurg 1977;38:477–80.

[92] Vanden Bossche H, Marichal P, Gorrens J, et al. Mode of action studies: Basis for the search of new antifungal drugs. Ann N Y Acad Sci 1988;544:191–207.

[93] Anstead G, Corcoran G, Lewis J, et al. Refractory coccidioidomycosis treated with posaconazole. Clin Infect Dis 2005;40:1770–6.

[94] Chin TWF, Loeb M, Fong IW. Effects of an acidic beverage (Coca-Cola) on absorption of ketoconazole. Antimicrob Agents Chemother 1995;39:1671–8.

[95] Daneshmend TK, Warnock DW, Ene MD. Influence of food on the pharmacokinetics of ketoconazole. Antimicrob Agents Chemother 1984;25:1–3.

[96] Defelice R, Galgiani JN, Campbell SC, et al. Ketoconazole treatment of nonprimary coccidioidomycosis. Evaluation of 60 patients during three years of study. Am J Med 1982;72:681–7.

[97] Catanzaro A, Einstein H, Levine B, et al. Ketoconazole for treatment of disseminated coccidioidomycosis. Ann Intern Med 1982;96:436–40.

[98] Graybill JR, Craven PC, Donovan W, et al. Ketoconazole therapy for systemic fungal infections: inadequacy of standard dosage regimens. Am Rev Respir Dis 1982;126: 171–4.

[99] Ross JB, Levine B, Catanzaro A, et al. Ketoconazole for treatment of chronic pulmonary coccidioidomycosis. Ann Intern Med 1982;96:440–3.

[100] Galgiani JN, Stevens DA, Graybill JR, et al, for the NIAID Mycoses Study Group. Ketoconazole therapy of progressive coccidioidomycosis. Comparison of 400 and 800 mg doses and observations at higher doses. Am J Med 1988;84:603–10.

[101] Pont A, Williams PL, Loose DS, et al. Ketoconazole blocks adrenal steroid synthesis. Ann Intern Med 1982;97:370–2.

[102] Pont A, Williams PL, Azhar S, et al. Ketoconazole blocks testosterone synthesis. Arch Intern Med 1982;142:2137–40.

[103] Como JA, Dismukes WE. Oral azole drugs as systemic antifungal therapy. N Engl J Med 1994;330:263–72.

[104] Barone JA, Koh JG, Bierman RH, et al. Food interaction and steady-state pharmacokinetics of itraconazole capsules in healthy male volunteers. Antimicrob Agents Chemother 1993;37:778–84.

[105] Barone JA, Moskovitz BL, Guarnieri J, et al. Enhanced bioavailability of itraconazole in hydroxyprolyl-beta-cyclodextrin solution versus capsules in healthy volunteers. Antimicrob Agents Chemother 1998;42:1862–5.

[106] Sharkey PK, Rinaldi MG, Dunn JF, et al. High dose itraconazole in the treatment of severe mycoses. Antimicrob Agents Chemother 1991;35:707–13.

[107] Catanzaro A, Cloud G, Stevens D, et al. Safety and tolerance of posaconazole (SCH56592) in patients with nonmeningeal coccidioidomycosis [abstract 1417]. Fortieth Interscience Conference on Antimicrobial Agents and Chemotherapy 2000;40.

[108] Antony S. Use of the echinocandins (caspofungin) in the treatment of disseminated coccidioidomycosis in a renal transplant recipient. Clin Infect Dis 2004;39:879–80.

[109] Kuberski TT, Servi RJ, Rubin PJ. Successful treatment of a critically ill patient with disseminated coccidioidomycosis, using adjunctive interferon-gamma. Clin Infect Dis 2004;38:910–2.

[110] Bar-Oz B, Moretti ME, Bishai R, et al. Pregnancy outcome after in utero exposure to itraconazole: a prospective cohort study. Am J Obstet Gynecol 2000;183:617–20.

[111] Galgiani JN, Ampel NM, Catanzaro A, et al. Practice guidelines for the treatment of coccidioidomycosis. Clin Infect Dis 2000;30:658–61.

[112] Hostetler JS, Catanzaro A, Stevens DA, et al. Treatment of coccidioidomycosis with SCH39304. J Med Vet Mycol 1994;32:105–14.

[113] Graybill JR. Treatment of coccidioidomycosis. Ann N Y Acad Sci 1988;544:481–7.

ELSEVIER
SAUNDERS

Infect Dis Clin N Am
20 (2006) 645–662

INFECTIOUS
DISEASE CLINICS
OF NORTH AMERICA

Endemic Mycoses: Blastomycosis, Histoplasmosis, and Sporotrichosis

Carol A. Kauffman, MD[a,b,*]

[a]*University of Michigan Medical School, Ann Arbor, MI 48109, USA*
[b]*Infectious Diseases Section, Veterans Affairs Ann Arbor Healthcare System,
2215 Fuller Road, Ann Arbor, MI 48105, USA*

The endemic mycoses are a diverse group of fungi that share several characteristics. They are able to cause disease in healthy hosts, they each occupy a specific ecologic niche in the environment, and they exhibit temperature dimorphism, existing as molds in the environment at temperatures of 25°C to 30°C, and as yeasts, or spherules in the case of coccidioidomycosis, at body temperatures. This article discusses histoplasmosis and blastomycosis. Sporotrichosis, which differs in that it is usually a localized lymphocutaneous infection, is included because it shares the characteristics of endemic mycoses. Coccidioidomycosis is discussed elsewhere in this issue. Paracocci-dioidomycosis, restricted to South America, and penicilliosis, found only in Southeast Asia, are not discussed because they are uncommonly seen in North America.

With the exception of sporotrichosis, infection follows inhalation of the organisms in the mold phase from the environment. The severity of infection is determined by the extent of the exposure to the organism and by the immune status of the patient. Hematogenous dissemination is common, and reactivation of infection years later is possible.

Early recognition of infection caused by one of the endemic mycoses is often difficult because they mimic many common pulmonary infections in the initial stages, and other types of systemic diseases in their later manifestations. Given the modern day propensity for travel and the ability of these fungi to remain dormant for many years, fungal infections restricted to certain geographic regions can manifest symptoms outside of that area,

* Infectious Diseases Section, Veterans Affairs Ann Arbor Healthcare System, 2215 Fuller Road, Ann Arbor, MI 48105.
   E-mail address: ckauff@umich.edu

0891-5520/06/$ - see front matter. Published by Elsevier Inc.
doi:10.1016/j.idc.2006.07.002   *id.theclinics.com*

requiring physicians to have some knowledge of the clinical manifestations of all of the common endemic mycoses.

Blastomycosis

Epidemiology

Blastomyces dermatitidis is endemic in the south central and north central United States, extending into Wisconsin, Minnesota, and the southern portions of Ontario, Manitoba, Saskatchewan, and Alberta. The organism is also found in the Mediterranean basin and parts of Africa. The natural habitat is assumed to be soil and decaying wood, although growth of the organism from soil is difficult. Several outbreaks have been described along waterways in Wisconsin [1,2]. The largest outbreak involved 95 students in northern Wisconsin who camped along a beaver pond and explored a beaver lodge. *B dermatitidis* was isolated from wood on the pond bank and the lodge [1].

Most patients who develop blastomycosis are men who spend time outdoors. Blastomycosis has been described to occur in hunters and their dogs, presumably because they share the same environment [3]. One recent study in the United States noted an increased risk among African-Americans, and another study in Canada noted an increased incidence among the Aboriginal population of Manitoba [4,5]. Whether these findings reflect a genetic predisposition or merely increased exposure in the environment is unclear.

Pathogenesis

Blastomycosis is acquired through inhalation of the conidia of the mold form of *B dermatitidis* into the alveoli, and extremely rarely through direct cutaneous inoculation [6]. The organisms change to the yeast form in the lungs and then multiply through budding. Many patients infected with *B dermatitidis* probably experience hematogenous dissemination of the organism before immunity develops. Hematogenous dissemination occurs without clinical manifestations, and only later will a few patients present with skin lesions or other organ involvement. The immune response to *B dermatitidis* likely includes neutrophils and cell-mediated immune mechanisms involving T cells and macrophages [7]. Patients who are immunosuppressed do not seem to be at greater risk for developing blastomycosis, but more severe disease is likely to occur and the mortality rate is higher in these patients [8].

Clinical manifestations

Pulmonary manifestations of blastomycosis range from asymptomatic infection in most patients to overwhelmingly severe infection with adult respiratory distress syndrome [9,10]. One common clinical presentation is an acute pneumonia believed to be caused by an atypical organism, such as mycoplasma or legionella, that does not respond to the usual antibacterial agents. Another common manifestation is a subacute to chronic pneumonia with symptoms of fever, night sweats, fatigue, productive cough, and dyspnea. Chest radiography often shows a mass-like lesion, but multiple nodular lesions, lobar infiltrates, and cavitary lesions are also seen [11]. The differential diagnosis of chronic pulmonary blastomycosis includes lung cancer, tuberculosis, histoplasmosis, and sarcoidosis. In contrast to histoplasmosis and sarcoidosis, hilar and mediastinal lymphadenopathy are less often noted with blastomycosis. Severe diffuse pneumonia is rare, but remains a major cause of death from blastomycosis. It is the initial manifestation in some patients, but occurs after mild to moderate systemic symptoms are present for weeks in others [10].

Many patients who have blastomycosis present with cutaneous rather than pulmonary manifestations. Pulmonary lesions are sometimes noted on chest radiographs in these patients, but in others the lesions have cleared and patients experience no pulmonary manifestations. The skin lesions are typically well-circumscribed nonpainful papules, nodules, or plaques that often become verrucous and develop punctate microabscesses in the center. However, they can be primarily ulcerated and painful. A single lesion or many may be present. Uncommonly and mostly in patients who are immunocompromised, hundreds of acute pustular lesions may appear, often associated with widespread visceral involvement. The skin lesions of blastomycosis can be mistaken for squamous cell carcinoma, atypical pyoderma gangrenosum, nontuberculous mycobacterial infections, and other fungal infections, especially coccidioidomycosis or paracoccidioidomycosis.

Other common manifestations of disseminated blastomycosis are genitourinary tract infection, septic arthritis, and osteomyelitis [12]. Bone and joint involvement can occur either in association with skin lesions or at sites distant from those lesions. Less commonly, laryngeal and oropharyngeal nodules, ocular infection, meningitis, and intracerebral abscesses occur [13,14].

Diagnosis

The definitive diagnostic test for blastomycosis is growth of the organism from an aspirate, tissue biopsy, sputum, or body fluid. *B dermatitidis* generally takes several weeks to grow in the mold phase at room temperature. Once growth has occurred, laboratories that use the highly specific and sensitive DNA probe for *B dermatitidis* can rapidly confirm the identity of the organism [15]. Conversion of the mold phase to the yeast phase for definitive identification is rarely performed now.

Standard serologic antibody assays for blastomycosis are neither sensitive nor specific and should not be performed. A urinary antigen enzyme immunoassay for *B dermatitidis* is now available [16]. A significant amount of cross-reactivity is noted in samples from patients who have histoplasmosis. Whether this assay will be as useful as the urinary *Histoplasma* antigen test for diagnosis requires more study.

Tissue biopsy with histopathologic examination and cytologic or wet-mount examination of body fluids allows early diagnosis of blastomycosis based on the distinctive morphology of the yeast form of *B dermatitidis*. The yeasts are large and thick-walled, and the buds are single and broad-based (Fig. 1). In patients who have pulmonary lesions, yeasts are readily found using calcofluor white or Papanicolaou's stains on sputum or bronchoalveolar lavage fluid. Tissues should be stained with methenamine silver or periodic acid–Schiff stains to visualize the organisms. To define the extent of disease in patients who have disseminated infection, prostatic massage with urine culture for fungi should be performed. A bone scan is recommended because of the propensity of the organism to seed into bone and because osteomyelitis requires prolonged therapy.

Treatment

Guidelines for treating blastomycosis were published in 2000 [17], and will be updated later in 2006. Recommendations are based on multicenter, nonrandomized, open-label treatment trials; reports from single institutions; and individual anecdotal experiences. Patients who experience any manifestation of dissemination, even if only one skin lesion, require systemic antifungal therapy to prevent progression of disease. Patients who have mild to moderate illness should be treated with an azole; those who have severe disease, including central nervous system (CNS) involvement, and those who are immunosuppressed should be treated with amphotericin B initially followed by an azole.

Itraconazole is the preferred azole agent for treating mild to moderate blastomycosis [17,18]. The dosage used is 200 mg once or twice daily for

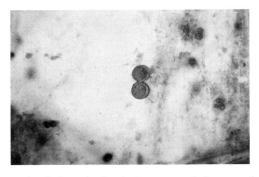

Fig. 1. Papanicolaou stain of a bronchoalveolar lavage sample from a patient who has chronic pneumonia showing a thick-walled yeast with a broad-based bud typical of *Blastomyces dermatitidis*.

6 to 12 months, depending on the clinical response. All skin lesions and pulmonary infiltrates should be resolved. Patients who have osteoarticular involvement generally undergo treatment for at least 12 months. Success rates for itraconazole therapy approach 90% to 95% [18]. Fluconazole is less effective, and a higher dosage of 800 mg daily is required [19,20]. Voriconazole has been reported to be effective in several cases of blastomycosis, including two that involved CNS infection [21–23]. Posaconazole will likely be effective, but data are not available. Until more data are available, neither agent should be used as initial therapy for blastomycosis.

The daily dosage of amphotericin B is 0.7 to 1.0 mg/kg or 3 to 5 mg/kg/d of a lipid formulation of amphotericin B [17]. For disseminated or severe pulmonary disease, therapy can be changed to itraconazole, 200 mg twice daily, after the patient's condition has improved. Although prior recommendations were to use amphotericin B for the entire course of therapy, this is rarely done now because of the considerable toxicity associated with this agent.

One treatment issue that remains controversial is the appropriate therapy for CNS blastomycosis. The length of treatment with amphotericin B is not established, nor is it clear whether fluconazole, with its better penetration into the CNS, or itraconazole, with its greater intrinsic activity, is the better agent for step-down therapy [17]. Early anecdotal data on voriconazole effectiveness in this circumstance are intriguing [21,22], but use of this agent currently cannot be recommended.

Another issue for which only anecdotal experience exists is whether corticosteroids should be used in patients who have severe pulmonary blastomycosis associated with adult respiratory distress syndrome. Given the high mortality of this complication and the possible benefits of corticosteroids, many experts favor using these agents along with amphotericin B for a period not exceeding 7 to 10 days.

Histoplasmosis

Epidemiology

The dimorphic fungus *Histoplasma capsulatum* is endemic in the Mississippi and Ohio River valleys, Central America, and certain areas of Southeast Asia and the Mediterranean basin. High concentrations of the mold phase of *H capsulatum* are found in soil that is rich in nitrogen, as occurs in areas in which large flocks of birds roost. Many caves also contain enormous numbers of *H capsulatum* growing luxuriantly on bat guano. Activities, such as landscaping; cleaning debris from attics, bridges, or barns; tearing down structures on which birds and bats may have roosted; and spelunking are associated with histoplasmosis [24]. Infection is so common in the endemic area that most persons have been infected before adulthood and never know. Outbreaks have been described involving anywhere from a handful of persons to hundreds of thousands in the case of the

Indianapolis outbreak traced back to the demolition of a large recreational park in the city [25].

Pathogenesis

The microconidia of *H capsulatum* are the infectious form. These small structures easily find their way into the alveoli where they are met by neutrophils and macrophages that phagocytize the organism. Inside the macrophage, the organism converts to the yeast phase and is able to survive within the cell [26]. The macrophage is responsible for the spread of the yeast to the hilar and mediastinal lymph nodes and subsequent hematogenous dissemination throughout the reticuloendothelial system. Only after several weeks, when specific cell-mediated immunity against *H capsulatum* develops, are sensitized T cells able to activate the macrophages and kill the organism. Histoplasmosis exemplifies the crucial importance of the cell-mediated immune system in host defense against fungi.

The extent of disease is determined by the inoculum of conidia inhaled into the lungs and the immune response of the host to the conidia. Healthy individuals develop severe life-threatening infection when exposed to a huge number of organisms, which can occur during demolition of an old building with years of accumulated guano or when spelunking in a bat-infested cave. On the other hand, in a markedly immunosuppressed host, such as a patient who has AIDS, a tiny inoculum can lead to severe disease with widespread disseminated infection.

Almost all persons infected with *H capsulatum* have asymptomatic hematogenous dissemination, but only rarely does this lead to symptomatic disease. *H capsulatum* has the propensity to remain as a latent infection in tissues and then reactivate years later if the host becomes immunosuppressed. Exposure to a heavy inoculum of *H capsulatum* can also lead to reinfection in an immune host, and in an immunosuppressed host who has waning of cell-mediated immunity, reinfection can occur with exposure to even a small inoculum from the environment.

Clinical manifestations

Pulmonary infection

Most patients infected with *H capsulatum* remain asymptomatic or have a mild respiratory illness that is not diagnosed as histoplasmosis. Patients who do have symptoms of an acute pulmonary infection may or may not seek medical attention, depending on the length and severity of the illness. The usual symptoms are fever, chills, fatigue, myalgias, dyspnea, nonproductive cough, and anterior chest discomfort. Most patients are initially treated for a bacterial pneumonia with antibiotics. When no response to this therapy occurs and chest radiography shows a patchy lobar or multilobar nodular infiltrate with mediastinal or hilar lymphadenopathy, the possibility of a fungal infection arises [27,28].

Patients who have had extensive exposure to *H capsulatum* and those who are immunosuppressed can develop severe life-threatening pneumonia. These patients generally experience high fevers, dyspnea, nonproductive cough, and prostration. Diffuse reticulonodular infiltrates are noted on chest radiograph, and adult respiratory distress syndrome can quickly develop. Early and aggressive antifungal treatment is essential to prevent a fatal outcome [27].

Most patients who have pulmonary histoplasmosis have a self-limited illness or show a good response to therapy. However, a small number, far fewer than 1%, develop complications related to mediastinal involvement with the infection. *Histoplasma* pericarditis is a benign self-limited condition that occurs in a small number of patients who have acute pulmonary infection [29]. Except in very rare cases, the organism cannot be grown from the pericardial fluid. The pericardial effusion and associated pleural effusion are apparently caused by an inflammatory reaction to adjacent mediastinal infection with *H capsulatum*. Positional chest pain, dyspnea, fever, and fatigue are common symptoms. The pericardial and pleural fluid is exudative and often bloody. Tamponade is rare, and the condition is self-limited.

Granulomatous mediastinitis is characterized by persistently enlarged mediastinal and hilar lymph nodes. The nodes may become very large and are frequently necrotic. They impinge on adjacent mediastinal structures, causing dysphagia, chest pain, and cough [30]. Esophageal traction diverticula and tracheoesophageal fistula can occur. Resolution may take months to years.

Fibrosing mediastinitis is an even more rare complication of pulmonary histoplasmosis and does not seem to be related to granulomatous mediastinitis. It occurs most often in young women. Pathologically, this condition is characterized by an excessive fibrotic response in the mediastinum, leading to entrapment of the great vessels or bronchi [31]. Patients experience dyspnea, cough, wheezing, and sometimes hemoptysis. Superior vena cava syndrome, heart failure, and pulmonary emboli can ensue, and the outcome is death after several years.

Chronic cavitary pulmonary histoplasmosis occurs almost entirely in older adults who have underlying emphysema [32]. Whether it is caused by new infection or reactivation of an earlier infection is unclear. This form of histoplasmosis mimics tuberculosis clinically and radiographically. Patients experience fever, fatigue, anorexia, weight loss, cough productive of purulent sputum, and hemoptysis. Chest radiographs show cavitary upper lobe infiltrates and fibrosis in the lower lung fields. This disease is progressive and fatal if not treated.

Disseminated infection

Acute disseminated histoplasmosis is seen mostly in patients who are immunosuppressed, including those who have undergone transplantation, those who have hematologic malignancies, and patients who have AIDS and who have CD4 counts less than 150/μL [33,34]. Young infants cannot handle primary infection with *H capsulatum* and develop overwhelming disseminated infection. Patient undergoing treatment with corticosteroids and those treated with tumor necrosis factor antagonists also are at risk for disseminated histoplasmosis [35]. Whether most patients have reactivation histoplasmosis or new exposure to the organism is unclear.

Symptoms include chills, fever, malaise, anorexia, weight loss, and dyspnea. Hypotension and sepsis syndrome with adult respiratory distress syndrome and disseminated intravascular coagulation and Addisonian crisis can occur with overwhelming infection. Physical examination usually shows an acutely ill individual who has fever, skin and mucous membrane lesions, and hepatosplenomegaly. Diffuse reticulonodular infiltrates or features of adult respiratory distress syndrome are noted on chest radiograph. Laboratory values show pancytopenia, elevated alkaline phosphatase, and an elevated erythrocyte sedimentation rate. Gastrointestinal involvement is probably more common than realized; symptoms are often nonspecific mild abdominal discomfort and intermittent diarrhea, but also can be those of an unremitting diarrhea with malabsorption [36].

Chronic progressive disseminated histoplasmosis occurs predominantly in middle-aged to elderly men who are not known to be immunosuppressed [33]. Patients often experience symptoms for months before being diagnosed. Symptoms include fever, night sweats, weight loss, and fatigue, and presentation with fever of unknown origin is common. Hepatosplenomegaly, painful ulcerations in the oral cavity and sometimes skin lesions that are papular, nodular, or ulcerated are noted on examination. Laboratory evaluation routinely shows increased erythrocyte sedimentation rate, pancytopenia, and elevated alkaline phosphatase. Diffuse reticulonodular pulmonary infiltrates are usually noted on chest radiograph. Symptoms and laboratory findings suggesting adrenal insufficiency should be sought.

CNS histoplasmosis is an uncommon manifestation of disseminated histoplasmosis [37]. Patients can present with obvious disseminated histoplasmosis with concomitant CNS involvement, or with isolated chronic meningitis with no symptoms or signs suggesting active disease elsewhere. Symptoms include headache, behavioral changes, signs of increased intracranial pressure, and focal neurologic deficits. Lumbar puncture shows lymphocytic meningitis with mildly decreased glucose and elevated protein. Focal lesions should be sought through MRI of the brain and the spinal cord.

Other focal involvement with *H capsulatum* is rare. Epididymitis, prostatitis, and osteoarticular infection have been reported [38], and reflect hematogenous dissemination of the organism during initial infection.

Diagnosis

Growth of *H capsulatum* from tissue or fluid samples is the definitive method to establish the diagnosis of histoplasmosis [39]. The organism takes weeks to grow in vitro, and cultures, especially those from sputum samples, can be overgrown with commensal fungi before *H capsulatum* is detected. Once growth occurs, probes specific for *H capsulatum* confirm the identification of the organism, obviating the need to convert from the mold to the yeast phase. Blood cultures, especially those using the lysis–centrifugation system (Isolator tube), frequently yield the organism in patients who have disseminated histoplasmosis.

Identification of the rather uniform-appearing 2- to 4-μm oval budding yeasts in tissue or fluid samples can yield the diagnosis long before culture results are known. This method is more sensitive for patients who have disseminated infection than for those who only have pulmonary disease. Biopsies should be performed on bone marrow, liver, lymph nodes, mucous membrane lesions, and cutaneous lesions. Methenamine silver or periodic acid–Schiff stains are required in most cases to show the tiny yeasts (Fig. 2). Patients who have severe infection may have yeasts visualized inside white blood cells on the peripheral blood smear. In contrast to blastomycosis, cytologic examination of bronchoalveolar lavage fluid or sputum generally does not show the tiny yeasts of *H capsulatum*.

Measuring the cell-wall polysaccharide antigen of *H capsulatum* in urine is a sensitive diagnostic tool for patients who have disseminated infection [40]. The greatest experience is with patients who have AIDS, but this enzyme immunoassay has also been very useful in patients who do not have AIDS. Antigen is rarely detected in patients who have chronic pulmonary histoplasmosis or granulomatous mediastinitis, but is positive in approximately 80% of those who have acute pulmonary histoplasmosis. Testing for antigen is more sensitive in urine than in serum. Cross-reactivity occurs with blastomycosis, paracoccidioidomycosis, and penicilliosis, but the latter two are rarely in the differential diagnosis.

Work is ongoing to develop a useful molecular assay, such as polymerase chain reaction, for detecting *H capsulatum* in blood and tissue samples taken from patients who have disseminated histoplasmosis. Although several

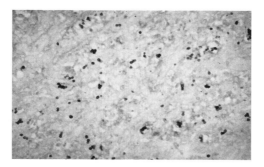

Fig. 2. Methenamine silver stain of omental tissue obtained at operation for bowel perforation in a patient who has AIDS and disseminated histoplasmosis. The typical yeasts of *Histoplasma capsulatum* are 2- to 4-μm oval structures with thin-based buds.

assays have been reported to be useful [41,42], none have evolved to routine clinical use.

Serology plays an important role in the diagnosis of certain forms of histoplasmosis [39]. The standard assays are complement fixation (CF) and immunodiffusion (ID). The ID test reports whether H or M antibodies are present, with the M band appearing sooner and lasting longer than the H band. The CF test reports the presence of mycelial-phase and yeast-phase antibodies. The sensitivity of the CF and ID assays is approximately 80%, and performing both assays increases the possibility of making a diagnosis [38]. Patients who have chronic cavitary pulmonary histoplasmosis and chronic progressive disseminated histoplasmosis almost always show positive results with both assays. Patients who have acute pneumonia may show a fourfold rise in CF titer or the appearance of an M band through ID. However, in patients who are immunosuppressed and who cannot mount an antibody response, serology is rarely useful and should not be relied on to help diagnose histoplasmosis.

Treatment

Guidelines for the treatment of histoplasmosis were published in 2000 [43] and will be updated in 2006. The guidelines are derived mostly from multicenter open-label treatment trials, reports from individual institutions, and anecdotal experience. As a general rule, patients who have severe histoplasmosis should be treated with an amphotericin B formulation, and those who have mild to moderate disease can be treated with an azole. The most appropriate azole is itraconazole [44,45]; fluconazole is less effective [46,47]. There is little experience with the use of voriconazole for treating histoplasmosis [23,48]. A preliminary report of seven patients showed success in six treated with posaconazole, and a further report detailed the clinical response of one patient [49,50]. These agents should not be considered primary therapy for histoplasmosis. The echinocandins are inactive and should not be used to treat histoplasmosis.

Most patients who have acute pulmonary histoplasmosis do not require therapy. For many patients, the diagnosis is established after their symptoms have abated. However, some patients experience symptoms that persist for weeks to months, and should be treated with itraconazole, 200 mg once or twice daily for 6 to 12 weeks. Patients who develop severe pneumonia and those who are immunosuppressed should undergo antifungal therapy for pulmonary histoplasmosis. Initial therapy should be with amphotericin B, 0.7 mg/kg/d, or a lipid formulation of amphotericin B, 3 to 5 mg/kg daily. After a favorable response is noted, therapy can be changed to oral itraconazole, 200 mg twice daily. Treatment should continue until the infiltrate has resolved, which for most patients will be at least 6 months. All patients who have chronic pulmonary histoplasmosis should undergo treatment to prevent progression of the infection. Itraconazole, 200 mg twice daily for 12 to 24 months is the preferred treatment.

Patients who have granulomatous mediastinitis are often treated with itraconazole, 200 mg twice daily for 3 to 6 months. No clinical trials show effectiveness of this approach; however, the side effects are minimal and some patients appear to benefit. Surgical resection of enlarged lymph nodes has been beneficial in some patients [27]. No effective antifungal therapy is available for fibrosing mediastinitis. The disease follows a relentless downhill course, especially when bilateral involvement is present. However, selected patients can experience dramatic relief of symptoms when stents are placed in obstructed great vessels and sometimes in bronchi [51].

Symptomatic disseminated histoplasmosis should be treated with antifungal agents. Patients who have mild to moderate disease can be treated with oral itraconazole, 200 mg twice daily. Those who have severe illness, are immunosuppressed, and have CNS infection should receive amphotericin B, 0.7 to 1 mg/kg/d. Many clinicians use lipid formulation amphotericin B (3–5 mg/kg/d) rather than amphotericin B deoxycholate, especially if patients have risk factors for renal toxicity or if therapy is expected to last for several weeks. One randomized, blinded trial conducted in patients who had AIDS and who had severe disseminated histoplasmosis showed that liposomal amphotericin B was superior to amphotericin B deoxycholate for initial therapy [52]. Therapy for most patients can be switched to oral itraconazole when their condition has stabilized and they are able to take oral medications. Most patients who have disseminated infection should undergo 12 months of therapy. The length of therapy depends on the severity of disease and whether the patient remains immunosuppressed. Although older adults who have the chronic progressive disseminated form of histoplasmosis are not overtly immunosuppressed, they respond slowly to therapy and should undergo treatment for at least 12 months.

Patients who have AIDS should receive suppressive therapy with itraconazole, 200 mg/d, after an initial 12 weeks of induction therapy at a dosage of itraconazole, 200 mg twice daily. When CD4 counts return to more than 200 cells/μL for at least 1 year, itraconazole suppression can be stopped safely [53]. Prophylaxis against histoplasmosis is effective for patients who have AIDS, have CD4 counts less than 150 cells/μL, and who live in endemic areas that have a high attack rate [54].

CNS histoplasmosis should be treated initially with amphotericin B, usually a lipid formulation at 3 to 5 mg/kg/d for 6 to 12 weeks. The length of therapy depends on patient response and the occurrence of side effects from amphotericin B. An oral azole agent should be given after amphotericin B therapy is completed. Fluconazole, 800 mg/d, or itraconazole, 200 mg twice daily, have both been recommended [37,43]. The length of therapy is unknown, but may be lifelong in some patients.

Sporotrichosis

Epidemiology

More than the other endemic mycoses, the source of infection with the dimorphic fungus *Sporothrix schenckii* is often known. A history usually reveals exposure to soil, moss, hay, or decaying material and trauma to the skin leading to direct inoculation of the organism. Infection is more common among men and occurs especially in gardeners or landscapers. Cases have been documented in persons exposed through Christmas tree farming, topiary production, and hay baling, and inoculation has occurred with motor vehicle accidents [55–58]. Less commonly, inhalation of *S schenckii* conidia from soil can lead to pulmonary infection.

Zoonotic sporotrichosis occurs with exposure to infected animals, most often cats, that develop ulcerated lesions that often contain large numbers of organisms [59]. An ongoing outbreak in Brazil involves mostly housewives and children who care for cats that are infected [60]. Infection has also been transmitted passively from uninfected animals that transfer the organism from soil through scratching or biting.

Pathogenesis

Sporotrichosis develops when *S schenckii* conidia from the mold phase are inoculated into the skin or subcutaneous tissues. The organism converts to the yeast form in the body. The clinical picture evolves as the organisms spread along lymphatics draining the primary inoculation site. Some *S schenckii* strains grow poorly at temperatures higher than 35°C and generally are associated with fixed cutaneous lesions that do not extend along lymphatics [61,62].

In patients who have underlying conditions, such as alcoholism, diabetes mellitus, chronic obstructive pulmonary disease, and HIV infection, dissemination of *S schenckii* to osteoarticular structures, lungs, meninges, and other organs can occur. The initial host response to *S schenckii* is composed of neutrophils and macrophages, which are able to ingest and kill the yeast phase of *S schenckii*. Cell-mediated immunity also appears to play a role in containing infection; visceral dissemination is rarely reported in the absence of severe defects in cell-mediated immunity [63]. At least one patient has been reported to develop disseminated sporotrichosis after undergoing treatment with a tumor necrosis factor antagonist [64].

Clinical manifestations

Sporotrichosis is primarily a cutaneous disease. After inoculation, a papule develops at the site within days to weeks. The primary lesion generally ulcerates, but remains only mildly tender. Nodules develop proximal to the primary lesion following the lymphatic distribution and often ulcerate, mimicking the primary lesion. The lesions of sporotrichosis must be differentiated from those caused by atypical mycobacteria, especially *M marinum*; *Nocardia*, particularly *N brasiliensis*; *Leishmania*; and tularemia [65]. In some patients, only the primary lesion, which can be either ulcerative or verrucous, occurs and slowly enlarges over weeks to months, persisting as a fixed cutaneous lesion until treated [62].

Involvement of other structures during infection with *S schenckii* is rare in normal hosts. Osteoarticular sporotrichosis occurs more frequently in patients who have alcoholism. Infection can occur secondary to contiguous spread, but is more likely caused by hematogenous spread to one or more joints. The joints most commonly affected are the knee, elbow, wrist, and ankle. Tenosynovitis is another manifestation and may present as carpal tunnel syndrome [66].

Pulmonary sporotrichosis occurs most often in patients who have chronic obstructive pulmonary disease or who abuse alcohol [67]. This form of sporotrichosis follows inhalation of the organism, rather than cutaneous inoculation. Patients present with fever, night sweats, weight loss, fatigue, dyspnea, cough with purulent sputum, and hemoptysis. Unilateral or bilateral nodular and cavitary lesions are seen on chest radiograph and mimic the findings of reactivation tuberculosis.

Reports exist of infection localized to the meninges, pericardium, eye, larynx, breast, epididymis, spleen, liver, bone marrow, and lymph nodes [55]. Disseminated sporotrichosis presenting as widespread ulcerative cutaneous lesions with or without concomitant visceral involvement is reported primarily in patients who have advanced HIV infection [68].

Diagnosis

The definitive diagnostic method to confirm sporotrichosis is growth of *S schenckii* from material aspirated from a lesion or a tissue biopsy specimen. At room temperature, growth of the mold is usually evident within a week. With visceral or osteoarticular involvement, tissue, rather than synovial fluid or sputum, provides the best yield for culture.

Histopathologic examination of biopsy material is less sensitive than culture methods. Typically, a mixed granulomatous and pyogenic process is noted, but the organisms may be difficult to find because they often are present in small numbers. In tissues, the yeasts are 3 to 5 μm in diameter, oval to cigar-shaped, and can show multiple buds (Fig. 3).

Serology has not been useful for diagnosing sporotrichosis, and antigen-based tests are not available.

Treatment

Guidelines for treating sporotrichosis have been published [69] and will be updated in 2006. The guidelines are based entirely on open-label

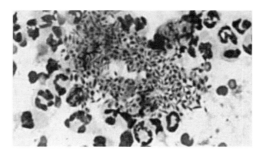

Fig. 3. Aspirate of an ulcerated lesion showing neutrophils and a cluster of cigar-shaped yeasts typical of *Sporothrix schenckii*.

treatment trials and anecdotal experience. Azole agents, and specifically itraconazole, have become standard therapy for most forms of sporotrichosis. Lymphocutaneous sporotrichosis is treated with itraconazole, 100 to 200 mg/d, until several weeks after all lesions have disappeared, which for most patients is 3 to 6 months [70,71]. Success rates of more than 90% can be expected. Fluconazole is less active against *S schenckii*, but has been effective at a daily dose of 400 mg [72]. In one small study, terbinafine at a dosage of 500 mg twice daily was effective for sporotrichosis [73]. Saturated solution of potassium iodide (SSKI) is the least costly effective therapy, but SSKI is associated with many side effects, including metallic taste, salivary gland swelling, rash, and fever [74]. The initial dosage is 5 to 10 drops three times daily in water or juice, and is increased each week to a maximum of 40 to 50 drops three times daily. Local hyperthermia, induced by various different warming devices or baths, has been reported to be effective for fixed cutaneous lesions of sporotrichosis [75].

Osteoarticular sporotrichosis is generally treated with itraconazole, 200 mg twice daily, for as long as 1 to 2 years. Unfortunately, joint function rarely returns to baseline. Other azoles are less effective, and SSKI is ineffective. Itraconazole, 200 mg twice daily, also is used to treat patients who have pulmonary sporotrichosis who are not acutely ill. For those who are seriously ill, amphotericin B, 0.7 to 1.0 mg/kg/d, or lipid formulation amphotericin B, 3 to 5 mg/kg/d, should be given initially, and itraconazole can be used after improvement occurs. Treatment generally is required for 1 to 2 years. Surgical resection is a useful adjunctive treatment, but most patients have severe chronic pulmonary disease and cannot tolerate surgery.

Patients who have disseminated sporotrichosis should be treated with amphotericin B, 0.7 to 1.0 mg/kg/d, or lipid formulation amphotericin B, 3 to 5 mg/kg/d. After patients have experienced a response to therapy, itraconazole, 200 mg twice daily, can be substituted for amphotericin B. Patients who have AIDS and disseminated sporotrichosis likely require lifelong therapy with itraconazole, 200 mg daily; no reports have addressed the issue of whether antifungal therapy can be stopped when CD4 counts return to normal with highly active antiretroviral therapy.

References

[1] Klein BS, Vergeront JM, DiSalvo AF, et al. Two outbreaks of blastomycosis along rivers in Wisconsin: isolation of *Blastomyces dermatitidis* from riverbank soil and evidence of its transmission along waterways. Am Rev Respir Dis 1987;136:1333–8.
[2] Baumgardner DJ, Buggy BP, Mattson BJ, et al. Epidemiology of blastomycosis in a region of high endemicity in North Central Wisconsin. Clin Infect Dis 1992;15:629–35.
[3] Armstrong CW, Jenkins SR, Kaufman L, et al. Common-source outbreak of blastomycosis in hunters and their dogs. J Infect Dis 1987;155:568–70.
[4] Cano MV, Ponce-de-Leon GF, Tippen S, et al. Blastomycosis in Missouri: epidemiology and risk factors for endemic disease. Epidemiol Infect 2003;131:907–14.
[5] Crampton TL, Light RB, Berg GM, et al. Epidemiology and clinical spectrum of blastomycosis diagnosed at Manitoba hospitals. Clin Infect Dis 2002;34:1310–6.
[6] Gray NA, Baddour LM. Cutaneous inoculation blastomycosis. Clin Infect Dis 2002;34: e44–9.
[7] Klein BS, Bradsher RW, Vergeront JM, et al. Development of long-term specific cellular immunity after acute *Blastomyces dermatitidis* infection: assessments following a large point-source outbreak in Wisconsin. J Infect Dis 1990;161:97–101.
[8] Pappas PG, Threlkeld MG, Bedsole GD, et al. Blastomycosis in immunocompromised patients. Medicine (Baltimore) 1993;72:311–25.
[9] Meyer KC, McManus EJ, Maki DG. Overwhelming pulmonary blastomycosis associated with the adult respiratory distress syndrome. N Engl J Med 1993;329:1231–6.
[10] Pappas PG. Blastomycosis. Semin Respir Crit Care Med 2004;25:113–21.
[11] Sheflin JR, Campbell JA, Thompson GP. Pulmonary blastomycosis: findings on chest radiographs in 63 patients. AJR Am J Roentgenol 1990;154:1177–80.
[12] Saccente M, Abernathy RS, Pappas PG, et al. Vertebral blastomycosis with paravertebral abscess: report of eight cases and review of the literature. Clin Infect Dis 1998;26:413–8.
[13] Hanson JM, Spector G, El-Mofty SK. Laryngeal blastomycosis: a commonly missed diagnosis. Report of two cases and review of the literature. Ann Otol Rhinol Laryngol 2000; 109:281–6.
[14] Friedman JA, Wijdicks EFM, Fulgham JR, et al. Meningoencephalitis due to *Blastomyces dermatitidis*: case report and literature review. Mayo Clin Proc 2000;75:403–8.
[15] Areno JP, Campbell GD, George RB. Diagnosis of blastomycosis. Semin Respir Infect 1997; 12:252–62.
[16] Durkin M, Witt J, LeMonte A, et al. Antigen assay with the potential to aid in the diagnosis of blastomycosis. J Clin Microbiol 2004;42:4873–5.
[17] Chapman SW, Bradsher RW Jr, Campbell GD Jr, et al. Practice guidelines for the management of patients with blastomycosis. Clin Infect Dis 2000;30:679–83.
[18] Dismukes WE, Bradsher RW, Cloud GC, et al. Itraconazole therapy for blastomycosis and histoplasmosis. Am J Med 1992;93:489–97.
[19] Pappas PG, Bradsher RW, Chapman SW, et al. Treatment of blastomycosis with fluconazole: a pilot study. Clin Infect Dis 1995;20:267–71.
[20] Pappas PG, Bradsher RW, Kauffman CA, et al. Treatment of blastomycosis with higher doses of fluconazole. Clin Infect Dis 1997;25:200–5.
[21] Lentnek AL, Lentnek IA. Successful management of *Blastomyces dermatitidis* meningitis. Infect Med 2006;23:39–41.
[22] Bakleh M, Aksamit AJ, Tleyjeh IM, et al. Successful treatment of cerebral blastomycosis with voriconazole. Clin Infect Dis 2005;40:e69–71.
[23] Perfect JR, Marr KA, Walsh TJ, et al. Voriconazole treatment for less-common, emerging, or refractory fungal infections. Clin Infect Dis 2003;36:1122–31.

[24] Cano M, Hajjeh RA. The epidemiology of histoplasmosis: a Review. Semin Respir Infect 2001;16:109–18.

[25] Wheat J. Histoplasmosis. Experience during outbreaks in Indianapolis and review of the literature. Medicine (Baltimore) 1997;76:339–54.

[26] Newman SL. Cell-mediated immunity to *Histoplasma capsulatum*. Semin Respir Infect 2001; 16:102–8.

[27] Wheat LJ, Conces D, Allen SD, et al. Pulmonary histoplasmosis syndromes: recognition, diagnosis, and management. Semin Respir Crit Care Med 2004;25:129–44.

[28] Gurney JW, Conces DJ. Pulmonary histoplasmosis. Radiology 1996;199:297–306.

[29] Picardi JL, Kauffman CA, Schwarz J, et al. Pericarditis caused by *Histoplasma capsulatum*. Am J Cardiol 1976;37:82–8.

[30] Goodwin RA, Loyd JE, Des Prez RM. Histoplasmosis in normal hosts. Medicine (Baltimore) 1981;60:231–66.

[31] Davis A, Pierson D, Loyd JE. Mediastinal fibrosis. Semin Respir Infect 2001;16:119–30.

[32] Goodwin RA, Owens FT, Snell JD, et al. Chronic pulmonary histoplasmosis. Medicine (Baltimore) 1976;55:413–52.

[33] Goodwin RA, Shapiro JL, Thurman GH, et al. Disseminated histoplasmosis: clinical and pathologic correlations. Medicine (Baltimore) 1980;59:1–33.

[34] McKinsey DS, Spiegel RA, Hutwagner L, et al. Prospective study of histoplasmosis in patients infected with human immunodeficiency virus: incidence, risk factors, and pathophysiology. Clin Infect Dis 1997;24:1195–203.

[35] Wood KL, Hage CA, Knos KS, et al. Histoplasmosis after treatment with anti-TNF-(alpha) therapy. Am J Respir Crit Care Med 2003;167:1279–82.

[36] Lamps LW, Molina CP, West B, et al. The pathologic spectrum of gastrointestinal and hepatic histoplasmosis. Am J Clin Pathol 2000;113:64–72.

[37] Wheat LJ, Musial CE, Jenny-Avital E. Diagnosis and management of central nervous system histoplasmosis. Clin Infect Dis 2005;40:844–52.

[38] Kauffman CA. Histoplasmosis. In: Dismukes WE, Pappas PG, Sobel JD, editors. Clinical mycology. Oxford University Press; 2003. p. 285–98.

[39] Wheat LJ. Laboratory diagnosis of histoplasmosis: a review. Semin Respir Infect 2001;16: 131–40.

[40] Wheat LJ, Garringer T, Brizendine E, et al. Diagnosis of histoplasmosis by antigen detection based upon experience at the histoplasmosis reference laboratory. Diagn Microbiol Infect Dis 2002;43:29–37.

[41] Bracca A, Tosello ME, Girardini JE, et al. Molecular detection of *Histoplasma capsulatum* var. *capsulatum* in human clinical samples. J Clin Microbiol 2003;41:1753–5.

[42] Bialek R, Feucht A, Aepinus C, et al. Evaluation of two nested PCR assays for detection of *Histoplasma capsulatum* DNA in human tissue. J Clin Microbiol 2002;40:1644–7.

[43] Wheat J, Sarosi G, McKinsey D, et al. Practice guidelines for the management of patients with histoplasmosis. Clin Infect Dis 2000;30:688–95.

[44] Dismukes WE, Bradsher RW Jr, Cloud GC, et al. Itraconazole therapy for blastomycosis and histoplasmosis. Am J Med 1992;93:489–97.

[45] Wheat J, Hafner R, Korzun AH, et al. Itraconazole treatment of disseminated histoplasmosis in patients with the acquired immunodeficiency syndrome. Am J Med 1995;98: 336–42.

[46] McKinsey DS, Kauffman CA, Pappas PG, et al. Fluconazole therapy for histoplasmosis. Clin Infect Dis 1996;23:996–1001.

[47] Wheat J, Mawhinney S, Hafner R, et al. Treatment of histoplasmosis with fluconazole in patients with acquired immunodeficiency syndrome. Am J Med 1997;103:223–32.

[48] Freifeld AG, Iwen PC, Lesiak BL, et al. Histoplasmosis in solid organ transplant recipients at a large midwestern transplant center. Transplant Infect Dis 2005;7:109–15.

[49] Clark B, Foster R, Tunbridge A, et al. A case of disseminated histoplasmosis successfully treated with the investigational drug posaconazole. J Infect 2005;51:e177–80.

[50] Restrepo A, Tobon A, Clark B, et al. Salvage treatment of histoplasmosis with posacona-zole. J Infect, in press.

[51] Doyle TP, Loyd JE, Robbins IM. Percutaneous pulmonary artery and vein stenting: a novel treatment for mediastinal fibrosis. Am J Respir Crit Care Med 2001;164:657–60.

[52] Johnson PC, Wheat LJ, Cloud GA, et al. Safety and efficacy of liposomal amphotericin B compared with conventional amphotericin B for induction therapy of histoplasmosis in patients with AIDS. Ann Intern Med 2002;137:105–9.

[53] Goldman M, Zackin R, Fichtenbaum CJ, et al. Safety of discontinuation of maintenance therapy for disseminated histoplasmosis after immunologic response to antiretroviral therapy. Clin Infect Dis 2004;38:1485–9.

[54] McKinsey DS, Wheat LJ, Cloud G, et al. Itraconazole prophylaxis against fungal infections in patients with advanced human immunodeficiency virus infection: randomized placebo-controlled double-blind study. Clin Infect Dis 1999;28:1049–56.

[55] Kauffman CA. Sporotrichosis. Clin Infect Dis 1999;29:231–7.

[56] Dixon DM, Salkin IF, Duncan RA, et al. Isolation and characterization of *Sporothrix schenckii* from clinical and environmental sources associated with the largest US epidemic of sporotrichosis. J Clin Microbiol 1991;29:1106–13.

[57] Hajjeh R, McDonnell S, Reef S, et al. Outbreak of sporotrichosis among tree nursery workers. J Infect Dis 1997;176:499–504.

[58] Dooley DP, Bostic PS, Beckius ML. Spook house sporotrichosis. A point-source outbreak of cutaneous sporotrichosis from hay bale props in a Halloween haunted-house. Arch Intern Med 1997;157:1885–7.

[59] Reed KD, Moore FM, Geiger GE, et al. Zoonotic transmission of sporotrichosis: case report and review. Clin Infect Dis 1993;16:384–7.

[60] Barros MBL, Schubach AAO, Valle ACF, et al. Cat-transmitted sporotrichosis epidemic in Rio de Janeiro, Brazil: description of a series of cases. Clin Infect Dis 2004;38:529–35.

[61] Kwon-Chung KJ. Comparison of isolates of *Sporothrix schenckii* obtained from fixed cutaneous lesions with isolates from other types of lesions. J Infect Dis 1979;139:424–31.

[62] Pappas PG, Tellez I, Deep AE, et al. Sporotrichosis in Peru: description of an area of hyper-endemicity. Clin Infect Dis 2000;30:65–70.

[63] Bolao F, Podzamczer D, Ventin M, et al. Efficacy of acute phase and maintenance therapy with itraconazole in an AIDS patient with sporotrichosis. Eur J Clin Microbiol Infect Dis 1994;13:609–12.

[64] Gottlieb GS, Lesser CF, Holmes KK, et al. Disseminated sporotrichosis associated with treatment with immunosuppressants and tumor necrosis factor–alpha antagonists. Clin Infect Dis 2003;37:638–40.

[65] Smego RA, Castiglia M, Asperilla MO. Lymphocutaneous syndrome. A review of non-Sporothrix causes. Medicine (Baltimore) 1999;78:38–63.

[66] Atdjian M, Granda JL, Ingberg HO, et al. Systemic sporotrichosis polytenosynovitis with median and ulnar nerve entrapment. JAMA 1980;243:1841–2.

[67] Pluss JL, Opal SM. Pulmonary sporotrichosis: review of treatment and outcome. Medicine (Baltimore) 1986;65:143–53.

[68] Al-Tawfiq JA, Wools KK. Disseminated sporotrichosis and *Sporothrix schenckii* fungemia as the initial presentation of human immunodeficiency virus infection. Clin Infect Dis 1998; 26:1403–6.

[69] Kauffman CA, Hajjeh R, Chapman SW. Practice guidelines for the management of patients with sporotrichosis. Clin Infect Dis 2000;30:684–7.

[70] Sharkey-Mathis PK, Kauffman CA, Graybill JR, et al. Treatment of sporotrichosis with itraconazole. Am J Med 1993;95:279–85.

[71] Restrepo A, Robledo J, Gomez I, et al. Itraconazole therapy in lymphangitic and cutaneous sporotrichosis. Arch Dermatol 1986;122:413–7.

[72] Kauffman CA, Pappas PG, McKinsey DS, et al. Treatment of lymphocutaneous and visceral sporotrichosis with fluconazole. Clin Infect Dis 1996;22:46–50.

[73] Chapman SW, Pappas P, Kauffman C, et al. Comparative evaluation of the efficacy and safety of two doses of terbinafine (500 and 1000 mg day^{-1}) in the treatment of cutaneous or lymphocutaneous sporotrichosis. Mycoses 2003;47:62–8.

[74] Kauffman CA. Old and new therapies for sporotrichosis. Clin Infect Dis 1995;21:981–5.

[75] Hiruma M, Kawada A, Noguchi H, et al. Hyperthermic treatment of sporotrichosis: experimental use of infrared and far infrared rays. Mycoses 1992;35:293–9.

ELSEVIER
SAUNDERS

Infect Dis Clin N Am
20 (2006) 663–678

INFECTIOUS
DISEASE CLINICS
OF NORTH AMERICA

Mycoses in Pediatric Patients

William J. Steinbach, MD[a],*, Thomas J. Walsh, MD[b]

[a]Department of Pediatrics, Division of Pediatric Infectious Diseases, and Department
of Molecular Genetics and Microbiology, Box 3499, Duke University Medical Center,
Durham, NC 27710, USA
[b]Immunocompromised Host Section, Pediatric Oncology Branch, CRC 1-5750, National
Cancer Institute, 10 Center Drive, Bethesda, MD 20892, USA

Fungal pathogens are an increasingly recognized complication of organ transplantation, childhood malignancies, neonatal medicine, and pediatric surgery. Fortunately the antifungal armamentarium available to clinicians has increased in the last several years to include new formulations of amphotericin B, antifungal triazoles, and the echinocandins. Important advances have been achieved in understanding the safety, tolerability, and pharmacokinetics of these antifungal agents in pediatric patients. Studies are ongoing as to the optimal use of these antifungal agents in the settings of prophylaxis, empiric therapy, and treatment of proven invasive fungal infections. Although data continue to accumulate on adult patients who have invasive fungal disease, there remains a paucity of pediatric interventional data. This discrepancy forces pediatricians to extrapolate many recommendations for use of antifungal agents in children from the studies conducted in adult patients. This article provides a brief overview of some of the unique differences in invasive fungal infections in children compared with those of adults and then focuses on the key differences in antifungal pharmacology and use in children. The specific pathogens are covered in greater detail elsewhere in this issue.

A worldwide survey of *Candida* isolates separated the results based by age and demonstrated that, although infection with *C albicans* was nearly uniform among all age groups, infection with *C parapsilosis* was more common in younger patients, whereas *C glabrata* was more prevalent in older patients [1]. Fluconazole was found to be less active against *C glabrata* in the youngest age group (≤ 1 year), whereas the species was more susceptible in the older cohorts. There were no highly resistant *C glabrata* isolates (minimum

---

* Corresponding author.
E-mail address: stein022@mc.duke.edu (W.J. Steinbach).

0891-5520/06/$ - see front matter. Published by Elsevier Inc.
doi:10.1016/j.idc.2006.06.006

inhibitory concentration [MIC] ≥ 64 $\mu g/mL$) in that youngest age group, but 5% to 9% of the isolates in the older groups were highly resistant [1]. This observation may be related to the greater exposure of older children to fluconazole for prophylaxis or therapeutic intervention.

Candidemia seems to have a somewhat different clinical presentation in children versus adult patients. In one prospective study the incidence of septic shock was greater in children versus adults (20% versus 10.8%, $P = .02$) with candidemia. Additionally, meningitis was found in 11.4% of infected children versus only 0.8% of infected adults ($P = .001$) [2]. A subsequent study confirmed the earlier epidemiologic reports of an increased proportion of *C parapsilosis* and decreased prevalence of *C glabrata* compared with that of adult patients [3]. This study also found that candidemia persisted longer in children compared with adult patients, and with a greater median number of positive blood cultures in pediatric candidemic patients.

The risk factors for candidemia in neonatal patients are different from those of older children. Risk factors have been clearly associated with a myriad of clinical aspects, including gestational age, birthweight, and others [4]. Birthweight in particular is consistently noted to be significantly correlated with disease development. In one study, infants with a birthweight of 400 to 750 grams possessed an odds ratio of 3.22 for developing candidiasis by the third day of life, compared with those infants born at 751 to 1000 grams [5]. Numerous organ systems can be involved in neonatal candidiasis, including most significantly a 49% concordance with urinary involvement in candidemia as reviewed in a large meta-analysis [6]. In a recent study of 4579 infants born at less than 1000 grams, 7% developed candidemia. Approximately 10% developed *Candida* meningitis, and yet half of those patients who developed meningitis had negative blood cultures [5].

Invasive aspergillosis in children offers some clinical differences from adult patients also [7]. Earlier reports have suggested that the species distribution of *Aspergillus* isolates for pediatric and adult patients is different. A large National Institute of Allergy and Infectious Diseases Bacteriology and Mycoses Study Group study reviewed 256 isolates of *Aspergillus* species from patients who had invasive aspergillosis from 24 medical centers [8], and *A fumigatus* yielded 67% (171/256) of isolates, whereas *A flavus* was the second most common isolate at 16% (41/256). This parallels the species distribution in the large voriconazole randomized clinical trial [9], in which 77% (85/110) were *A fumigatus* and 6% (7/110) were *A flavus*. In two large pediatric studies from Toronto [10] and St. Jude [11], however, *A flavus* was the predominant pathogen. In Toronto, 65% (17/26) of isolates were *A flavus*, followed by 15% (4/26) *A fumigatus* as the second most common pediatric *Aspergillus* isolate. At St. Jude, 72% (28/39) isolates were *A flavus*, followed by 38% (15/39) *A fumigatus* isolates. These differences may reflect greater environmental distribution of *A flavus* in these institutions.

In two more recent studies, however, the pediatric epidemiology paralleled previous adult studies. In the pediatric voriconazole compassionate release study, the species distribution was predominantly with patients infected with *A fumigatus* (26/42), followed by *A flavus* (6/42), and *A nidulans* (3/42) [12]. In a French pediatric study with amphotericin B lipid complex (ABLC) the most common isolates were *A fumigatus* (11/23), *A flavus* (6/23), *A niger* (1/23), and unspeciated *Aspergillus* spp (5/23) [13]. The differences in environmental exposure also parallel the differences in the site of infection, because the earlier studies with *A flavus* predominance cited a large percentage of cutaneous disease [10,11], whereas the later treatment studies contained mostly patients who had pulmonary aspergillosis [12,13].

The diagnostic features of invasive aspergillosis seem to also be different in children. In adult series of pulmonary aspergillosis, approximately 50% of cases show cavitation and 40% air crescent formation [14]. In one 10-year review of 27 consecutive pediatric patients (mean age, 5 years), there was central cavitation of small nodules in 25% of children and no evidence of air crescent formation within any area of consolidation [15]. In another pediatric report there was a 22% rate (6/27) of cavitation on chest radiography [16], and in a separate report there was a 43% rate (6/14) of cavitation on CT [17]. In these later two pediatric series, the mean ages were greater than the report of lower rates of cavitation and no air crescent formation, suggesting that there is a spectrum of radiologic disease presentation that is directly related to age. Perhaps cavitation and air crescent formation is more likely in the older child and adult than in the younger child.

Diagnosis of pediatric invasive aspergillosis with the enzyme immunoassay for galactomannan (GM) that is approved for use in adult patients is potentially difficult, because studies have shown repeated differences in pediatric and adult values. In one prospective study from Europe (1995–1998) of 450 adult allogeneic HSCT patients (3883 samples) and 347 children with hematologic malignancies (2376 samples), the false-positive rate in adult patients was 2.5% (10 of 406) and in children it was 10.1% (34 of 338) [18]. In another European study of 797 episodes, including 48 pediatric patients, the false-positive rate in the fever of unknown origin group was 0.9% in adults and 44.0% ($P < .0001$) in children. Additionally, the specificity of the test was lower in children, at 47.6% compared with 98.2% ($P < .0001$) in adult patients [19]. The causes of the false-positive results in these studies were not elucidated.

Galactomannan testing in children is associated with false-negative results in some specific pediatric patients, such as those who have chronic granulomatous disease (CGD). One report details a non-neutropenic 4-year-old child who had CGD and invasive aspergillosis diagnosed by lung biopsy who had persistent false-negative serum GM testing [20]. Another study evaluated patients who had CGD (n = 10), Job syndrome (n = 6), and invasive aspergillosis, and found GM antigenemia was detected in 4/15 cases of CGD and Job syndrome versus 24 of 30 cases of all other immunocompromised conditions ($P = .0004$) [21].

Antifungal options for pediatric and neonatal patients

There are several general reviews of antifungal pharmacology and spectrum of antifungal activity available [22–24]. One of the largest practical clinical issues facing those who care for children who have invasive fungal infections, however, is the lack of dedicated pediatric data. This problem is driven in part by the smaller number of patients available to perform complicated studies of pharmacology and dosing. During the past 15 years, however, there have been several studies dedicated to the systematic understanding of the safety, tolerability, and pharmacology of antifungal agents in pediatric patients. There are numerous precedents in medicine to suggest that dosing of antifungals would be different in children versus adults. Going beyond the concept of the correct dosage of antifungal is the obvious extension addressing efficacy in children, for which there are limited data. Here the authors' focus on some of the current thoughts on antifungal pharmacology and dosing in children.

Polyenes

Amphotericin B

Despite the availability of conventional amphotericin B deoxycholate for more than half a century, there are no studies comparing different dosages for the treatment of documented infections. Although opinions abound to this day, the optimal therapeutic dosage for this nephrotoxic agent for treatment of invasive fungal infections is not established. Although a higher dosage is likely to be more nephrotoxic, this does not necessarily translate into improved efficacy. Because of greater nephronal reserve, pediatric patients tend to tolerate the glomerular toxicity better than do adults; however, tubular toxicity reflected by hypokalemia in pediatric patients may be severe. The available pharmacokinetic data in pediatric patients suggest that the dosages of amphotericin B deoxycholate confer similar exposure to those of adults and do not require adjustment in children.

A multicenter maximum-tolerated dose study of liposomal amphotericin B (L-AmB) in adult patients using dosages from 7.5 to 15 mg/kg/d found a nonlinear plasma pharmacokinetic profile with a maximal concentration at 10 mg/kg/d and no demonstrable dose-limiting nephrotoxicity, infusion-related toxicity, or improvement in efficacy [25]. A recent randomized clinical trial comparing L-AmB at a standard dose of 3 mg/kg/d versus a higher dose of 10 mg/kg/d in adults failed to show any improvement in efficacy and only yielded more nephrotoxicity with the higher dose [26]. A pharmacokinetic study of L-AmB conducted in 39 children observed no dose-related trends in adverse events and a maximally-tolerated dose of 10 mg/kg/d (Gilead Sciences, data on file), similar to adult data. A 56-center prospective study evaluated the safety and efficacy of L-AmB administered to 260 adults, 242 children (<15 years), and 43 infants younger than

2 months of age [27]. In general, the infants and children tolerated the largest doses of L-AmB administered for the longest period of time (median, 16 days) [27], dispelling historical notions that children were unable to tolerate such a potentially toxic antifungal agent.

There are no large randomized controlled studies comparing amphotericin B deoxycholate and a lipid formulation of amphotericin B for treatment of documented invasive mycoses [28–32]. The few randomized studies, although informative, are limited by a heterogenous patient population and small sample size (large beta error). Although mortality was slightly lower in patients treated with L-AmB compared with AmB in one study with a small number of patients [33], another study showed no difference in response in treatment of documented invasive aspergillosis with amphotericin B colloidal dispersion versus deoxycholate amphotericin B [34]; amphotericin B deoxycholate was, however, more nephrotoxic. Although amphotericin B-induced nephrotoxicity is associated with excess mortality in adults, its impact in pediatric patients is not well defined. A study of 56 infants who had candidiasis, including 52 preterm infants, showed no differences in mortality or time to resolution of candidemia between neonates receiving conventional amphotericin B (n = 34), L-AB (n = 6), or amphotericin B colloidal dispersion (n = 16) [35]. The decision to prescribe a lipid formulation of amphotericin B therefore should be based on the potential of reducing nephrotoxicity or infusion-related toxicity rather than anticipated therapeutic benefit.

Among six children with hepatosplenic candidiasis (HSC) who received 2.5 mg/kg of ABLC for 6 weeks for a total dosage of 105 mg/kg, the mean serum creatinine (0.85 ± 0.12 mg/dL at baseline) was stable at the end of therapy at 0.85 ± 0.18 mg/dL and at 1-month follow-up at 0.72 ± 0.12 mg/dL [36]. Plasma pharmacokinetics suggested steady state was achieved by day 7 of therapy. The five evaluable patients responded to ABLC with complete or partial resolution of physical findings and of lesions of HSC. During the course of ABLC infusions and follow-up, there was no progression of HSC, breakthrough fungemia, or post-therapy recurrence. Hepatic lesions continued to resolve after the completion of administration of ABLC.

A more recent study of the pharmacokinetics of ABLC in neonates who had invasive candidiasis demonstrated that this compound has a similar pharmacokinetic profile to that of adults [37]. ABLC also was active in treatment of candidemia in these infants.

In non-comparative studies, ABLC has been found to be an effective antifungal agent in children. In an open-label pediatric trial, complete or partial therapeutic response was observed in 70% (38/54) of patients, including 56% (14/25) of those who had aspergillosis and 81% (22/27) of those who had candidiasis [38]. A retrospective study of 46 children treated with ABLC reported an overall response rate of 83% (38/46), including 78% (18/23) against aspergillosis and 89% (17/19) against candidiasis [13].

There are few published data on the use of lipid formulations of amphotericin B in neonates. One study that included 40 preterm neonates (mean birthweight, 1090 g; mean gestational age, 28.4 weeks) noted that L-AmB was associated with clinical resolution in more than 70% of patients who had candidiasis [39]; other uncontrolled studies have confirmed the high response rates. For example, in three other studies, 83% to 100% of neonates who had candidiasis cleared their infections [40].

Amphotericin B nephrotoxicity is generally less severe in infants and children than in adults, likely because of the greater nephronal reserve in children. Reports of reduced nephrotoxicity with a lipid formulation in adults also have been observed in children [38,41] and neonates [42].

Triazoles

Fluconazole

The pharmacokinetics of fluconazole differ between adults and children. In an early study of the safety, tolerance, and pharmacokinetics of fluconazole in children who had neoplastic diseases, the plasma half-life was found to be approximately one half that of adults, indicating the need for a higher dosage of fluconazole in pediatric patients [43]. A subsequent review of five separate fluconazole pharmacokinetic studies that included 101 infants and children ranging in age from 2 weeks to 16 years [44] demonstrated that fluconazole clearance is more rapid in children than in adults. The mean plasma half-life was approximately 20 hours in children, compared with 30 hours in adults. To achieve comparable drug exposure, the daily fluconazole dosage therefore needs to be approximately doubled for children older than 3 months of age to 6 to 12 mg/kg/day.

The volume of distribution of fluconazole is greater and more variable in neonates than in infants and children. There is also a slow elimination of fluconazole, however, with a mean half-life of 88.6 hours at birth, decreasing to approximately 55 hours by 2 weeks of age. Neonates therefore should be treated with a higher dose of fluconazole to compensate for their increased volume of distribution, but the frequency of dosing needs to be decreased because of their slow elimination. Specifically, during the first 2 weeks of life, fluconazole should be dosed every 72 hours; this dosing interval can be reduced to 48 hours during the next 2 weeks of life [44]. The pharmacologic consequence of such a long half-life is that patients require at least 8 days to reach steady-state [45].

Side effects of fluconazole are uncommon. Among 26 pediatric oncology patients receiving fluconazole, there was no nausea or vomiting related to fluconazole, whereas three patients had an asymptomatic increase in hepatic aminotransferase values after 4 to 6 doses (one patient at 2 mg/kg/d and two patients at 8 mg/kg/day), which returned to normal within 2 weeks after discontinuation of the drug [43]. In another study of 24 immunocompromised children, elevated transaminases were observed in only two cases [46].

Another review of 562 children confirmed that pediatric results mirror the excellent safety profile seen in adults. The most common side effects were gastrointestinal upset (7.7%) (vomiting, diarrhea, nausea) or a skin rash (1.2%) [47].

Clinical and mycologic response was observed in 97% of 40 neonates and infants who had candidiasis treated with fluconazole. These children had been either nonresponsive or intolerant to standard antifungal therapy [48]. In another report, 80% of 40 neonates who had invasive candidiasis were successfully treated with 6 mg/kg/d of fluconazole. Although three of these patients relapsed, they ultimately were cured with an increased dose of fluconazole (10 mg/kg/d) [49]. Finally, a prospective randomized study that compared fluconazole to amphotericin B in 24 infants who had candidemia noted a survival benefit among those treated with fluconazole (67%) compared with those who received amphotericin B (55%) [50].

Fluconazole also has been evaluated for neonatal antifungal prophylaxis. A prospective, placebo-controlled, randomized, double-blind evaluation of prophylactic fluconazole has been conducted in 100 low birthweight (<1000 g) infants. Six weeks of fluconazole therapy resulted in a statistically significant reduction in the frequency of fungal colonization (22% versus 60%; $P = .002$) and a decrease in the development of invasive fungal infection (0% versus 20%) [51]. The risk for developing a fungal infection in the fluconazole-prophylaxis infants was 0.20 (95% CI, 0.04–0.36, $P = .008$), but overall mortality was unaffected. A subsequent study evaluated only twice-weekly prophylaxis and found that fluconazole at the lower total dose led to lower colonization and disease compared with placebo and no emergence of fluconazole resistance [52]. Whether fluconazole should be used in prophylaxis in low-birthweight infants in a given institution depends on the frequency of invasive candidiasis in the NICU.

Itraconazole

In a study of 26 pediatric oncology patients (ages 6 months to 12 years), itraconazole oral solution produced a maximum concentration lower than in adults, whereas other pharmacokinetic properties such as half-life are similar to that of adults [53]. In this study, itraconazole at 5 mg/kg once daily resulted in plasma concentrations substantially lower than that historically reported in adults, especially in the children less than 2 years old [53]. The reason for this difference may have been related to the effects of chemotherapy on mucosal integrity and bioavailability. Another study of children aged 1.7 to 14.3 years showed that a split dosing of 2.5 mg/kg twice daily yielded peak and trough plasma concentrations similar to adults, but there was less exposure in the children younger than 5 years old [54].

The safety, pharmacokinetics, and pharmacodynamics of cyclodextrin itraconazole (CD-ITRA) oral suspension also were investigated in an open sequential dose-escalation study in 26 HIV-infected children and adolescents (5–18 years of age; mean CD4+ count, 128/μL) with oropharyngeal candidiasis (OPC) [55]. Patients received either 2.5 mg/kg daily or 2.5 mg/kg twice daily of CD-ITRA for a total of 15 days. Apart from mild to moderate gastrointestinal disturbances in three patients (11.5%), CD-ITRA was well tolerated; however, two patients (7.6%) discontinued treatment prematurely because of study-drug–related adverse events. A significantly higher percentage ($P < .05$) of patients in the 2.5 mg/kg twice-daily cohort achieved a complete clinical and mycologic response at end of therapy, indicating dose-dependent antifungal efficacy. Pharmacodynamic modeling revealed significant correlations between plasma concentrations and antifungal efficacy. Based on this documented safety and efficacy, a dosage of 2.5 mg/kg twice daily was recommended for treatment of OPC in pediatric patients older than 5 years of age [55].

A double-blind trial of 63 patients who had HIV infection in Thailand with itraconazole versus placebo showed development of systemic fungal infection decreased from 16.7% of patients given placebo versus 1.6% taking itraconazole, with only one infection with *Penicillium marneffei* in the itraconazole treatment arm [56].

Voriconazole

A multicenter study of the safety, tolerability, and plasma pharmacokinetics of the parenteral formulation of voriconazole in immunocompromised pediatric patients (2–11 years of age) demonstrated that children require higher dosages of voriconazole than adults to attain similar serum concentrations over time, because the drug exhibits nonlinear pharmacokinetics in adults, but exhibits linearity in children at the dosages between 3 and 4 mg/kg/dose [57]. Body weight was more influential than age in accounting for the observed variability in voriconazole pharmacokinetics. As observed in adults, elimination capacity correlated with CYP2C19 genotype. This study concluded that pediatric patients have a higher elimination capacity per kilogram of body weight of voriconazole than do adult healthy volunteers and that dosages of 4 mg/kg may be necessary to achieve exposures consistent with those in adults following 3 mg/kg, whereas dosages ≥ 5 mg/kg would be necessary to exposures comparable to that of 4 mg/kg in adults.

A subsequent pharmacokinetic study was performed to evaluate dosages of 4 to 8 mg/kg [58]. Although there was a large inter-patient variation in the individual pharmacokinetic parameters, the population-based pharmacokinetic model of these data support a dosage of 7 mg/kg in pediatric patients to approach an exposure achieved by 4 mg/kg in adults.

The largest pediatric report of voriconazole is an open-label, compassionate-use evaluation of the drug in 58 children who had proven or probable invasive fungal infection refractory to or intolerant of conventional antifungal therapy [12]. Voriconazole was administered as a loading dose of 6 mg/kg every 12 hours on the first day of therapy, followed by 4 mg/kg every 12 hours on subsequent days. When possible, the conversion to oral therapy was made with a dose of 100 or 200 mg twice a day for patients weighing less than 40 kg and greater than or equal to 40 kg, respectively. Almost three quarters of the patients had invasive aspergillosis. The most common treatment-related adverse reactions were transaminase or bilirubin elevation in 13.8% of patients, rash in 13.8%, abnormal vision (photophobia or blurred vision) in 5.1%, and photosensitivity reactions in 5.1% of patients. Only three patients discontinued voriconazole because of toxicity. Complete or partial response was observed in 43% of children who had aspergillosis, 50% with candidemia and 63% with scedosporiosis.

Voriconazole has not been formally tested in neonates. Because of reports of visual adverse events in adults and pediatric patients, there is concern over the unknown interactions with the developing retina and there are no planned clinical trials in this age group.

Posaconazole

Posaconazole has dose-proportional pharmacokinetics up to 800 mg/d, with bioavailability greatest when administered in divided doses, and has a large apparent volume of distribution with slow elimination, suggesting an extensive distribution into tissues [59]. Although approved in the European Union, posaconazole is currently only used as a compassionate release agent in the United States as an oral formulation, but an intravenous prodrug is also under development.

One retrospective study analyzed the pharmacokinetic profile of posaconazole for 12 pediatric patients (<18 years old) with resistant or refractory invasive fungal infections. These patients received a maintenance dose of 800 mg/d of posaconazole oral suspension given in two or three divided daily doses, compared with adult patients (18–64 years old) who received a maintenance dose of 800 mg/d and who were used as a comparison. The overall success rate and adverse event profile were similar for pediatric and adult patients [60]. Although only preliminary data, these results suggest that posaconazole pharmacokinetics are similar in adults and the children examined in this study.

Experience with posaconazole in children is limited. A recent open-label study of eight patients who had chronic granulomatous disease and invasive mold infection treated with posaconazole salvage therapy included seven pediatric patients. All patients had received itraconazole prophylaxis and had prior antifungal therapy with voriconazole, caspofungin, or a lipid formulation of amphotericin B [61]. There was a complete response with posaconazole in 7 of 8 patients, including 6 of 7 pediatric patients. Two other pediatric patients were enrolled in another open-label study of 23 patients who had zygomycosis. The overall success rate of therapy in this second study was 70% [62], but there were no pediatric-specific outcomes reported. Posaconazole may have an important role in antifungal management in the future; however, further studies of the pharmacokinetics, safety, and efficacy in pediatric patients have yet to be performed.

Echinocandins

Caspofungin

Caspofungin was evaluated in a pharmacokinetic study conducted in 39 children between the ages of 2 and 17 years. Data were analyzed on the basis of weight (1 mg/kg/d) and body surface area (50 or 70 mg/m^2/day) [63]. When compared with plasma concentrations attained in adults treated with 50 mg/day, the weight-based approach resulted in suboptimal plasma concentrations, whereas the 50 mg/m^2/day dose yielded similar plasma concentrations in children. Caspofungin's half-life is approximately one third less in children than in adults. Additionally, pediatric patient concentrations descend more rapidly compared with adults. The nuances in children continue, however, because body surface area dosing is consistent across pediatric ages; yet, there are statistically significant decreases in end-of-infusion concentrations of caspofungin with increasing age. Based on this initial study, subsequent dosing in children has been proposed to include a loading dose of 70 mg/m^2 followed by daily maintenance dosing of 50 mg/m^2.

A multicenter retrospective survey in Germany analyzed 53 immunocompromised pediatric patients considered to require caspofungin therapy [64] for refractory infection (n = 35), intolerance of standard agents (n = 7), or as the best perceived therapeutic option (n = 11). In 13 evaluable patients who had proven infection, complete responses (4 of 13), partial responses (6 of 13), or stabilization (2 of 13) were observed. This was compared with 11 evaluable patients who had probable infection, in whom complete responses (3 of 11), partial responses (1 of 11), or stabilization (3 of 11) were observed. Most patients (11 of 13) on empiric therapy completed without breakthrough fungal infection. Overall survival was 72% at end of therapy and 64% (44 evaluable patients) at 3 months post-end of therapy [64].

Several pediatric clinical studies using caspofungin are currently in progress. These include a multicenter, open-label comparative study evaluating the safety, tolerability, and efficacy of caspofungin in children who have documented *Candida* or *Aspergillus* infections and a pharmacokinetic and safety study in children between the ages of 3 and 24 months who have new-onset fever and neutropenia. Although there are good pharmacokinetic data to show the importance of an increased dose of caspofungin in a child versus an adult patient, the data on efficacy and the range of usefulness of the drug in children who have invasive fungal infections are largely limited to case reports and case series data. It is hoped these ongoing phase IV studies will allow greater insight into pediatric uses of caspofungin.

There have been limited reports of caspofungin use in neonates who have invasive candidiasis. The first case series of caspofungin for rescue therapy in treatment of refractory invasive candidiasis in neonates was reported by Odio and colleagues [65]. The population consisted of one term and nine premature neonates who had invasive candidiasis caused by *Candida albicans*, *Candida parapsilosis*, *Candida tropicalis*, and *Candida glabrata*.

Despite initial therapy with amphotericin B deoxycholate, blood cultures remained positive in all patients for 13 to 49 days. Invasive candidiasis progressed to meningitis and enlarging renal *Candida* bezoars in the kidney of one patient and an enlarging atrial vegetation in another infant. A caspofungin dosage of 1 mg/kg/d for 2 days followed by 2 mg/kg/d resulted in all positive blood cultures clearing between 3 and 7 days. The atrial vegetation and the renal *Candida* bezoars also resolved without attributable clinical adverse events. In the largest report, caspofungin was added to amphotericin B, fluconazole, or 5-fluorocytosine for 13 infants who had a median birthweight of 800 grams whose candidemia persisted despite conventional antifungal therapy. After addition of caspofungin, blood sterilization occurred in a mean of 3 days [66].

Micafungin

Several pediatric studies of micafungin have been completed. A phase I single-dose, multicenter, open-label neonatal study evaluated three dosages (0.75 mg/kg/d, 1.5 mg/kg/d, and 3 mg/kg/d) in two infant weight groups (500–1000 g and >1000 g). The mean serum concentration of micafungin was lower in the smaller infants, and the serum half-life was shorter and clearance more rapid. For instance, in the 500- to 1000-gram neonates, the half-life was 5.5 hours with a clearance of 97.3 mL/h/kg. In the neonates weighing more than 1000 grams, the half-life increased to 8 hours, whereas clearance decreased to 55.9 mL/h/kg. This compares with children (ages 2–8 years) in whom half-life extended to 12 hours and clearance was slowest at 32.2 mL/h/kg [67].

A phase I study in persistently febrile neutropenic pediatric patients (2–17 years old) found that doses up to 4 mg/kg/d were well tolerated with no side effects. A total of 78 children (mean age, 7.1 years) received at least one dose of micafungin with no signs of nephrotoxicity or hepatotoxicity. The micafungin pharmacokinetics were dose-proportional over the range tested and mean half-life values were constant on days 1 and 4 [68]. Dosing in children younger than age 8 years seems to yield a clearance 1.3 to 1.5 times greater of micafungin, resulting in the likely need for an increased dose in this age cohort. In general, the terminal half-life of micafungin does not change appreciably in pediatric versus adult patients, and the volume of distribution is only slightly higher in children [69]. Despite these early pharmacokinetic studies and the recent FDA approval, there is no accepted dosage for micafungin in pediatric patients.

A recent study of micafungin in combination with a second antifungal agent in pediatric and adult bone marrow transplant recipients who had invasive aspergillosis revealed an overall complete or partial response of 39.1% in adult patients and 37.5% in pediatric (n = 16) patients [70]. Other studies have demonstrated the efficacy of micafungin in the primary therapy of esophageal candidiasis [71], and as rescue therapy in those failing to respond to first-line antifungals [72]. In an open-label non-comparative study of new or refractory candidemia that included 15.1% (18 of 119) pediatric patients, the overall complete or partial response was 85.1% (86 of 101) in adult patients but only 72.2% (13 of 18) in pediatric patients [73], possibly because of inadequate dosing in children.

A study comparing prophylaxis in 882 stem-cell transplant recipients found that micafungin (80%) was more effective in preventing yeast and mold infections than fluconazole (73.5%) [74]. This study included 84 patients younger than age 16 years and found the success in those patients was 69.2% (27 of 39) in the micafungin arm and 53.3% (24 of 45) in the fluconazole arm. These values are lower than the results for patients aged 16 to 64 years in whom micafungin was 81.1% effective and fluconazole was 75.7% effective.

These few clinical studies comparing micafungin in adult and pediatric patients suggest further investigation into the nuances of pediatric efficacy is warranted. At present there are no reports of micafungin in neonates, but a large phase III trial comparing micafungin versus amphotericin B deoxycholate for neonatal candidiasis is currently underway.

Anidulafungin

A phase I/II dose escalation study of anidulafungin involving five centers enrolled children who had persistent neutropenia who were at risk for invasive fungal infection, and data were determined in 12 patients (0.75 mg/kg/d) and 7 patients (1.5 mg/kg/d) following the first and fifth dose of anidulafungin. No drug-related serious adverse events were observed; one patient had fever and one patient had rash/facial erythema that resolved with slowing the infusion rate. Anidulafungin in pediatric patients was well tolerated and can be dosed based on body weight. Pediatric patients receiving 0.75 mg/kg/d or 1.5 mg/kg/d have pharmacokinetics similar to adult patients receiving 50 or 100 mg/d, respectively [75]. This important fact separates anidulafungin from the pharmacokinetic values observed with caspofungin, which necessitated a higher dosing based on body surface area.

Summary

For more than 40 years, there has been limited progress in the treatment of invasive fungal infections. There are now numerous nuances to choosing the appropriate antifungal agent. Important advances have been achieved in understanding the safety, tolerability, and pharmacokinetics of these agents. One of the most important aspects for successful management of pediatric invasive fungal infections is an understanding of the differences in the pharmacokinetics of the drug in children and adults to offer optimal dosing strategies. Unfortunately there have been few antifungal studies conducted in children. Consequently most information for the pediatrician has been extrapolated from adult data. The breadth of antifungal data in children is expanding, however, with newer studies underway. Through the efforts of dedicated clinicians and collaboration, pediatric indications and dosing strategies will eventually be discovered that directly benefit pediatric patients.

References

[1] Pfaller MA, Diekema DJ, Jones RN, et al. Trends in antifungal susceptibility of *Candida* spp. isolated from pediatric and adult patients with bloodstream infections: SENTRY Antimicrobial Surveillance Program, 1997 to 2000. J Clin Microbiol 2002;40:852.

[2] Krupova Y, Sejnova D, Dzatkova J, et al. Prospective study on fungemia in children with cancer: analysis of 35 cases and comparison with 130 fungemias in adults. Support Care Cancer 2000;8:427.

[3] Pasqualotto AC, Nedel WL, Machado TS, et al. A 9-year study comparing risk factors and the outcome of paediatric and adults with nosocomial candidaemia. Mycopathologia 2005; 160:111.

[4] Benjamin DKJ, Garges H, Steinbach WJ. Candida bloodstream infection in neonates. Semin Perinatol 2003;27:375.

[5] Benjamin DKJ, Stoll BJ, Fanaroff AA, et al. Neonatal candidiasis among extremely low birth weight infants: risk factors, mortality rates, and neurodevelopmental outcomes at 18 to 22 months. Pediatrics 2006;117:84.

[6] Benjamin DKJ, Poole C, Steinbach WJ, et al. Neonatal candidemia and end-organ damage: a critical appraisal of the literature using meta-analytic techniques. Pediatrics 2003; 112(3 Pt 1):634.

[7] Steinbach WJ. Pediatric aspergillosis: disease and treatment differences in children. Pediatr Infect Dis J 2005;24:358.

[8] Perfect JR, Cox GM, Lee JY, et al. The impact of culture isolation of *Aspergillus* species: a hospital-based survey of aspergillosis. Clin Infect Dis 1824;2001:33.

[9] Herbrecht R, Denning DW, Patterson TF, et al. Voriconazole versus amphotericin B for primary therapy of invasive aspergillosis. N Engl J Med 2002;347:408.

[10] Walmsley S, Devi S, King S, et al. Invasive *Aspergillus* infections in a pediatric hospital: a ten year review. Pediatr Infect Dis J 1993;12:673.

[11] Abbasi S, Shenep JL, Hughes WT, et al. Aspergillosis in children with cancer: a 34-year experience. Clin Infect Dis 1999;29:1210.

[12] Walsh TJ, Lutsar I, Driscoll T, et al. Voriconazole in the treatment of aspergillosis, scedosporiosis and other invasive fungal infections in children. Pediatr Infect Dis J 2002; 21:240.

[13] Herbrecht R, Auvrignon A, Andres E, et al. Efficacy of amphotericin B lipid complex in the treatment of invasive fungal infections in immunosuppressed paediatric patients. Eur J Clin Microbiol Infect Dis 2001;20:77.

[14] Gefter WB, Albelda SM, Talbot GH, et al. Invasive pulmonary aspergillosis and acute leukemia: limitations in the diagnostic utility of the air crescent sign. Radiology 1985;157:605.

[15] Thomas KE, Owens CM, Veys PA, et al. The radiological spectrum of invasive aspergillosis in children: a 10-year review. Pediatr Radiol 2003;33:453.

[16] Allan BT, Patton D, Ramsey NKC, et al. Pulmonary fungal infections after bone marrow transplantation. Pediatr Radiol 1988;18:118.

[17] Taccone A, Occhi M, Garaventa A, et al. CT of invasive pulmonary aspergillosis in children with cancer. Pediatr Radiol 1993;23:177.

[18] Sulahian A, Tabouret M, Ribaud P, et al. Comparison of an enzyme immunoassay and latex agglutination test for detection of galactomannan in the diagnosis of invasive aspergillosis. Eur J Clin Microbiol Infect Dis 1996;15:139.

[19] Herbrecht R, Letscher-Bru V, Oprea C, et al. *Aspergillus* galactomannan detection in the diagnosis of invasive aspergillosis in cancer patients. J Clin Oncol 2002;7:1898.

[20] Verweij PE, Weemaes CM, Curfs JHAJ, et al. Failure to detect circulating *Aspergillus* markers in a patient with chronic granulomatous disease and invasive aspergillosis. J Clin Microbiol 2000;38:3900.

[21] Walsh TJ, Schaufele RL, Sein T, et al. Reduced expression of galactomannan antigenemia in patients with invasive aspergillosis and chronic granulomatous disease or Job's syndrome. Program and Abstracts of the 40th Annual Meeting of the Infectious Diseases Society of America, Chicago, IL, October 24–27, 2002.

[22] Groll AH, Piscitelli S, Walsh TJ. Clinical pharmacology of systemic antifungal agents: a comprehensive review of agents in clinical use, current investigational compounds, and putative targets for antifungal drug. Adv Pharmacol 1998;44:343–500.

[23] Steinbach WJ, Stevens DA. Review of newer antifungal and immunomodulatory strategies for invasive aspergillosis. Clin Infect Dis 2003;37(Suppl 3):S157.

[24] Walsh TJ, Viviani MA, Arathoon E, et al. New targets and delivery systems for antifungal therapy. Med Mycol 2000;38:335.

[25] Walsh TJ, Goodman JL, Pappas P, et al. Safety, tolerance, and pharmacokinetics of high-dose liposomal amphotericin B (AmBisome) in patients infected with *Aspergillus* species and other filamentous fungi: maximum tolerate dose study. Antimicrob Agents Chemother 2001;45:3487.

[26] Cornely OA, Maertens J, Bresnik M, et al. Liposomal amphotericin B as initial therapy for invasive filamentous fungal infections: a randomized, prospective trial of a high loading regimen vs. standard dosing (AmBiLoad trial). 47th American Society of Hematology Annual Meeting, Atlanta, GA, October 10–13, 2005.

[27] Anak S. Safety and efficacy of AmBisome in patients with fungal infections. A post marketing multicentre surveillance study in Turkey. In: Focus on fungal infections 14. New Orleans, LA, March 24–26, 2004.

[28] Dismukes WE. Introduction to antifungal agents. Clin Infect Dis 2000;30:653.

[29] Dix SP, Andriole VT. Lipid formulations of amphotericin B. Curr Clin Top Infect Dis 2000; 20:1.

[30] Graybill JR, Tollemar J, Torres-Rodriguez JM, et al. Antifungal compounds: controversies, queries and conclusions. Med Mycol 2000;38:323.

[31] Walsh TJ, Hiemenz JW, Seibel NL, et al. Amphotericin B lipid complex for invasive fungal infections: analysis of safety and efficacy in 556 cases. Clin Infect Dis 1998;26:1383.

[32] Wong-Beringer A, Jacobs RA, Guglielmo BJ. Lipid formulations of amphotericin B: Clinical efficacy and toxicities. Clin Infect Dis 1998;27:603.

[33] Leenders ACAP, Daenen S, Jansen RLH, et al. Liposomal amphotericin B compared with amphotericin B deoxycholate in the treatment of documented and suspected neutropenia-associated invasive fungal infections. Br J Haematol 1998;103:205.

[34] Bowden R, Chandrasekar P, White MH, et al. A double-blind, randomized, controlled trial of amphotericin B colloidal dispersion versus amphotericin B for the treatment of invasive aspergillosis in immunocompromised patients. Clin Infect Dis 2002;35:359.

[35] Linder N, Klinger G, Shalit I, et al. Treatment of candidaemia in premature infants: comparison of three amphotericin B products. J Antimicrob Chemother 2003;52:663.

[36] Walsh TJ, Whitcomb P, Piscitelli S, et al. Safety, tolerance, and pharmacokinetics of amphotericin B lipid complex in children with hepatosplenic candidiasis. Antimicrob Agents Chemother 1997;41:1944.

[37] Würthwein G, Groll AH, Hempel G, et al. Population pharmacokinetics of amphotericin B lipid complex in neonates. Antimicrob Agents Chemother 2005;49:5092.

[38] Walsh TJ, Seibel NL, Arndt C, et al. Amphotericin B lipid complex in pediatric patients with invasive fungal infections. Pediatr Infect Dis J 1998;18:702.

[39] Scarcella A, Pasquariello MB, Guigliano B, et al. Liposomal amphotericin B treatment for neonatal fungal infections. Pediatr Infect Dis J 1998;17:146.

[40] Weitkamp JH, Poets CF, Sievers R, et al. Candida infection in very low birth-weight infants: outcome and nephrotoxicity of treatment with liposomal amphotericin B (AmBisome). Infection 1998;26:11.

[41] Sandler ES, Mustafa MM, Tkaczewski I, et al. Use of amphotericin B colloidal dispersion in children. J Pediatr Hematol Oncol 2000;22:242.

[42] Al Arishi H, Frayha HH, Kalloghlian A, et al. Liposomal amphotericin B in neonates with invasive candidiasis. Am J Perinatol 1998;15:643.

[43] Lee JW, Seibel NI, Amantea MA, et al. Safety, tolerance, and pharmacokinetics of fluconazole in children with neoplastic diseases. J Pediatr 1992;120:987.

[44] Brammer KW, Coates PE. Pharmacokinetics of fluconazole in pediatric patients. Eur J Clin Microbiol Infect Dis 1994;13:325.

[45] Debruyne D. Clinical pharmacokinetics of fluconazole in superficial and systemic mycoses. Clin Pharmacokinet 1997;33:52.

[46] Vscoli CE, Castagnola M, Fioredda B, et al. Fluconazole in the treatment of candidiasis in immunocompromised children. Antimicrob Agents Chemother 1991;35:365.

[47] Novelli V, Holzel H. Safety and tolerability of fluconazole in children. Antimicrob Agents Chemother 1999;43:1955.

[48] Fasano C, O'Keeffe J, Gibbs D. Fluconazole treatment of neonates and infants with severe fungal infections not treatable with conventional agents. Eur J Clin Microbiol Infect Dis 1994;13:325.

[49] Huttova M, Hartmanova I, Kralinsjy K, et al. *Candida* fungemia in neonates treated with fluconazole: report of forty cases, including eight with meningitis. Pediatr Infect Dis J 1998;17:1012.

[50] Driessen M, Ellis JB, Cooper PA, et al. Fluconazole vs. amphotericin B for the treatment of neonatal fungal septicemia: a prospective randomized trial. Pediatr Infect Dis J 1996;15:1107.

[51] Kaufman D, Boyle R, Hazen KC, et al. Fluconazole prophylaxis against fungal colonization and infection in preterm infants. N Engl J Med 2001;345:1660.

[52] Kaufman D, Boyle R, Hazen KC, et al. Twice weekly fluconazole prophylaxis for prevention of invasive *Candida* infection in high-risk infants of < 1000 grams birth weight. J Pediatr 2005;147:172.

[53] de Repentigny L, Ratelle J, Leclerc J-M, et al. Repeated-dose pharmacokinetic of an oral solution of itraconazole in infants and children. Antimicrob Agents Chemother 1998;42:404.

[54] Schmitt C, Perel Y, Harousseau JL, et al. Pharmacokinetics of itraconazole oral solution in neutropenic children during long-term prophylaxis. Antimicrob Agents Chemother 2001;45:1561.

[55] Groll AH, Wood L, Roden M, et al. Safety, pharmacokinetics, and pharmacodynamics of cyclodextrin itraconazole in pediatric patients with oropharyngeal candidiasis. Antimicrob Agents Chemother 2002;46:2554.

[56] Chariyalertsak S, Supparatpinyo K, Sirisanthana T, et al. A controlled trial of itraconazole as primary prophylaxis for systemic fungal infections in patients with advanced human immunodeficiency virus infection in Thailand. Clin Infect Dis 2002;34:277.

[57] Walsh TJ, Karlsson MO, Driscoll T, et al. Pharmacokinetics and safety of intravenous voriconazole in children after single- or multiple-dose administration. Antimicrob Agents Chemother 2004;48:2166.

[58] Walsh TJ, Driscoll T, Groll A, et al. Pharmacokinetics, safety, and tolerability of voriconazole in hospitalized children. 46th Annual Interscience Conference on Antimicrobial Agents and Chemotherapy. San Francisco, CA.

[59] Ullmann AJ, Cornely OA, Burchardt A, et al. Pharmacokinetics, safety, and efficacy of posaconazole in patients with persistent febrile neutropenia or refractory invasive fungal infection. Antimicrob Agents Chemother 2006;50:658.

[60] Krishna G, Wexler D, Courtney R, et al. Posaconazole plasma concentrations in pediatric patients with invasive fungal infections. Program of the 44th Interscience Conference on Antimicrobial Agents and Chemotherapy, Washington, DC, October 30-November 2, 2004.

[61] Segal BH, Barnhart LA, Anderson VL, et al. Posaconazole as salvage therapy in patients with chronic granulomatous disease and invasive filamentous fungal infection. Clin Infect Dis 2005;40:1684.

[62] Greenberg RN, Anstead G, Herbrecht R, et al. Posaconazole experience in the treatment of zygomycosis. Program and Abstracts of the 43rd Annual Interscience Conference on Antimicrobial Agents and Chemotherapy, Chicago, IL, September 14–17, 2003.

[63] Walsh TJ, Adamson PC, Seibel NL, et al. Pharmacokinetics, safety, and tolerability of caspofungin in children and adolescents. Antimicrob Agents Chemother 2005;49:4536.

[64] Lehrnbecher T, Attarbaschi A, Schuster F, et al. Caspofungin in immunocompromised pediatric patients without therapeutic alternative: a multicenter survey. Program of the 44th Interscience Conference on Antimicrobial Agents and Chemotherapy, Washington, DC, October 30-November 2, 2004.

[65] Odio CM, Araya R, Pinto LE, et al. Caspofungin therapy of neonates with invasive candidiasis. Pediatr Infect Dis J 2004;23:1093.

[66] Natarajan G, Lulic-Botics M, Rongkavilt C, et al. Experience with caspofungin in the treatment of persistent fungemia in neonates. J Perinatol 2005;25:770–7.

[67] Heresi GP, Gerstmann DR, Blumer JL, et al. Pharmacokinetic study of micafungin in premature neonates. Pediatric Academic Society Meeting, Seattle, WA.

[68] Seibel NL, Schwartz C, Arrieta A, et al. Safety, tolerability, and pharmacokinetics of micafungin (FK463) in febrile neutropenic pediatric patients. Antimicrob Agents Chemother 2005;49:3317.

[69] Townsend R, Bekersky I, Buell DN, et al. Pharmacokinetic evaluation of echinocandin FK463 in pediatric and adult patients. Focus on Fungal Infections 11. Washington, DC.

[70] Ratanatharathorn V, Flynn P, Van Burik JA, et al. Micafungin in combination with systemic antifungal agents in the treatment of refractory aspergillosis in bone marrow transplant patients. Program and abstracts of the American Society of Hematology 44th Annual Meeting, Philadelphia, December 6–10, 2002.

[71] Suleiman J, Della Negra M, Llanos-Cuentas A, et al. Open label study of micafungin in the treatment of esophageal candidiasis. Program and abstracts of the 42nd Interscience Conference on Antimicrobial Agents and Chemotherapy. San Diego, CA, September 27–30, 2002.

[72] Ullmann AJ, Van Burik JA, McSweeney P, et al. An open phase II study of the efficacy of micafungin (FK463) alone and in combination for the treatment of invasive aspergillosis in adults and children. 13th European Congress of Clinical Microbiology and Infectious Diseases, Glasgow, UK, May 10–13, 2003.

[73] Ostrosky-Zeichner L, Anaissie E, Kontoyannis D, et al. Micafungin, an echinocandin antifungal agent for the treatment of new and refractory candidemia. Focus on fungal infections 13. Maui, HI, March 19–21, 2003.

[74] van Burik JA, Ratanatharathorn V, Stepan DE, et al. Micafungin versus fluconazole for prophylaxis against invasive fungal infections during neutropenia in patients undergoing hematopoietic stem cell transplantation. Clin Infect Dis 2004;39:1407.

[75] Benjamin DKJ, Driscoll T, Seibel NL, et al. Safety and pharmacokinetics of intravenous anidulafungin in children with neutropenia at high risk for invasive fungal infections. Antimicrob Agents Chemother 2006;50:632.

ELSEVIER
SAUNDERS

Infect Dis Clin N Am
20 (2006) 679–697

INFECTIOUS
DISEASE CLINICS
OF NORTH AMERICA

Pharmacokinetics and Pharmacodynamics of Antifungals

David Andes, MD[a,b,*]

[a]Department of Medicine, Infectious Diseases Section, University of Wisconsin,
600 Highland Avenue, H4/572, Madison, WI 53792, USA
[b]Department of Medical Microbiology and Immunology, University of Wisconsin,
600 Highland Avenue, H4/572, Madison, WI 53792, USA

The role of pharmacokinetics and pharmacodynamics has gained increasing recognition as critical for selection and dosing of antimicrobial therapeutics, including antifungal agents. The study of pharmacokinetics involves understanding the interaction of a drug with the host, including measurements of absorption, distribution, metabolism and elimination. The study of antimicrobial pharmacodynamics provides insight into the link between drug pharmacokinetics, in vitro susceptibility, and treatment efficacy. Pharmacokinetic/pharmacodynamic (PK/PD) investigations have been valuable for defining optimal antifungal dosing regimens and developing in vitro susceptibility breakpoints. Numerous in vitro, animal, and clinical studies have been instrumental in characterizing the pharmacodynamic activity of the triazoles, polyenes, flucytosine, and echinocandins against *Candida* species. Several studies have begun to apply these principles to optimize therapy against filamentous fungi. The principles that have been used to characterize pharmacodynamic characteristics of single antifungal drugs are also beginning to be used to examine the more complex relationship encountered with combinations therapy.

Understanding of PK/PD principles can provide useful information for the clinician, clinical trial development, and for development of microbiology laboratory guidelines [1–3]. Antifungal pharmacodynamics allows the clinician to choose the most potent drug and provides a guide to the most efficacious and safe dose and interval of administration for a particular pathogen and infection site. For the pharmaceutical industry, preclinical

Funding: NIH/NIAID AI01767-01A1, AI067703-01, AI65728-01A1.
* Department of Medicine, Infectious Diseases Section, University of Wisconsin, 600 Highland Avenue, H4/572, Madison, WI 53792, USA.
E-mail address: dra@medicine.wisc.edu

PK/PD investigations help to predict the likelihood of success of a compound in development and can guide dosing regimen design for clinical trials. Understanding the relationship between antifungal drug exposure, in vitro potency (minimum inhibitory concentration [MIC]), and efficacy can be instructive for determining appropriate susceptibility breakpoints (ie, should an organism with MIC X be classified as susceptible or resistant?) [4–6].

Pharmacokinetics

Pharmacokinetic studies describe how the body handles a drug, including absorption, distribution, binding to serum and tissue proteins, metabolism, and elimination. Comparison of antifungals is frequently based on their pharmacokinetic properties [7]. Antifungal drug concentrations have been well characterized in numerous body fluids and tissues, including serum, urine, cerebrospinal fluid, vitreous, epithelial lining fluid or bronchoalveolar lavage, brain, lung, and kidney. The pharmacokinetic goal of antifungal therapy is to achieve adequate drug concentrations at the site of infection. This begs the rather simplistic question, where is the fungus relative to the antifungal drug? The site of infection for fungal pathogens can range from the bloodstream, where one would expect serum measurements to be of importance, to various tissue sites for which tissue drug concentrations may be of greater interest. Most pathogenic fungi exist primarily in extracellular fluid, however, even at tissue sites of infection. Serum measurements thus serve as a reliable tissue concentration surrogate. The body sites for which tissue antifungal concentrations have been suggested to be most important include the brain parenchyma and the vitreous space in the eye [8–13]. Outcomes of infection at other tissue sites have correlated well with serum concentrations. The same is true for body fluid kinetics. For example, despite marked differences in antifungal measurements in urine and CSF, therapeutic outcome seems more dependent on extracellular parenchymal tissue concentrations (serum). For example, Groll and colleagues examined the relationship between CSF and brain kinetics of several amphotericin B (AmB) preparations and efficacy [8]. The CSF concentrations of four polyene compounds were remarkably similar. Brain tissue concentrations of liposomal AmB (AmBisome), however, were from 6- to 10-fold higher than the other polyene preparations. The burden of *Candida* in the brains of rabbits following therapy correlated well with brain tissue penetration of the various drugs. The relationship between urine antifungal pharmacokinetics and efficacy in fungal pyelonephritis has been similarly examined [13]. For example, marked differences in urine kinetics have been demonstrated among the triazole antifungals. Nearly all of the absorbed fluconazole is secreted as active drug into the urine. Conversely, almost none of the absorbed itraconazole or voriconazole is secreted into this body fluid [14,15]. Outcomes in the kidneys, however, have been linked more closely to serum levels than urine. It has been theorized that tissue concentrations in extracellular space in the renal parenchyma are more relevant than urine concentrations for this infection.

Another pharmacokinetic factor shown to impact the availability of antimicrobial compounds in tissue is binding to serum proteins such as albumin [16]. In general it is accepted that only unbound (free) drug is pharmacologically active. This is related to the limited ability of protein-bound drug to diffuse across tissue and cellular membranes to reach the drug target. The relevance of protein binding has been most clearly demonstrated for drugs from the triazole class, in which there are marked differences in degree of binding among the drugs in this class. The studies demonstrating these findings are discussed later.

Defining antifungal drug pharmacodynamic characteristics

Predictive parameter (how often do I give the drug?)

Pharmacodynamics examines the relationship between pharmacokinetics and outcome. An added dimension of antimicrobial pharmacodynamics is consideration of the drug exposure relative to a measure of in vitro potency or the minimum inhibitory concentration (MIC) [1,3]. Three traditional pharmacodynamic parameters have been used to describe these relationships, including the peak concentration in relation to the MIC ($C_{max}/$MIC), the area under the concentration curve in relation to the MIC (24 h area under the concentration curve [AUC]/MIC), and the time that drug concentrations exceed the MIC expressed as a percentage of the dosing interval (%T > MIC) (Fig. 1). Knowledge of which of the three pharmacodynamic parameters describes antifungal activity provides the basis for determining the frequency with which a drug is most efficaciously

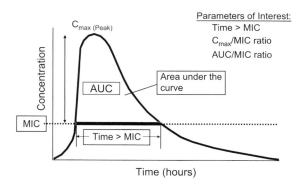

Fig. 1. Pharmacokinetics of antimicrobial dosing relative to organism MIC. (*From* Andes D. Clinical pharmacodynamics of antifungals. Infect Dis Clin N Am 2003;17:635–49; with permission.)

administered. For example, if the C_{max}/MIC parameter relationship strongly correlates with activity of drug A, the optimal dosing schedule would provide large infrequent doses. Conversely, if the %T > MIC better describes drug activity, a dosing strategy may include smaller more frequent drug administration to prolong the period of time that drug levels exceed the MIC.

Two types of experimental studies have been used to examine these relationships. The first study design involves investigation of the antifungal drug activity over time. Two outcomes are commonly noted. First is the impact of increasing drug concentrations on the rate and extent of organism killing. When higher concentrations enhance killing, the drug is referred to as concentration dependent. The second study endpoint includes examination of antifungal activity after drug concentrations decrease to below the organism MIC. For some drugs there is a period of prolonged growth suppression following an initial supra-MIC exposure. This period of growth suppression is termed a post-antifungal effect (PAFE). Three combinations of these time kill endpoint characteristics have been observed and each combination is predictive of one of the pharmacodynamic parameters. The C_{max}/MIC is associated with concentration-dependent killing and prolonged PAFEs. The %T > MIC is associated with concentration-independent killing and short PAFEs. The AUC/MIC is associated with prolonged PAFEs and either concentration-dependent or -independent killing.

The second study type used to determine which pharmacodynamic parameter is predictive of efficacy is termed dose fractionation. Traditional dose escalation studies use a single dosing interval. With only a single dosing interval, escalating doses increase the values of all three parameters. Dose fractionation studies examine efficacy of various dose levels that are administered by using three or more dosing intervals. In examining treatment results, if the regimens with shorter dosing intervals are more efficacious, the time-dependent parameter (T > MIC) is the more important parameter. If the large, infrequently administered dosing regimens are more active, the peak level in relation to the MIC is most predictive. Finally, if the outcome is similar with each of the dosing intervals, the outcome depends on the total dose or the AUC for the dosing regimen.

Parameter magnitude (how much drug do I give?)

Knowledge of the pharmacodynamic characteristics of a compound allows one to better design a dosing interval strategy. This knowledge can also be useful to design studies to determine the amount of drug or parameter magnitude that is required for treatment efficacy [1,2,17]. These studies can be used to help answer numerous questions related to the exposure response relationship. For example, what pharmacodynamic magnitude of a drug is needed to treat a *Candida* infection? Is this pharmacodynamic magnitude the same as that needed to treat a drug-resistant *Candida* infection? Is the magnitude similar for other fungal species, for different infection sites, in different animal species? The answers to these questions have been explored and most successfully addressed using various in vivo infection models. The results of these studies have demonstrated that the magnitude of a pharmacodynamic parameter associated with efficacy is similar for drugs within the same class, provided that free drug levels are considered. Furthermore, these data show that the parameter magnitude associated with efficacy is independent of the animal species, dosing interval, site of infection, and most often, the infecting pathogen. Most important, correlation of human pharmacokinetics and clinical trial outcome with several antifungal agents has suggested that the pharmacodynamic parameter magnitude that produces efficacy in animal models also predicts efficacy in humans. The pharmacodynamic evaluation of each antifungal drug class and the clinical implications of these studies are detailed here.

Triazole pharmacodynamics

Predictive pharmacodynamic parameter

In vitro and in vivo time kill studies have been undertaken with all of the clinically available triazole compounds [18–26]. Studies have shown that over a wide triazole concentration range (starting below the MIC [sub-MIC] to those more than 200-fold in excess of the MIC), growth of *Candida* organisms are similarly inhibited [22]. In other words, increasing drug concentrations do not enhance antifungal effect. Furthermore, in vitro studies demonstrated organism regrowth soon after drug removal [20,21]. In vivo studies, however, demonstrated prolonged growth suppression after levels in serum decreased to below the MIC [22–25]. These prolonged in vivo PAFEs have been theorized to be caused by the profound sub-MIC activity of these drugs (ie, effect of the triazoles after concentrations fall below the MIC in vivo). The time kill combination of concentration-independent killing and prolonged PAFEs suggest that the 24 AUC/MIC parameter is most closely tied to treatment effect. Dose fractionation studies in several in vivo models with each of the triazole compounds have corroborated these results [22–25,27]. The earliest fluconazole dose fractionation studies with fluconazole examined the impact of dividing four total dose levels into one, two, or four doses over a 24-hour period [27]. The results clearly demonstrated that outcome depended on the total amount of drug or AUC rather than the dosing interval. Subsequent studies with fluconazole, posaconazole, ravuconazole, and voriconazole similarly demonstrated that outcome was independent of fractionation of the total drug exposure supporting the 24-hour AUC/MIC as the pharmacodynamic parameter driving treatment efficacy [22–25]. These later observations demonstrate that the pharmacodynamic parameter associated with efficacy was similar within the triazole drug class.

Predictive pharmacodynamic magnitude

The usefulness of knowing which parameter predicts efficacy is being able to then determine the magnitude of that parameter needed for successful outcome. The most efficient experimental way to define the magnitude of the predictive parameter is to examine treatment efficacy against organisms with widely varying MICs. For example, the efficacy of posaconazole over a more than 1000-fold AUC range was studied in therapy against 12 *C albicans* with MICs varying nearly 100-fold [24]. Results from these studies showed that the AUC/MIC exposure associated with treatment efficacy was similar across the group of strains. Similar studies have now been undertaken with four triazole compounds that include more than nearly 40 drug/organism combinations for which MICs and dose levels varied more than 1000-fold each (Fig. 2) [22–25]. The consistency of data with these triazoles demonstrates that when protein binding is considered (ie, free drug concentrations), the antifungal pharmacodynamic target is similar among drugs within a mechanistic class (triazoles).

Several host, pathogen, and infection site factors have also been investigated to determine if and how they might impact the pharmacodynamic magnitude necessary for efficacy. For example, intuitively one may expect that more drug would be required to achieve an efficacy endpoint in absence of host neutrophils. Data from two murine candidiasis models differing only in the presence (or absence) of neutrophils, however, found a similar AUC/MIC associated with fluconazole efficacy [22,27]. Study with several triazoles has also investigated the impact of resistance mechanism on antifungal pharmacodynamics [22–25,28]. The triazole AUC/MIC associated with

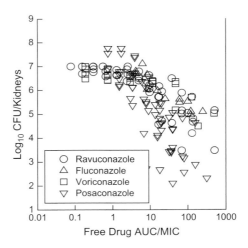

Fig. 2. Relationship between the 24-hour AUC/MIC parameter and efficicay of four triazoles against *Candida* in mice. (*From* Andes D. Clinical pharmacodynamics of antifungals. Infect Dis Clin N Am 2003;17:635–49; with permission.)

efficacy in these studies was similar for susceptible *C albicans* and those with reduced susceptibility caused by target site mutations and over expression of several drug efflux pumps. Finally, pharmacodynamic analysis of triazole studies can be used to examine the impact of treatment in different animal species. Study results in mice, rats, and rabbits are remarkably similar, suggesting that the pharmacodynamic magnitude target associated with treatment outcome is similar in different mammals [2]. One may expect differences in pharmacokinetics in different animal species to impact the pharmacodynamic target. Consideration of drug exposures in pharmacodynamic terms (relative to MIC of the organism), however, corrects for interspecies kinetic differences. Simply put, the drug target is in the organism and not in the host and thus host pharmacokinetic differences should not change the antimicrobial exposure the organism needs to see for effect. This knowledge allows one to use results from preclinical animal pharmacodynamic target studies to estimate antifungal dosing efficacy in humans.

The important next question is what endpoint in these preclinical animal models is relevant to treatment outcome in patients. Numerous microbiologic and survival endpoints are routinely examined using these in vivo infection models. The most reproducible endpoint that has correlated well with outcome following triazole therapy in patients is the drug exposure associated with 50% of the maximal effect (ED50) [2]. For each of the triazoles examined in pharmacodynamic animal model studies, the 24-hour AUC/MIC necessary to produce the ED50 corresponds to a value near 25. For the non-pharmacokinetically oriented, this is essentially the same as averaging a drug concentration near the organism MIC for a 24-hour period ($1 \times \text{MIC} \times 24\ \text{h} = \text{AUC/MIC of } 24$).

Clinical impact

The logical next step is to determine if and how the experimental pharmacodynamic studies relate to outcome in patients. Data from antibacterial pharmacodynamics provide a compelling precedence for the predictive value of animal model pharmacodynamics and clinical therapeutic efficacy [1]. The complexities surrounding patients who have fungal disease are well known and undoubtedly contribute to outcome independent of antifungal pharmacodynamics. The most important confounding host variable is the underlying host immune deficiency, which has been shown to be perhaps the most important factor influencing patient survival [29,30].

Despite this limitation, there are a several data sets that allow one to consider the relationship between antifungal dose, organism MIC, and clinical outcome. The largest of these is summarized in the Clinical Laboratory Standards Institute (CLSI) antifungal susceptibility breakpoint guideline publication [6]. Data from six fluconazole trials include nearly 500 episodes of oropharyngeal candidiasis in which the organism MIC, drug dose, and clinical outcomes were available. One can use the organism MIC and dose in these patients to estimate a 24-hour AUC-MIC value and then examine the relationship between this value and treatment success. When the 24-hour fluconazole AUC/MIC exceeded a value of 25, clinical treatment success was observed in 91% to 100% of patients. When this pharmacodynamic value decreased to less than 25, however, treatment failures were reported in 27% to 35% of cases. The association between the 24-hour AUC/MIC and outcome is similar to that observed in animal model pharmacodynamic studies. The fluconazole AUC/MIC magnitude of near 25 is supportive of the susceptibility breakpoint guidelines suggested in the CLSI publication. Of additional interest in this publication was the proposal of a new susceptibility category, termed "susceptible-dose dependent," in which the organism is considered susceptible if a higher drug dose is used. In this particular case a fluconazole dose escalation to 400 or 800 mg/d achieves a 24-hour AUC-MIC value of approximately 25 for organisms with MICs up to 16 and 32 mg/L, respectively. There are numerous additional publications of smaller series of patients (in total more than 1000 patients) with oropharyngeal candidiasis in which treatment failures were associated with an elevated MIC and the fluconazole drug dose was provided [31–50]. For nearly all treatment failures reported, the estimated fluconazole AUC/MIC value would have decreased to less than a value of 25, again in line with predictions from animal models.

Pharmacodynamic analysis of studies in patients who have candidemia and deep *Candida* infection is more difficult. Most of the larger trials in treatment of candidemia provide a paucity of data with organisms for which the MIC is elevated. In this case it is difficult to show a relationship between MIC and outcome, because the AUC/MIC values are above a value at which one expects failures related to drug therapy. For example, in the large candidemia trial examining the efficacy of fluconazole, among the *C albicans* isolates from patients treated with fluconazole the MIC for more than 90% of organisms was less than 1 mg/L, where the 24-hour AUC/MIC value is many fold higher than that expected to be associated with treatment failure [51]. In addition, outcome in candidemia can be impacted not only by antifungal therapy and underlying host immune state, but also by management of intravascular catheters, adding yet another confounding variable. Four studies, however (in total more than 600 patients), of invasive candidiasis allow consideration of fluconazole dose, MIC, and outcome [6,52–54]. Examination of data from these studies also demonstrates a strong relationship between MIC, fluconazole AUC, and outcome. Taken together these studies showed that clinical success was observed in 70% of patients when the fluconazole AUC/MIC ratio was 25 or greater and was 47% when the value decreases to less than 25. When the pharmacokinetics of fluconazole in humans are considered, these AUC/MIC ratios would support in vitro susceptibility breakpoints of 8 mg/L for doses of 200 mg/d and susceptibility breakpoints of 16 to 32 mg/L for doses of 400 to 800 mg/d for candidemia and mucosal disease.

Most recently attempts have been made to similarly correlate the pharmacokinetics of the recently approved triazole, voriconazole, with MIC, and outcome [5]. If one considers the kinetics of voriconazole in humans, an intravenous dose of 4 mg/kg every 12 hours would produce free drug AUCs of approximately 20 μg·h/ml. Given a pharmacodynamic target of a free drug AUC/MIC ratio of 20–25, one could predict that these voriconazole dosing regimens could successfully be used for treatment of infections caused by *Candida* spp. for which MICs are as high as 1 mg/L. Indeed, maximal efficacy was observed with *C albicans* isolates for which MICs were less than 1. The highest failure rates (45%) were observed with *C glabrata* isolates for which many MICs were greater than 1 mg/L. These data were used in the development of susceptibility breakpoints for voriconazole [5].

Unfortunately there are no complete clinical databases (kinetics, MIC, and outcome) to examine these relationships for voriconazole or other antifungals in treatment of filamentous fungal infections. There is, however, an accumulating body of evidence from which one can attempt to draw pharmacodynamic information. There have been more than 40 reported patients who have developed breakthrough infections while receiving voriconazole [55–59]. A common feature of nearly all of these cases was infection with an organism for which the voriconazole MIC was greater than 1 mg/mL. Unfortunately voriconazole serum concentrations were not available for these patients. A recent case series did, however, identify a relationship between voriconazole serum concentration and patient outcome [59]. Patients who have concentrations less than 2 mg/L were more likely to die from invasive fungal infection (mostly aspergillosis) than those who had serum concentrations exceeding this value. Considering free drug concentrations and the MICs of organisms involved in these case series, one can estimate that treatment failure was associated with 24-hour free drug AUC/MIC values less than 20 to 50. Again, these values are similar to those with fluconazole for treatment of *Candida* infections in clinical trials.

Polyene pharmacodynamics

Predictive pharmacodynamic parameter

In vitro polyene time kill studies have been undertaken with numerous yeast and filamentous fungal pathogens [18,20,21,60]. Each of these studies has demonstrated marked concentration-dependent killing and maximal antifungal activity at concentrations exceeding the MIC from 2- to 10-fold. Several of these in vitro models have demonstrated prolonged persistent growth suppression following drug exposure and removal (PAFE) [18,20,21]. In vivo time kill studies with AmB and each of the lipid preparations against several *Candida* species have also demonstrated an enhanced rate and extent of killing with increasing AmB concentrations [61,62]. Maximal killing was similarly observed with doses that produce serum concentrations exceeding the MIC from 4- to 10-fold. The AmB products also produced prolonged in vivo PAFEs. The duration of these persistent effects was also linearly related to the concentration of the AmB exposure. For example, the longest periods of in vivo growth suppression were nearly an entire day (>20 h) following a single high dose of AmB in neutropenic mice. For drugs displaying this pattern of activity the C_{max}/MIC ratio has most often been the PK/PD parameter predictive of efficacy [1].

Dose fractionation studies with AmB in vivo against *Candida* and *Aspergillus* demonstrated superior efficacy when administered as large doses as infrequently as every 3 days [61,63]. In the study against *Candida*, the total drug required to produce microbiologic efficacy was nearly eightfold less when administered every 3 days compared with daily dosing. The results of these experiments corroborate the importance of the C_{max}/MIC pharmacodynamic parameter.

Predictive pharmacodynamic magnitude

In vivo study with AmB against multiple *Candida* species in a neutropenic disseminated candidiasis model observed a net static effect (growth inhibition) when the C_{max}/MIC ratio approached values of 2 to 4 [61]. Maximal microbiologic efficacy was observed with ratios near 10. Similar investigation of efficacy in a murine pulmonary aspergillosis model found near maximal efficacy with C_{max}/MIC exposures in the range of 2 to 4 [63]. These most recent studies with aspergillus address a critical gap in knowledge and suggest that at least for AmB, pharmacodynamic relationships are similar among fungal species.

It is generally accepted that the lipid formulations of AmB are not as potent as conventional AMB on a mg/kg basis [62]. Each of the lipid formulations is complexed to a different lipid and exhibits unique pharmacokinetic characteristics. For example, the liposomal formulation of AmB achieves high serum concentrations relative to those achieved by the other formulations. Conversely, following administration of the lipid complex formulation of AmB, serum levels are low, yet the distribution to certain organs, such as the lungs, is reported to exceed those of the other formulations. Recently murine candidiasis models (lung, kidney, and liver) were used to discern if pharmacokinetic differences in serum or tissue could explain these in vivo potency differences [62]. Similar to prior in vivo experiments, the lipid formulations were 4.3- to 5.9-fold less potent than conventional AmB. The pharmacokinetic differences in serum accounted for much of the difference in potency between conventional AmB and the lipid complex formulation. The differences in the kinetics in the various end organs between AmB and the liposomal product were better at explaining the disparate potencies at these infection sites. Groll and colleagues performed a similar investigation with *Candida* in a rabbit CNS infection model. There was a poor relationship between CSF concentrations and microbiologic efficacy [8]. The brain tissue C_{max}/MIC ratio, however, was a reliable predictor of outcome. The liposomal formulation of AmB seemed to provide a pharmacokinetic/outcome advantage over the other formulations in this CNS infection model.

Clinical impact

The pharmacokinetics of AmB and the various lipid formulations have been carefully characterized in serum and tissues for several patient populations. Several investigations have attempted to demonstrate a correlation between AmB MIC and outcome. Most of these studies have found it difficult to discern MIC impact, likely related to the narrow MIC range observed with current testing methods [64]. The author is aware of only a single investigation that has attempted to correlate individual patient level pharmacokinetics, MIC, and outcome with polyenes [65]. This recently published study examined liposomal AmB kinetics and outcome of invasive fungal infections in pediatric patients. In this small study, data from a subset of patients provided detailed kinetics, MIC, and outcome. The results demonstrate a statistically significant relationship between C_{max}/MIC ratio and outcome. Maximal efficacy was observed with liposomal AmB serum C_{max}/MIC ratios greater than 40. This value is similar to that observed in the animal model studies described earlier when using serum liposomal AmB measurements. This small study demonstrates that pharmacodynamic investigation with a drug from the polyene class can produce meaningful results that are congruent with those from preclinical infection models.

Flucytosine pharmacodynamics

Predictive pharmacodynamic parameter

In vitro and in vivo studies have examined the pharmacodynamics of flucytosine [21,66–69]. Results from these models have been consistent. Increasing drug concentrations in vitro and larger doses in vivo produced minimal concentration-dependent killing of *Candida* species and soon after exposure organism growth resumes. Dose fractionation studies in vivo against *Candida* spp demonstrated that efficacy was optimal when drug was administrated in smaller dose levels more frequently [66,70]. Tenfold less drug was needed for efficacy when administered using the most fractionated dosing strategy by prolonging the time of the antifungal exposure. The time course and dose fractionation results in therapy against *C albicans* suggest the $\%T > MIC$ would be the most predictive parameter [66]. Recent study of flucytosine in an in vivo *Aspergillus* model also suggests that the most fractionated regimen (every 6 as opposed to every 12 or 24 hours) was most effective [69].

Predictive pharmacodynamic magnitude

Maximal efficacy from in vivo candidiasis and aspergillosis models has been observed when flucytosine levels exceeded the MIC for only 20% to 40% of the dosing interval [66,69]. These data also suggest a concordance of pharmacodynamic relationships among fungal species.

Clinical impact

Although no clinical studies have examined the relationship between flucytosine pharmacokinetics, MIC, and efficacy, there are several investigations that demonstrate a strong relationship between flucytosine kinetics and toxicity [71]. These studies have shown that bone marrow toxicity is observed when levels in serum exceed 50 to 60 mg/L. If one were to consider the human kinetics of the most frequently recommended flucytosine dosing of 150 mg/kg/d divided into four doses, each dose of 37.5 mg/kg would remain higher than the MIC for 90% of *C albicans* isolates tested for 12 to 14 hours [72]. Use of significantly smaller amounts of drug would allow flucytosine administration with much less concern about related toxicities. Whether higher concentrations would be optimal for cryptococcal CNS infection remains an important unanswered question.

Echinocandin pharmacodynamics

Predictive pharmacodynamic parameter

In vitro time course studies with each of the available echinocandin drugs have demonstrated concentration-dependent killing and prolonged PAFEs similar to those observed with the polyenes [18,73]. In vivo studies have confirmed these pharmacodynamic characteristics [74,75]. Following single escalating doses of the new echinocandin, aminocandin, marked killing of *C albicans* was observed when drug levels in serum were more than four times the MIC. The extent of killing increased as concentrations relative to the MIC approached a factor of 10. Early dose fractionation studies with the first echinocandin derivative, cilofungin, also demonstrated enhanced efficacy by maximizing serum and tissue concentrations [75]. Subsequent investigations in vivo with newer derivatives against *C albicans* and *A fumigatus* found that efficacy was maximized by providing large, infrequently administered doses [74,76,77]. The total amount of drug necessary to achieve various microbiologic outcomes over the treatment period was 4.8- to 7.6-fold smaller when the dosing schedule called for large single doses than when the same amount of total drug was administered in two to six doses [74]. The concentration-dependent killing pattern and results from dose fractionation studies would suggest that either the C_{max}/MIC or AUC/MIC would best represent the driving pharmacodynamic parameter [1]. In vivo studies using serum kinetics suggest that the C_{max}/MIC was better predictive of efficacy [74]. A tissue kinetic study, however, also demonstrated the importance of the AUC/MIC parameter [76].

Predictive pharmacodynamic magnitude

Study against multiple *C albicans* strains in a murine model demonstrated maximal efficacy when the total drug C_{max}/MIC of aminocandin approached a value of 10 (net inhibitory outcomes were observed with values near 3) [74]. In a pulmonary aspergillosis model, caspofungin efficacy was similarly maximized at a C_{max}/MEC ratio in the range of 10 to 20 [77]. These data support the principle that pharmacodynamic relationships are similar for drugs within the same mechanistic drug class (echinocandins) and for different fungal species.

Clinical impact

Most clinical studies with echinocandins have not been extensively examined from the pharmacodynamic standpoint. Several observations, however, can be gleaned from the dose/effect data evident from the group of clinical studies as a whole [78–81]. Accumulating evidence with several of the echinocandins in trials of esophageal candidiasis and candidemia suggest that increasing drug concentrations improves efficacy. A recently presented study with micafungin for esophageal candidiasis is the first to examine not only dose escalation but alternative dosing intervals [82]. The results suggest efficacy can be optimized with a dosing strategy that maximizes the C_{max} and allows dosing less frequently than daily. It will be interesting to see if this strategy can be used in treatment of systemic fungal infections.

Combination

Despite the recent boom in antifungal drug development, patient outcome associated with invasive fungal infections remains less than acceptable. It has been theorized that combination of two or more antifungal compounds with different mechanisms of action could improve efficacy. The success of the combination of amphotericin and flucytosine for cryptococcal meningitis serves as a critical proof of principle [83]. Numerous in vitro and in vivo infection models have been used to investigate various combinations against *Candida* and *Aspergillus* [84–86]. The results have been variable, ranging from reduced to an enhanced effect. Prior study with antibacterial combination studies has demonstrated that consideration of pharmacodynamics can help to decipher these often complex relationships [87]. Even if two drugs together can enhance outcome, it is possible or even likely that this positive interaction is not evident at all drug concentration combinations. Recent in vitro antifungal combination studies using pharmacodynamic analysis have shown this to be the case [67,88,89]. Examination of a wide variety of concentration combinations in these studies provides a means to determine not only if drug A and drug B interact in a helpful way, but they allow estimation of the optimal concentrations of each compound. In vivo pharmacodynamic studies should be useful to design clinical trials investigating antifungal drug combination therapy.

Summary

Application of pharmacodynamic principles to antifungal drug therapy of *Candida* and *Aspergillus* infections has provided an understanding of the relationship between drug dosing and treatment efficacy. Observations of the pharmacodynamics of triazoles and AmB have correlated with the results of clinical trials and have proven useful for validation of in vitro susceptibility breakpoints. Although there remain many unanswered questions regarding antifungal pharmacodynamics, available data suggest usefulness in the application of pharmacodynamics to antifungal clinical development. Future application of these principles should aid in the design of optimal combination antifungal therapies.

References

[1] Craig WA. Pharmacokinetic/pharmacodynamic parameters: rationale for antibacterial dosing of mice and men. Clin Infect Dis 1998;26:1–12.

[2] Andes D. In vivo pharmacodynamics of antifungal drugs in treatment of candidiasis. Antimicrob Agents Chemother 2003;47:1179–86.

[3] Drusano GL. Antimicrobial pharmacodynamics: critical interactions of 'bug and drug'. Nat Rev Microbiol 2004;2:289–300.

[4] National Committee for Clinical Laboratory Standards. Reference method for broth dilution antifungal susceptibility testing for yeast; approved standard. Document M27-A. Wayne, PA: National Committee for Clinical Laboratory Standards; 1997.

[5] Pfaller MA, Diekema DJ, Rex JH, et al. Correlation of MIC with outcome for *Candida* species tested against voriconazole: analysis and proposal for interpretive breakpoints. J Clin Microbiol 2006;44:819–26.

[6] Rex JH, Pfaller MA, Galgiani JN, et al. Development of interpretive breakpoints for antifungal susceptibility testing: conceptual framework and analysis of in vitro and in vivo correlation data for fluconazole, itraconazole, and *Candida* infections. Clin Infect Dis 1997;24: 235–47.

[7] Smith J, Andes D. Pharmacokinetics of antifungal drugs; implications for drug selection. Infect Med 2006;23:328–33.

[8] Groll AH, Giri N, Petraitis V, et al. Comparative efficacy and distribution of lipid formulations of amphotericin B in experimental *Candida albicans* infection of the central nervous system. J Infect Dis 2000;182:274–82.

[9] Gauthier GM, Nork TM, Prince R, et al. Subtherapeutic ocular penetration of caspofungin and associated treatment failure in *Candida albicans* endophthalmitis. Clin Infect Dis 2005; 41:27–8.

[10] Savani DV, Perfect JR, Cobo LM, et al. Penetration of new azole compounds into the eye and efficacy in experimental *Candida* endophthalmitis. Antimicrob Agents Chemother 1987;31:6–10.

[11] Fisher JF, Taylor AT, Clark J, et al. Penetration of amphotericin B into the human eye. J Infect Dis 1983;147:164.

[12] Sorensen KN, Sobel RA, Clemons KV, et al. Comparison of fluconazole and itraconazole in a rabbit model of coccidioidal meningitis. Antimicrob Agents Chemother 2000;44:1512–7.

[13] Perfect JR, Savani DV, Durack DT. Comparison of itraconazole and fluconazole in treatment of cryptococcal meningitis and candida pyelonephritis in rabbits. Antimicrob Agents Chemother 1986;29:579–83.

[14] Purkins L, Wood N, Ghahramani P, et al. Pharmacokinetics and safety of voriconazole following intravenous- to oral-dose escalation regimens. Antimicrob Agents Chemother 2002; 46:2546–53.

[15] Brammer KW, Farrow PR, Faulkner JK. Pharmacokinetics and tissue penetration of fluconazole in humans. Rev Infect Dis 1990;12(Suppl 3):S318–26.

[16] Craig WA, Suh B. Protein binding and the antimicrobial effects: methods for the determination of protein binding. In Lorian V, editor. Antibiotics in laboratory medicine. 4th editor. Williams & Wilkins Co.; Baltimore, MD; 1996. p. 367–402.

[17] Dudley MN, Ambrose PG. Pharmacodynamics in the study of drug resistance and establishing in vitro susceptibility breakpoints: ready for prime time. Curr Opin Microbiol 2000;3: 515–21.

[18] Ernst EJ, Klepser ME, Pfaller MA. Postantifungal effects of echinocandin, azole, and polyene antifungal agents against *Candida albicans* and *Cryptococcus neoformans*. Antimicrob Agents Chemother 2000;44:1108–11.

[19] Klepser ME, Malone D, Lewis RE, et al. Evaluation of voriconazole pharmacodynamics using time-kill methodology. Antimicrob Agents Chemother 2000;44:1917–20.

[20] Ernst EJ, Klepser ME, Pfaller MA. Postantifungal effects of echinocandin, azole, and polyene antifungal agents against *Candida albicans* and *Cryptococcus neoformans*. Antimicrob Agents Chemother 2000;44:1008–11.

[21] Turnidge JD, Gudmundsson S, Vogelman B, et al. The postantibiotic effect of antifungal agents against common pathogenic yeasts. J Antimicrob Chemother 1994;34:83–92.

[22] Andes D, Van Ogtrop M. Characterization and quantitation of the pharmacodynamics of fluconazole in a neutropenic murine disseminated candidiasis infection model. Antimicrob Agents Chemother 1999;43:2116–20.

[23] Andes D, Marchillo K, Stamstad T, et al. In vivo pharmacokinetics and pharmacodynamics of a new triazole, voriconazole, in a murine candidiasis model. Antimicrob Agents Chemother 2003;47:3165–9.

[24] Andes D, Marchillo K, Conklin R, et al. Pharmacodynamics of a new triazole, posaconazole, in a murine model of disseminated candidiasis. Antimicrob Agents Chemother 2004; 48:137–42.

[25] Andes D, Marchillo K, Stamstad T, et al. In vivo pharmacodynamics of a new triazole, ravuconazole, in a murine candidiasis model. Antimicrob Agents Chemother 2003;47:1193–9.

[26] Lewis RE, Wiederhold NP, Klepser ME. In vitro pharmacodynamics of amphotericin b, itraconazole, and voriconazole against *Aspergillus*, *Fusarium*, and *Scedosporium* spp. Antimicrob Agents Chemother 2005;49:945–51.

[27] Louie A, Drusano GL, Banerjee P, et al. Pharmacodynamics of fluconazole in a murine model of systemic candidiasis. Antimicrob Agents Chemother 1998;42:1105–9.

[28] Andes D, Forrest A, Lepak A, et al. Antimicrobial dosing regimen impact on the evolution of drug resistance in vivo: fluconazole and *Candida albicans*. Antimicrob Agents Chemother 2006;50:2374–83.

[29] Pappas PG, Rex JH, Sobel JD, et al. Guidelines for treatment of candidiasis. Clin Infect Dis 2004;38:161–89.

[30] Stevens DA, Kan LV, Judson MA, et al. practice guidelines for diseases caused by *aspergillus*. Clin Infect Dis 2000;30:696–709.

[31] Baily GG, Perry FM, Denning DW, et al. Fluconazole resistant candidiasis in an HIV cohort. AIDS 1994;8:787–92.

[32] Barchiesi F, Hollis RJ, McGough DA, et al. DNA subtypes and fluconazole susceptibilities of *Candida albicans* isolates from the oral cavities of patients with AIDS. Clin Infect Dis 1995;20:634–40.
[33] Bart-Delabesse E, Boiron P, Carlotti A, et al. Candida albicans genotyping in studies with patients with AIDS developing resistance to fluconazole. J Clin Microbiol 1993;31:2933–7.
[34] Boken DJ, Swindells S, Rinaldi MG. Fluconazole-resistant *Candida albicans*. Clin Infect Dis 1993;17:1018–21.
[35] He X, Tiballi RN, Zarins LT, et al. Azole resistance in oropharyngeal *Candida albicans* strains isolated from patients infected with human immunodeficiency virus. Antimicrob Agents Chemother 1994;38:2495–7.
[36] Heinic GS, Stevens DA, Greenspan D, et al. Fluconazole-resistant *Candida* in AIDS patients: report of two cases. Oral Surg Oral Med Oral Pathol 1993;76:711–5.
[37] Newman SL, Flanigan TP, Fisher A, et al. Clinically significant mucosal candidiasis resistant to fluconazole treatment in patients with AIDS. Clin Infect Dis 1994;19:684–6.
[38] Pfaller MA, Rhine-Chalberg J, Redding SW, et al. Variations in fluconazole susceptibility and electrophoretic karyotype among oral isolates of *Candida albicans* from patients with AIDS and oral candidiasis. J Clin Microbiol 1994;32:59–64.
[39] Redding S, Smith J, Farinacci G, et al. Resistance to *Candida albicans* to fluconazole during treatment of oropharyngeal candidiasis in patients with AIDS: documentation of in vitro susceptibility testing and DNA subtype analysis. Clin Infect Dis 1994;18:240–2.
[40] Reynes J, Mallie M, Andre D, et al. Traitement et prophylxie secondarire par fluconazole des candidoses oropharyngees des suets VIH +. Analyse mycologique des echecs. Pathol Biol 1992;40:513–7.
[41] Rodriguez-Tudela JL, Laguna F, Martinez-Suarez JV, et al. Fluconazole resistance of *Candida albicans* isolates from AIDS patients receiving prolonged antifungal therapy [abstract 1204]. Program and abstracts of the 32nd Interscience Conference on Antimicrobial Agents and Chemotherapy, New Orleans (LA), October 17–20, 1992.
[42] Ruhnke M, Eigler A, Engelmann E, et al. Correlation between antifungal susceptibility testing of *Candida* isolates from patients with HIV infection and clinical results after treatment with fluconazole. Infection 1994;22:132–6.
[43] Ruhnke M, Eigler A, Tennagen I, et al. Emergence of fluconazole-resistant strains of *Candida albicans* in patients with recurrent oropharyngeal candidosis and human immunodeficiency virus infection. J Clin Microbiol 1994;32:2092–8.
[44] Sandven P, Bjorneklett A, Maeland A. Norwegian Yeast Study Group. Susceptibility testing of Norwegian *Candida albicans* strains to fluconazole: emergence of resistance. Antimicrob Agents Chemother 1993;37:2443–8.
[45] Sangeorzan JA, Bradley SF, He X, et al. Epidemiology of oral candidiasis in HIV infected patients: colonization, infection, treatment, and emergence of fluconazole resistance. Am J Med 1994;97:339–46.
[46] Ghannoum MA, Rex JH, Galgiani JN. Susceptibility testing of fungi: current status of correlation of in vitro data with clinical outcome. J Clin Microbiol 1996;34:489–95.
[47] Cartledge JD, Midgley J, Petrou M, et al. Unresponsive HIV-related oro-oesophageal candidosis: an evaluation of two new in vitro azole susceptibility tests. J Antimicrob Chemother 1997;40:517–23.
[48] Dannaoui E, Colin S, Pichot J, et al. Evaluation of the ETEST for fluconazole susceptibility testing of *Candida albicans* isolates from oropharyngeal candidiasis. Eur J Clin Microbiol Infect Dis 1997;16:228–32.
[49] Revankar SG, Dib OP, Kirkpatrick WR, et al. Clinical evaluation and microbiology of oropharyngeal infection due to fluconazole resistant *Candida* in human immunodeficiency virus-infected patients. Clin Infect Dis 1998;26:960–3.
[50] Quereda C, Polanco AM, Giner C, et al. Correlation between in vitro resistance to fluconazole and clinical outcome of oropharyngeal candidiasis in HIV-infected patients. Eur J Clin Microbiol Infect Dis 1996;15:30–7.

[51] Rex JH, Bennett JE, Sugar AM, et al. A randomized trial comparing fluconazole with amphotericin B for the treatment of candidemia in patients without neutropenia. Candidemia Study Group and the National Institute. N Engl J Med 1994;17(331):1325–30.

[52] Takakura S, Fujihara N, Saito T, et al. Clinical factors associated with fluconazole resistance and short-term survival in patients with *Candida* bloodstream infection. Eur J Clin Microbiol Infect Dis 2004;23:380–8.

[53] Lee SC, Fung CP, Huang JS, et al. Clinical correlates of antifungal macrodilution susceptibility test results for non-AIDS patients with severe *Candida* infections treated with fluconazole. Antimicrob Agents Chemother 2000;44:2715–8.

[54] Clancy CJ, Yu VL, Morris AJ, et al. Fluconazole MIC and the fluconazole dose/MIC ratio correlate with therapeutic response among patients with candidemia. Antimicrob Agents Chemother 2005;49:3171–7.

[55] Alexander B, Schell WA, Miller JL, et al. Candida glabrata fungemia in transplant patients receiving voriconazole after fluconazole. Transplantation 2005;27:868–71.

[56] Imhof A, Balajee SA, Fredricks DN, et al. Breakthrough fungal infections in stem cell transplant recipients receiving voriconazole. Clin Infect Dis 2004;39:743–6.

[57] Marty FM, Cosimi LA, Baden L. Breakthrough zygomycosis after voriconazole treatment in recipients of hematopoietic stem-cell transplants. N Engl J Med 2004;350:950–2.

[58] Siwek GT, Dodgson KJ, de Magalhaes-Silvermanet M, et al. Invasive zygomycosis in hematopoietic stem cell transplant recipients receiving voriconazole prophylaxis. Clin Infect Dis 2004;39:584–7.

[59] Smith J, Safdar N, Knasinski V, et al. Consideration of voriconazole therapeutic drug monitoring. Antimicrob Agents Chemother 2006;50:1570–2.

[60] Gunderson SM, Hoffman H, Ernst EJ, et al. In vitro pharmacodynamic characteristics of nystatin including time-kill and postantifungal effect. Antimicrob Agents Chemother 2000; 44:2887–90.

[61] Andes D, Stamstad T, Conklin R. Pharmacodynamics of amphotericin B in a neutropenic-mouse disseminated-candidiasis model. Antimicrob Agents Chemother 2001;45:922–6.

[62] Andes D, Safdar N, Marchillo K, et al. Pharmacokinetic-pharmacodynamic comparison of amphotericin B (AMB) and two lipid-associated AMB preparations, liposomal AMB and AMB lipid complex, in murine candidiasis models. Antimicrob Agents Chemother 2006; 50:674–84.

[63] Wiederhold NP, Tam VH, Chi J, et al. Pharmacodynamic activity of amphotericin B deoxycholate is associated with peak plasma concentrations in a neutropenic murine model of invasive pulmonary aspergillosis. Antimicrob Agents Chemother 2006;50:469–73.

[64] Park BJ, Arthington-Skaggs BA, Hajjeh RA, et al. Evaluation of amphotericin B interpretive breakpoints for *Candida* bloodstream isolates by correlation with therapeutic outcome. Antimicrob Agents Chemother 2006;50:1287–92.

[65] Hong Y, Shaw PJ, Nath CE, et al. Population pharmacokinetics of liposomal amphotericin B in pediatric patients with malignant diseases. Antimicrob Agents Chemother 2006;50: 935–42.

[66] Andes D, Van Ogtrop M. In vivo characterization of the pharmacodynamics of flucytosine in a neutropenic murine disseminated candidiasis model. Antimicrob Agents Chemother 2000;44:938–42.

[67] Hope WW, Warn PA, Sharp A, et al. Surface response modeling to examine the combination of amphotericin B deoxycholate and 5-fluorocytosine for treatment of invasive candidiasis. J Infect Dis 2005;192:673–80.

[68] Te Dorsthorst DTA, Verweij PE, Meis JFGM, et al. In vitro interactions between amphotericin B, itraconazole, and flucytosine against 21 clinical *Aspergillus* isolates determined by two drug interaction models. Antimicrob Agents Chemother 2004;48:2007–13.

[69] Te Dorsthorst DTA, Verweij PE, Meis GFJM, et al. Efficacy and Pharmacodynamics of flucytosine monotherapy in a nonneutropenic murine model of invasive aspergillosis. Antimicrob Agents Chemother 2005;49:4220–6.

[70] Karyotakis NC, Anaissie EJ. Efficacy of continuous flucytosine infusion against *Candida lusitaniae* in experimental hematogenous murine candidiasis. Antimicrob Agents Chemother 1996;40:2907–8.

[71] Francis P, Walsh TJ. Evolving role of flucytosine in immunocompromised patients: new insights into safety, pharmacokinetics, and antifungal therapy. Clin Infect Dis 1992;15: 1003–18.

[72] Polak A, Eschenhof E, Fernex M, et al. Metabolic studies with 5-fluorocytosine-6–14C in mouse, rat, rabbit, dog and man. Chemotherapy 1976;22:137–53.

[73] Ernst EJ, Roling EE, Petzold CR, et al. In vitro activity of micafungin (FK-463) against *Candida* spp.: microdilution, time-kill, and postantifungal-effect studies. Antimicrob Agents Chemother 2002;46:3846–53.

[74] Andes D, Marchillo K, Lowther J, et al. In vivo pharmacodynamics of HMR 3270, a glucan synthase inhibitor, in a murine candidiasis model. Antimicrob Agents Chemother 2003;47: 1187–92.

[75] Walsh TJ, Lee JW, Kelly P, et al. Antifungal effects of the nonlinear pharmacokinetics of cilofungin, a 1, 3-3-glucan synthetase inhibitor, during continuous and intermittent intravenous infusions in treatment of experimental disseminated candidiasis. Antimicrob Agents Chemother 1991;35:1321–8.

[76] Louie A, Deziel M, Liu W, et al. Pharmacodynamics of caspofungin in a murine model of systemic candidiasis: importance of persistence of caspofungin in tissues to understanding drug activity. Antimicrob Agents Chemother 2005;49:5058–68.

[77] Wiederhold NP, Kontoyiannis DP, Chi J, et al. Pharmacodynamics of caspofungin in a murine model of invasive pulmonary aspergillosis: evidence of concentration-dependent activity. J Infect Dis 2004;190:1464–71.

[78] Pfaller MA, Diekema DJ, Boyken L, et al. Effectiveness of anidulafungin in eradicating *Candida* species in invasive candidiasis. Antimicrob Agents Chemother 2005;49:4795–7.

[79] de Wet N, Llanos-Cuentas A, Suleiman J, et al. A randomized, double-blind, parallel-group, dose-response study of micafungin compared with fluconazole for the treatment of esophageal candidiasis in HIV-positive patients. Clin Infect Dis 2004;39:842–9.

[80] Krause DS, Reinhardt J, Vazquez JA, et al. Phase 2, randomized, dose-ranging study evaluating the safety and efficacy of anidulafungin in invasive candidiasis and candidemia. Antimicrob Agents Chemother 2004;48:2021–4.

[81] Ostrosky-Zeichner L, Kontoyiannis D, Raffalli J, et al. International, open-label, noncomparative, clinical trial of micafungin alone and in combination for treatment of newly diagnosed and refractory candidemia. Eur J Clin Microbiol Infect Dis 2005;24:654–61.

[82] Buell D, Kovanda L, Drake T, et al. Alternate day dosing of micafungin in treatment of esophageal candidiasis. ICAAC 2006;M719:419.

[83] Bennett JE, Dismukes WE, Duma RJ, et al. A comparison of amphotericin B alone and combined with flucytosine in the treatment of cryptococcal meningitis. N Engl J Med 1979;301: 126–31.

[84] MacCallum DM, Whyte JA, Odds FC. Efficacy of caspofungin and voriconazole combinations in experimental aspergillosis. Antimicrob Agents Chemother 2005;49: 3697–701.

[85] Kirkpatrick WR, Perea S, Coco BJ, et al. Efficacy of caspofungin alone and in combination with voriconazole in a guinea pig model of invasive aspergillosis. Antimicrob Agents Chemother 2002;46:2564–8.

[86] Warn PA, Sharp A, Morrissey G, et al. Activity of aminocandin (IP960) compared with amphotericin B and fluconazole in a neutropenic murine model of disseminated infection caused by a fluconazole-resistant strain of *Candida tropicalis*. J Antimicrob Chemother 2005;56: 590–3.

[87] Mouton JW, Van Ogtrop JW, Andes D, et al. Use of pharmacodynamic indices to predict efficacy of combination therapy in vivo. Antimicrob Agents Chemother 1999;43: 2473–8.

[88] Meletiadis J, Verweij PE, te Dorsthorst DTA, et al. Assessing in vitro combinations of antifungal drugs against yeasts and filamentous fungi: comparison of different drug interaction
models. Med Mycol 2005;43:133–52.
[89] Lewis RE, Kontoyiannis DP. Micafungin in combination with voriconazole in *Aspergillus*
species: a pharmacodynamic approach for detection of combined antifungal activity in vitro.
J Antimicrob Chemother 2005;56:887–92.

ELSEVIER
SAUNDERS

Infect Dis Clin N Am
20 (2006) 699–709

INFECTIOUS
DISEASE CLINICS
OF NORTH AMERICA

Antifungal Susceptibility Testing

Annette W. Fothergill, MA, MBA, MT(ASCP),
CLS(NCA)[a], Michael G. Rinaldi, PhD[a,b],
Deanna A. Sutton, PhD, MT, SM(ASCP),
SM, RM(NRM)[a]

[a]Fungus Testing Laboratory, Department of Pathology, University of Texas Health Science
Center at San Antonio, 7703 Floyd Curl Drive, San Antonio,
TX 78229, USA
[b]Clinical Microbiology and Mycology Reference Laboratory Merton Minter Drive,
Audie L. Murphy Veterans Administration Health System,
San Antonio, TX 78229, USA

Historically, antifungal susceptibility testing was conducted by various methods that were primarily based on both broth and agar diffusion or disk diffusion procedures. These methods produced results as diverse as the methods themselves. In 1982, the Clinical and Laboratory Standards Institute (CLSI, at that time named the National Committee of Clinical Laboratory Standards, NCCLS) established a subcommittee to review antifungal susceptibility testing. Their findings were documented 3 years later in NCCLS M20-CR (committee report) and stated that approximately 20% of the responding hospital and reference laboratories were indeed conducting antifungal susceptibility testing as part of their patient care program. Testing was predominately by variations of a broth method and was limited to yeast fungi. In addition, the intra-laboratory agreement between laboratories was unacceptable, with results for a given isolate ranging from susceptible to resistant for the same isolate. Following this report the subcommittee determined that it was necessary to develop a standard method for antifungal susceptibility testing. The goal of the subcommittee was to develop a method that was reproducible between laboratories as opposed to developing a method that correlated the minimum inhibitory concentration (MIC) with patient outcome. The subcommittee reported that the

E-mail address: fothergill@uthscsa.edu (A.W. Fothergill).

standard should be based on a broth method that used a synthetic medium for testing.

Yeast testing

Following the recruitment of several laboratories from across the United States, a preliminary standard was introduced 7 years following the initial committee report. This standard, M27-P [1], provided guidelines and stipulated the parameters that are still in effect. These parameters include use of RPMI-1640 as the test medium, an inoculum prepared spectrophotometrically to a final test concentration of 0.5 to 2.5 × 10^3 CFU/mL, an incubation temperature of 35°C for 48 hours, and the criteria for determining the endpoint or MIC. The MIC is defined as optically clear or the absence of growth for amphotericin B and a 50% reduction in growth for the azoles tested by the microtiter method. Azoles tested by the macro-broth method, however, have endpoints at the concentration at which an 80% reduction in growth occurs. With input from the scientific community, this method has undergone review and has been amended to its current version of M27-A2 [2]. While this method was being developed in the United States, the European community began work on a standard method also. The EUCAST (European Community Antifungal Susceptibility Testing) method, although similar, incorporated some revisions to the CLSI method to include the addition of a higher concentration of glucose to the RPMI-1640. This addition facilitates the rate of fungal growth allowing the MIC to be determined at 24 hours as opposed to the M27-A2 48 hours. Studies have shown that the two methods are equivalent despite these differences [3], and that a given set of isolates can expect the same categoric placement regardless of the method used. Two other methods have evolved from the initial yeast procedure. These methods are described in M38-A for mold testing [4] and M44-A for yeast disk diffusion testing [5].

Realizing that M27-A2 is labor intensive and not practical for busy clinical laboratories, the CLSI introduced M44-A. This method is a disk diffusion method that is similar to the routine Kirby-Bauer method used globally for bacterial susceptibility testing. To date, only fluconazole and voriconazole have been evaluated. This method uses the same Mueller-Hinton agar that is required for bacterial testing but stipulates the addition of methylene blue-glucose to assist with fungal growth and to enhance visualization of the zone diameters. Methylene blue-glucose solution is added to the surface of the Mueller-Hinton agar and is permitted to air-dry before adding the yeast inoculum. Many laboratories find that M44-A fits into their workflow more easily than M27-A2 and is much less costly. Much work has been done to provide quality control limits to ensure this method has the same validity as the original M27-A2 [6].

Since approved methods have been developed, the industry has introduced kits to assist laboratories with antifungal susceptibility testing. Systems that have been evaluated include the Yeast One system by Trek Diagnostics and the ETEST by AB Biodisk. These methods are easy to incorporate into the routine laboratory and give equivalent results to M27-A2 [7–9]. In addition, automated methods are under development. Before launching an antifungal susceptibility program, institutions should consider the volume of testing they can expect. The method is inherently variable and reproducibility can be a problem. Another problem is determining who is available to discuss interpretation of the testing. To date, interpretive guidelines are provided only for fluconazole, itraconazole, voriconazole, and 5-fluorocytosine. Unfortunately breakpoints do not exist for amphotericin B or the echinocandins. The interpretive categories for 5-fluorocytosine are the same categories used to interpret bacterial testing. These categories include susceptible (S), intermediate (I), and resistant (R). Azole testing, however, requires a change in these categories. For azoles, the categories include susceptible (S) and resistant (R) with susceptible-dose-dependent (SDD) being substituted for the intermediate category. The SDD category relates to yeast testing only and is not interchangeable with the intermediate category associated with bacterial and 5-fluorocytosine breakpoints. This category is in recognition that yeast susceptibility depends on achieving maximum blood levels. By maintaining blood levels with higher doses of antifungal, an isolate with an SDD endpoint may be successfully treated with a given azole [2]. One main problem with antifungal susceptibility testing is the correlation of the MIC with patient outcome. In an article written by Rex and Pfaller [10], the "90-60" rule is discussed. From this rule, some assumptions can be made between the MIC and patient outcome. This rule states that infections caused by isolates that have MICs considered susceptible respond favorably to appropriate therapy approximately 90% of the time, whereas infections caused by isolates with MICs considered resistant respond favorably approximately 60% of the time. As a result of this, physicians are frequently more interested in determining potential resistance than in determining the susceptibility of a given isolate.

Amphotericin B is often held up as the standard to which other antifungals are measured. Amphotericin B is easily tested and acceptable results are obtained for most fungal species. One acceptable deviation from the standard is the use of antibiotic medium 3 (M3) as opposed to RPMI-1640. Isolates tested in RPMI-1640 give amphotericin B MICs that are tightly clustered around 1.0 µg/mL. This does not allow the distinction of susceptible isolates from potentially resistant ones. Antibiotic medium 3 provides a wider distribution of MIC values and isolates with low MICs can easily be distinguished from those with much higher MICs. As a result, clinicians must determine which medium is being used when evaluating results. Another concern documented in M27-A2 regards lot-to-lot variability with

M3. This, however, has not been the authors' experience over a 25-year history of antifungal susceptibility testing.

Mold testing

The M38-A method was released in 2002 to accommodate mold testing. This method is virtually identical to M27-A2 with the exception of the inoculum size. The inoculum size continues to be determined spectrophotometrically but to a higher final test concentration of 1 to 5×10^4 CFU/mL. The guideline provides target percent transmission (%T) readings based on conidial size and these are listed by species. Species such as *Aspergillus* spp, *Paecilomyces* spp, and *Sporothrix* spp are measured at 80%T to 82%T, whereas species with larger conidia, such as *Fusarium* spp, *Rhizopus* spp, and *Scedosporium* spp are standardized to 68%T to 70%T. Although efforts are underway to determine the correct %T for most clinically-significant fungi, the list is not yet complete. When testing other fungi not specifically discussed in the M38-A, laboratories must determine the correct %T through trial and error to achieve the correct final concentration.

During the tenure of the M27-A2 committee, it was recognized that the scientific community preferred the microtiter method to the macrobroth method. As a result, the macrobroth method is not discussed in M38-A. This poses a problem when the testing of endemic fungi such as *Histoplasma capsulatum*, *Blastomyces dermatitidis*, or *Coccidioides immitis* is necessary. Mold testing may be conducted by the macrobroth method, because early studies have shown that the two methods are equivalent. Other fungi that may benefit from testing by the macrobroth method are those fungi that grow very slowly. It is difficult to hold microtiter tests longer than 72 hours due to of dehydration. Many of the less frequently encountered fungi may require as long as 120 to 144 hours before growth is detected in the drug-free growth control well. For this reason, isolates that are known to be slow growers should be tested by way of the macrobroth method.

Endpoint determination is also much more difficult with molds than with the yeast fungi. Although a reduction in turbidity is easily visualized for the yeast fungi, it is not so easily recognized when testing the molds. Because of the unique growth patterns of the mold fungi in the macrobroth system, one looks for a decrease in volume of growth rather than a reduction in turbidity as for the yeasts. In *Aspergillus* spp, for example, growth is seen as a cottony clump in the broth. To determine an endpoint, the reader must assess the amount of growth for each concentration and call the endpoint at that concentration that has at least 50% smaller volume of growth. Many individuals are not comfortable with this subjective endpoint determination and prefer to leave mold testing to reference centers.

Interpretation of results

Perhaps the biggest dilemma facing the clinician is determining how best to use the results obtained by the laboratory. Although breakpoints have not been offered for any drug in M38-A or for amphotericin B in M27-A2, the value most often quoted in the literature as a guideline to potential resistance to amphotericin B is any MIC greater than 1.0 μg/mL [11]. Few isolates have such high MICs when tested against amphotericin B. Notable exceptions include *Pseudallescheria boydii* (*Scedosporium apiospermum*), *Scedosporium prolificans*, *Paecilomyces lilacinus*, *Fusarium* spp, and some species of *Aspergillus* other than *A fumigatus*, most notably *A terreus*. All of these species give MIC values that are extremely elevated. One yeast that has been reported to possess resistance to amphotericin B is *Candida lusitaniae*. Early reports labeled this isolate as amphotericin B-resistant [12,13], but susceptibility studies reveal that less than 10% of *C lusitaniae* isolates tested have MICs that may be considered resistant (Table 1). This species does, however, possess the ability to develop resistance more readily than other *Candida* spp.

It is more difficult to determine the MIC for azoles than for amphotericin B. The endpoint by the microtiter method is the concentration at which a 50% reduction in turbidity can be visualized. Two problems exist with determining this endpoint visually. A 50% reduction in growth is difficult to discern by eye and results are somewhat subjective. A reduction of only 50% is far more growth than can easily be distinguished from lesser percentages of reduction. The difference is subtle. For this reason, a spectrophotometric plate reader should be considered. The other problem is caused by the static nature of the azoles. The earlier azoles, such as fluconazole and itraconazole, act to inhibit fungi but do not typically possess lethal activity. Because of this static nature, trailing may be observed in yeast fungi. The trailing effect occurs when a distinct reduction is seen at a lower concentration but at a point at which significant growth continues through the highest concentration. This pattern may be misinterpreted as resistance by some, thereby accentuating the need for accurate determination of the percent reduction in growth for correct categoric placement. Some of the newer azoles, such as voriconazole and posaconazole, do seem to possess some cidal activity.

Although the azoles as a group possess similar mechanisms of action, they clearly have differing spectra of activity. Fluconazole shows good activity against the yeast fungi but is not the drug of choice for most common mold infections, such as aspergillosis. Most yeast fungi show favorable MIC patterns when tested against fluconazole, but some exceptions do exist. *Candida krusei* is recognized for intrinsic resistance, and testing against fluconazole is not recommended. Of primary concern is acquired resistance. The most notorious species for acquiring resistance to fluconazole following prolonged therapy are *C albicans* and *C glabrata*. It is not as common to

Table 1
Susceptibility trends for selected *Candida* species

(N)	MIC_{50} (µg/mL)	MIC_{90} (µg/mL)
Candida albicans		
Amphotericin B (1344)	0.25	0.25
Caspofungin (1188)	0.06	0.125
Fluconazole (2147)	0.25	2.0
Voriconazole (716)	≤0.015	1.0
Candida glabrata		
Amphotericin B (985)	0.25	5
Caspofungin (1039)	0.125	25
Fluconazole (1676)	8.0	64
Voriconazole (723)	0.5	2
Candida parapsilosis		
Amphotericin B (619)	0.125	0.25
Caspofungin (606)	0.25	1.0
Fluconazole (858)	0.5	2.0
Voriconazole (334)	0.03	0.125
Candida tropicalis		
Amphotericin B (300)	0.25	25
Caspofungin (265)	0.06	06
Fluconazole (452)	1.0	16
Voriconazole (175)	0.06	1
Candida lusitaniae		
Amphotericin B (130)	0.25	0.5
Caspofungin (88)	0.125	0.25
Fluconazole (197)	0.5	2.0
Voriconazole (67)	0.03	0.25
Candida krusei		
Amphotericin B (142)	0.25	0.5
Caspofungin (141)	0.25	0.25
Fluconazole (0)[a]	—	—
Voriconazole (123)	0.5	1.0

Abbreviations: MIC, minimum inhibitory concentration; *N*, number tested.

[a] M27-A2 does not recommend testing of *C Krusei* against flyconazole.

Selected MIC_{50} and MIC_{90} *in vitro* Fungus Testing Laboratory data for the most common yeast species against amphotericin B, caspofungin, fluconazole, and voriconazole.

observe resistance in *C albicans*, but some reports list *C glabrata* resistance as high as 15% of the species population [14]. *Cryptococcus* spp are generally susceptible and acquired resistance has not been documented.

Itraconazole has activity against yeast and mold fungi. It is useful in treating aspergillosis, blastomycosis, coccidioidomycosis, histoplasmosis, and candidiasis. In addition, itraconazole possesses perhaps the lowest endpoints against the dematiaceous fungi and may be considered the drug of choice for treatment of infections caused by isolates from this group. Some species within this group include *Bipolaris* spp, *Alternaria* spp, and *Exophiala* spp. Any time one is evaluating drugs from the same class, cross-resistance is of concern. Comparison of resistance patterns between itraconazole and fluconazole reveal similar percentages of resistance among *Candida* species.

Voriconazole is the newest approved azole and is noted for its activity against *Aspergillus* spp, *S apiospermum*, and *Fusarium solani*. This is remarkable because *S apiospermum* and *F solani* are notoriously resistant to all other antifungal agents. Of note is that voriconazole seems to possess lethal rather than static activity against the aspergilli. Susceptibility patterns for voriconazole against the yeast are similar to itraconazole and fluconazole with a notable exception. There is an extremely low incidence of resistance for *C krusei* against voriconazole with intrinsic resistance reported for fluconazole and approximately 10% of isolates reported as resistant to itraconazole (A. Fothergill, Fungus Testing Laboratory, unpublished data, 2001–2005).

One other azole is of interest and is awaiting approval by the Food and Drug Administration (FDA). Posaconazole is approved in Europe, and FDA action is anticipated in the near future. This agent has a broad spectrum of activity. Clinical trials are underway to assess activity against aspergillosis, candidiasis, fusariosis, coccidioidomycosis, and zygomycosis (mucormycosis). Favorable results against species such as *Rhizopus* and *Mucor* show that this drug may provide alternative therapy to amphotericin B for infections caused by this group of fungi that historically has been difficult to treat. Resistance with the yeast fungi has not been observed, but some cross-resistance may be expected to occur.

The echinocandins are the newest class of antifungals to be released for use within the United States. Currently available agents include caspofungin, micafungin, and anidulafungin. These agents share excellent activity against *Candida* and *Aspergillus* spp [15–19]. This class has not yet been evaluated by the CLSI subcommittee and a standard for testing does not exist. Most yeast studies have involved testing in RPMI-1640 with the MIC being the lowest concentration exhibiting a 50% reduction in turbidity. Alternative reports have tested the echinocandins in M3 with the endpoint being the lowest concentration that is optically clear. Results using the two media are significantly different, with M3 results typically fourfold dilutions lower than those obtained with RPMI-1640. Investigational animal studies do not support the high results seen with RPMI and some researchers feel that the M3 result is more representative of a true MIC.

Mold testing requires a different endpoint determination for the echinocandins. The MIC is not an appropriate endpoint; therefore, the minimum effective concentration (MEC) is used. Molds tested against the echinocandins result in visible growth through all concentrations. The growth that is present is abnormal and the effect of the drug is obvious. The MEC is the lowest concentration at which this growth defect is visualized.

Resistance has not been widely reported for this class of antifungal. There are, however, a few occurrences of isolates with high MICs. *Candida parapsilosis* and *C guilliermondii* are two species with notoriously increased MICs. Some clinical isolates of *C albicans* and *C glabrata* exist with elevated

MICs, but it is unclear if these isolates are truly resistant in vivo. Susceptibility data for selected yeast and drugs are presented in Table 1.

Combination testing

Combination testing is one of the hottest topics discussed by clinicians
faced with patients who have refractory fungal disease. Historically the
only antifungal combination was amphotericin B plus 5-fluorocytosine. Additionally, amphotericin B plus rifampin was believed to have some value in
treating certain infections. These combinations have been replaced by combining amphotericin B with some of the newer antifungal agents. It is not
uncommon to test amphotericin B plus azoles or echinocandins. Other combinations include azoles plus echinocandins or azoles plus terbinafine. The
azole plus terbinafine combinations have resulted in perhaps the most synergistic results.

Perhaps the most sought after information is the potential for antagonism as a result of the combination. Although synergistic activity is desir-
able, the physician may be most concerned by the potential to treat with
two agents whose activity is decreased because of negative antifungal/anti-
fungal interactions. The potential for antagonism is real but has not been
proven in humans. Animal studies to date have given conflicting results.
Theoretically all drugs tested in combination, with the exception of azoles
and amphotericin B, should result in indifferent or possible synergistic results. Because of the mechanisms of action of azoles and amphotericin B,
however, there may be antagonism when combining these drugs. Although
antagonism may not be noted initially, it should only be expressed once inhibition of the 14 alpha-demethylase by the azole results in depletion of ergosterol in the fungal cell wall, thus eliminating the target for amphotericin
B. Because staggered introduction is required to detect it, evaluation using
checkerboard methods may not detect antagonism. As a result, clinicians
are discouraged from concomitant use of azoles and amphotericin B. A
more rational approach may be to initiate use of amphotericin B followed
by azole therapy when the patient's condition has stabilized [20].

Currently the best that the laboratory can offer is an estimation of which
pathogens are more likely to respond to given antifungals alone and in combination. Combination testing is accomplished in the classic checkerboard
dilution scheme. All testing parameters remain the same, including medium,
inoculum, and incubation. The checkerboard arrangement places single
doubling concentrations of drug A along the X-axis and single concentrations of drug B along the Y-axis. Within the checkerboard, every possible
concentration combination of the two drugs is tested. The final result is
the lowest concentration of drug A plus the lowest concentration of drug
B in which the endpoint criteria are met. Although the result can be determined mathematically, it is still a confusing matter. The MIC of each drug
within the combination is expressed as a fraction of each drug alone. The

Table 2
Aspergillus spp combination testing results

	Synergistic	Indifferent	Antagonistic
AMB+RIF			
A fumigatus	0	10(4)	0
A flavus	0	2	0
A terreus	0	2(1)	0
AMB+CAS			
A fumigatus	0	25(4)	0
A flavus	0	2(1)	0
A terreus	0	3	0
A niger	0	1	0
AMB+ITRA			
A fumigatus	0	7	1
A flavus	0	2(1)	0
A terreus	0	2	0
Emericilla nidulans	0	1	0
AMB+VORI			
A fumigatus	0	15(2)	2
A flavus	0	1	3
A terreus	0	2(1)	0
A niger	0	3	0
VORI+CAS			
A fumigatus	0	14(2)	0
A terreus	0	4(1)	0
A niger	0	3	0

Selected *in vitro* Fungus Testing Laboratory data for combination testing of aspergili. Numbers in parentheses indicate tests that had lower MICs as a result of the combination, formerly know as additive, as opposed to no change in the MIC as a result of the combination.

fractions are then added to arrive at the fractional inhibitory concentration index (FICI) [21].

Synergism is achieved when the FICI is less than 0.6 and antagonism occurs with FICI greater than 1. Indifference is noted when the FICI falls between 0.6 and 0.9. Early writings included another category, but this category has fallen from favor for current reporting. The term "additivism" is considered to provide a confusing connotation and therefore has been eliminated [22]. An FICI that would have placed results in this category are now considered indifferent. Sample results for aspergilli are presented in Table 2.

Summary

Antifungal susceptibility testing has been in routine use now for more than 15 years and has become a useful tool for clinicians who are faced with difficult treatment decisions. Although most clinicians order susceptibility testing, much confusion still exists regarding the use of the results. Sufficient data have been generated to determine susceptibility trends for specific fungi against specific agents, but correlation data are minimal. Despite the lack of correlation data, antifungal susceptibility testing continues to provide useful information to assist with patient care.

References

[1] NCCLS. Reference method for broth dilution antifungal susceptibility testing of yeasts; proposed standard NCCLS document M27-P. Wayne (PA): National Committee for Clinical Laboratory Standards; 1992.

[2] NCCLS. Reference method for broth dilution antifungal susceptibility testing of yeasts; approved standard NCCLS document M27–A2. Wayne (PA): National Committee for Clinical Laboratory Standards; 2002.

[3] Espinel-Ingroff A, Barchiesi F, Cuenca-Estrella M, et al. International and multicenter comparison of EUCAST and CLSI M27–A2 broth microdilution methods for testing susceptibilities of Candida spp to fluconazole, itraconazole, posaconazole, and voriconazole. J Clin Microbiol 2005;43(8):3884–9.

[4] NCCLS. Reference method for broth dilution antifungal susceptibility testing of conidial-forming filamentous fungi; approved standard NCCLS M38-A. Wayne (PA): National Committee for Clinical Laboratory Standards; 2002.

[5] NCCLS. Reference method for antifungal disk diffusion susceptibility testing of yeasts; approved guideline NCCLS document M44-A. Wayne (PA): National Committee for Clinical Laboratory Standards; 2004.

[6] Barry A, Bille J, Brown S, et al. Quality control limits from fluconazole disk susceptibility tests on Mueller-Hinton agar with glucose and methylene blue. J Clin Microbiol 2003; 41(7):3410–2.

[7] Espinel-Ingroff A, Pfaller M, Messer SA, et al. Multicenter comparison of the Sensititre YeastOne colorimetric antifungal panel with the NCCLS M27–A2 reference methods for testing new antifungal agents against clinical isolates of Candida spp. J Clin Microbiol 2004;42(2): 718–21.

[8] Maxwell MJ, Messer SA, Hollis RJ, et al. Evaluation of ETEST method for determining fluconazole and voriconazole MICs for 279 clinical isolates of Candida species infrequently isolated from blood. J Clin Microbiol 2003;41(3):1087–90.

[9] Maxwell MJ, Messer SA, Hollis RJ, et al. Evaluation of ETEST method for determining voriconazole and amphotericin B MICs for 162 clinical isolates of Cryptococcus neoformans. J Clin Microbiol 2003;41(1):97–9.

[10] Rex JH, Pfaller MA. Has antifungal susceptibility testing come of age? Clin Infect Dis 2002; 35(8):982–9.

[11] Chaturvedi V, Ramani R, Rex JH. Collaborative study of antibiotic medium 3 and flow cytometry for identification of amphotericin B-resistant Candida isolates. J Clin Microbiol 2004;42(5):2252–4.

[12] Pappagianis D, Collins MS, Hector R, et al. Development of resistance to amphotericin B in Candida lusitaniae infecting a human. Antimicrob Agents Chemother 1979;16:123–6.

[13] Merz WG. Candida lusitaniae: frequency of recovery, colonization, infection, and amphotericin B resistance. J Clin Microbiol 1984;20:1194–5.

[14] Pfaller MA, Messer SA, Hollis RJ, et al. Trends in species distribution and susceptibility to fluconazole among blood stream isolates of Candida species in the United States. Diagn Microbiol Infect Dis 1999;33:217–22.

[15] Messer SA, Diekema DJ, Boyken L, et al. Activities of micafungin against 315 invasive clinical isolates of fluconazole-resistant Candida spp. J Clin Microbiol 2006;44(2):324–6.

[16] Odds FC, Motyl M, Andrade R, et al. Interlaboratory comparison of results of susceptibility testing with caspofungin against Candida and Aspergillus species. J Clin Microbiol 2004; 42(8):3475–82.

[17] Pfaller MA, Boyken L, Hollis RJ, et al. In vitro susceptibilities of *Candida* spp to caspofungin; four years of global surveillance. J Clin Microbiol 2006;44(3):760–3.

[18] Pfaller MA, Boyken L, Hollis RJ, et al. In vitro activities of anidulafungin against more than 2,500 clinical isolates of *Candida* spp, including 315 isolates resistant to fluconazole. J Clin Microbiol 2005;43(11):5424–7.

[19] Pfaller MA, Diekema DJ, Boyken L, et al. Effectiveness of anidulafungin in eradicating *Candida* species in invasive candidiasis. Antimicrob Agents Chemother 2005;49(11):4795–7.

[20] Lewis RE, Kontoyiannis DP. Rationale for combination antifungal therapy. Pharmacotherapy 2001;21(8 Pt 2):149S–64S.

[21] Johnson MD, MacDougal C, Ostrosky-Zeichner L, et al. Mini review: combination antifungal therapy. Antimicrob Agents Chemother 2004;48(3):693–715.

[22] Greco WR, Bravo G, Parsons JC. The search for synergy; a critical review from a response surface perspective. Pharmacol Rev 1995;47:331–85.

ELSEVIER
SAUNDERS

Infect Dis Clin N Am
20 (2006) 711–727

INFECTIOUS
DISEASE CLINICS
OF NORTH AMERICA

Non–Culture-Based Diagnostics for Opportunistic Fungi

Monique A.S.H. Mennink-Kersten, PhD[a,b], Paul E. Verweij, MD, PhD[a,b],*

[a]*Department of Medical Microbiology, Radboud University, Nijmegen Medical Center,
P.O. Box 9101, 6500 HB Nijmegen, The Netherlands*
[b]*Nijmegen University Center for Infectious Diseases, P.O. Box 9101,
6500 HB Nijmegen, The Netherlands*

Diagnostic markers are becoming available for the diagnosis of opportunistic mycoses. The markers differ in the range of fungi that are detected. Detection of genomic fungal DNA has largely been studied using in-house–made polymerase chain reaction (PCR) systems, although recently commercial formats have become available. The diagnostic value of PCR systems remains to be determined, although in-house assays indicate that circulating fungal DNA is an early marker of invasive fungal disease. Commercial systems that detect the *Aspergillus* cell wall antigen galactomannan (GM, Platelia Aspergillus) and 1,3-β-D-glucan (BG, Fungitell), which are present in a broad range of fungi and plants, have been approved by the US Food and Drug Administration (FDA). In a meta-analysis of diagnostic trials, the Platelia Aspergillus was shown to be moderately accurate for diagnosing invasive aspergillosis in patients who have hematologic malignancy, although a significant variation between trials was observed. Some factors that have impact on the performance of the assay have been identified, including exposure to mold-active antifungal agents and the underlying disease of the patient. Also, factors that might cause false reactivity have been identified, including certain β-lactam antibiotics and intestinal bacteria.

The clinical experience with BG is limited, although several studies show high sensitivity in patients who have invasive aspergillosis and invasive candidiasis. Glucans, however, are widely distributed throughout the environment, and some studies have identified patient groups that might react

---

* Corresponding author.
E-mail address: p.verweij@mmb.umcn.nl (P.E. Verweij).

0891-5520/06/$ - see front matter © 2006 Elsevier Inc. All rights reserved.
doi:10.1016/j.idc.2006.06.009   *id.theclinics.com*

positively, including those undergoing hemodialysis with cellulose membranes and those receiving intravenous treatment with immunoglobulins. BG has also been detected in amoxicillin-clavulanic acid and the blood of patients treated with this antibiotic. With increasing experience with this assay, more insight will be obtained in the characteristics and potential sources of false reactivity.

With the availability of multiple diagnostic markers, strategic studies are warranted that help us to determine the value of the different diagnostic markers in various risk groups and the optimal sequence or combination.

Opportunistic mycoses remain an important cause of morbidity and mortality in immunocompromised patients. Common causes of invasive fungal infections include the yeast *Candida* and the mold *Aspergillus*, although a broad range of yeasts and molds have been described to be able to cause invasive fungal disease in humans. Zygomycetes especially have gained interest because of the observed increasing frequency in some centers [1].

Although the outcome of invasive fungal disease strongly depends on the underlying condition of the patient and the recovery of the host defenses, the timing of therapeutic intervention seems also to be important. Recently the time of initiation of antifungal therapy in patients who have candidemia was shown to have significant impact on mortality, with those patients being treated within 12 hours of obtaining a blood culture having a 20% lower mortality rate than those in whom antifungal therapy was delayed until 12 to 24 hours or later [2].

Early identification of patients who require antifungal therapy is therefore an important goal and requires diagnostic tools that not only have good performance characteristics, but also become positive in an early phase of the infection. Until the last two decades, the diagnostic arsenal mainly depended on microscopy and culture of biologic samples. Culture of fungi generally lacks sensitivity and specificity and becomes positive in advanced stages of the infection when the fungal burden is high. Although the sensitivity of blood cultures for detection of yeast is high (approximately 80%), the time to detection in commercial blood culture vials varies between 18 and 74 hours depending on the *Candida* species, which is beyond the 12-hour window in which treatment should be commenced to achieve a survival benefit [2,3]. This underscores the need for additional diagnostic tools.

Within the last two decades substantial effort has been made to identify markers that are released by fungi and can be detected in clinical samples. These efforts have focused on the detection of genomic fungal DNA and on cell wall components. Both these types of markers can be detected in the blood of patients who have invasive fungal disease, although only systems that detect cell wall components have been made commercially available and have undergone clinical validation. Systems that detect genomic fungal DNA include mainly in-house–developed formats that are not widely available. They provide evidence that fungal DNA can be an early marker of invasive fungal disease [4], but until the tests are standardized, it remains difficult to determine the value of this approach. Recently, however, some commercial PCR formats have become available and the results of the technical and clinical validation studies are eagerly awaited. Antigen detection systems have been developed for numerous fungi, including *Aspergillus*, *Candida*, *Cryptococcus*, and several endemic mycoses. For *Candida*, several systems have been commercialized, such as the Platelia Candida (BioRad), which detects mannan antigen and anti-mannan antibodies. This and other assays, however, are not widely available or are awaiting approval. In this review, the authors discuss two surrogate markers that have been approved by the FDA, the *Aspergillus* antigen galactomannan (GM) and the cell wall component 1,3-β-D-glucan (BG).

Requirements of non–culture-based diagnostic systems

In general, the requirements needed for an optimal diagnostic tool are, besides good performance characteristics and early detection of invasive fungal disease, detection of a broad range of fungi and identification to the species level. Patients are at risk for infection by a broad range of fungi, but the choice of antifungal drug is driven by the fungal genus and species. The markers differ in the range of fungi that can be detected (Table 1). Only systems for genomic fungal DNA can be designed to detect many relevant fungi and to identify fungi to the species level. The systems based on cell wall components at best can identify to the genus level. There is presently no non–culture-based antigen system that detects Zygomycetes. Although antigens are released during growth of Zygomycetes, among those are not GM or BG, and consequently invasive zygomycosis remains undetected when patients are monitored using these antigen detection systems.

Table 1
Opportunistic fungi that can be detected by different surrogate marker systems

Fungus	GM	BG	PCR[a]
A. fumigatus	+	+	+
Non-fumigatus *Aspergillus*	+	+	+
Fusarium	−	+	+
Zygomycetes	−	−	+
Candida	−	+	+
Cryptococcus	+[b]	±[c]	+
Penicillium	+	+	+
Paecilomyces	+	+	+

Abbreviations: GM, galactomannan; BG, 1,3-β-D-glucan.

[a] Detection of genomic fungal DNA by PCR techniques. In principle the PCR can be designed to detect any fungus, although the clinical experience is limited for fungi other than *Aspergillus, Candida,* and *Cryptococcus.*

[b] The *Cryptococcus* cell wall component galactoxylomannan is suggested to contain one or multiple epitopes that cross-react with aspergillus GM [19].

[c] The *Cryptococcus* cell wall contains 1,3-β-D-glucan; however, only a small amount is released [45]. In approximately 25% of patients who have invasive cryptococcosis, circulating BG can be detected [48].

The test systems preferably should give a quantitative result, which enables the detection of trends of the levels when repeated samples are taken. This property is present in all markers, including GM and BG, and for both markers the course of the antigen titer during antifungal therapy was found to correspond with clinical response [5,6].

Most studies that have evaluated the performance of surrogate markers have relied on repetitive sampling of patients. If the period of high risk for invasive fungal disease is well established and the patient is admitted to the hospital, this approach can be followed. In addition, the pretest probability of the disease has to be high to achieve an acceptable positive predictive value. With prevalence of invasive aspergillosis typically being between 0.05 and 0.10, the positive predictive value of GM surveillance was 0.25 and 0.49, respectively, in published studies [7]. Approaches that rely on surveillance might be feasible for invasive aspergillosis in specific host groups, but not for invasive *Candida* infection. For *Aspergillus*, the risk is high in patients who have neutropenia, hematologic malignancy (most notably acute myeloid leukemia and myelodysplastic syndrome), and stem cell transplant recipients, and the vast majority of studies with surrogate markers, especially GM, have been performed in these patient groups. *Candida*, however, is less common in patients who have hematologic malignancy and occurs more frequently in other, more heterogeneous patient groups, such as critically ill patients. Whether prospective monitoring is a feasible approach in these patients remains to be established.

Although antigen detection has become an important tool in the diagnosis and management of patients who have invasive mycoses, the results should be interpreted in the context of the presence of risk factors in the host, appropriate signs and symptoms, or radiologic imaging.

Galactomannan

Aspergillus contains mannoproteins in the outer cell wall layer, and one of the structures present is the carbohydrate galactomannan. Although the name suggests that GM is a single molecule, recent studies indicate that this is not the case, and that GM is a family of molecules that are referred to as galactofuranose (gal*f*)-antigens [8]. The gal*f*-antigens contain galactofuranose residues that react with the rat IgM monoclonal antibody (EB-A2) that is used in the Platelia Aspergillus enzyme immunoassay (PA-ELISA, BioRad). It was recently shown that a galactofuranose residue is also present in fungal glycoproteins, including phospholipase C and phytase, which consequently also react with the EB-A2 antibody [8]. That *Aspergillus* releases several substances that contain galactofuranose epitopes might have a positive effect on the sensitivity of the PA-ELISA in clinical practice, but it remains unclear how *Aspergillus* releases antigen during infection, which factors have impact on this release, and in which form the antigens circulate in the blood.

Until recently the PA-ELISA was used in the United States with a threshold of 0.5, whereas the rest of the world used a threshold of 1.5, despite the fact identical assays were used. This difference is historical, because the kit first became available in Europe in 1995. At that time a threshold of 1.5 was chosen by the manufacturer without underlying evidence supporting that choice. Since then several publications have indicated that a lower cut-off could be used [9,10]. In fact, even in the publication that first described the PA-ELISA, a threshold of 0.7 was recommended [11]. Recently the threshold was re-evaluated based on receiver-operator-curve (ROC) analyses of data from two centers from Europe, confirming that 0.5 was the optimal cut-off, which is now recommended by the manufacturer worldwide [12].

Clinical studies

In approximately two thirds of patients who have hematologic malignancy, circulating antigen can be detected before diagnosis is made by other means, although considerable variability of sensitivity has been reported even within the group of patients who have hematologic malignancy [13]. The sensitivity varied between 33% and 100% in individual prospective trials with a specificity generally greater than 85%. A recent meta-analysis calculated an overall sensitivity of 0.71 (95% CI, 0.68–0.74) and a specificity of 0.89 (95% CI, 0.88–0.90) for proven cases [7]. The investigators concluded that the assay has a moderate accuracy for diagnosing invasive aspergillosis, at least in hematology patients [7]. There are many reasons for variability in performance, which were recently reviewed [13]. Factors that have emerged that cause false-negative reactivity include exposure to mold-active antifungal agents [14,15]. In one study the sensitivity of the assay was reduced to only 20% in patients receiving mold-active antifungal drugs, as compared with 87.5% in the non-exposed control subjects [15]. Also, the underlying condition of the patient has impact on the performance of the PA-ELISA. The highest sensitivity is found in patients who have hematologic malignancy, especially those who are neutropenic. In liver transplant recipients the sensitivity was only 56%, and in lung transplant patients it was 30% [16,17]. In patients who have chronic granulomatous disease (CGD), circulating antigen is often not detected, although the number of cases reported is limited [18]. The pathogenesis of invasive aspergillosis is different between these patient groups, with rapid angioinvasion in the neutropenic host as opposed to abscess formation in the patient who have CGD. This might affect the release and leakage of GM from the site of infection to the circulation.

Causes of false reactivity

The GM antigen is widely distributed through the environment and is heat stable. It has been found in foods and beverages, and as shown in Table 1, it is not exclusively produced by *Aspergillus* species, but also by *Penicillium*,

Paecilomyces, and *Cryptococcus* [19]. The proportion of patients who show false-positive reactivity with serum decreases with age. In neonates, as many as 83% of patients might show false-positive serum reactivity [20], whereas this rate is approximately 10% in pediatric patients [21] and 2.5% in adults [22,23]. The integrity of the gut might play a role in this respect, because feces was found to be highly reactive with the PA-ELISA. Cases have been reported that link GM serum reactivity to ingestion of GM-containing beverages [24] or that describe associations between neutropenia (loss of intestinal integrity caused by mucosal barrier injury) and transient antigenemia [25]. Translocation of the antigen as source of false serum reactivity, however, has not been proven.

Besides the presence of environmental GM in feces, the β-1,5-galactofuranose residue is present in bifidobacteria, which are part of the gastrointestinal microflora [26,27]. These bacteria have lipoglycans in their cell wall with the gal*f*-epitope detectable as a surface antigen. When secreted, they may form micelles with multiple gal*f*-epitopes exposed to the outside [27]. In vitro, these bacteria and their culture supernatants showed significant reactivity with the PA-ELISA [27]. As the intestinal bacterial flora of neonates predominantly contains bifidobacteria, it was suggested that translocation of these bacteria or the cross-reacting antigen might contribute to the high false serum reactivity observed in this patient group [26,27].

Serum reactivity has been observed in patients who receive β-lactam antibiotics, including piperacillin/tazobactam, amoxicillin/clavulanic acid, ampicillin, and phenoxymethyl-penicillin [28–34]. These antibiotics have been shown to contain PA-ELISA–reactive material [28,30–34]. This is likely to be GM, because the fungus *Penicillium* is used in the production process of the aforementioned antibiotics, and *Penicillium* is known to release GM and other gal*f*-antigens. There is not always a relationship between the concentration in the lot and the GM indices found in the patient's serum [30,34]. Repeated administration of the piperacillin tazobactam combination (GM index: 0.75) over 7 days resulted in accumulation of circulating antigen to positive GM index levels [32]. Other investigators found three patterns of serum reactivity in patients receiving positive lots. Persisting GM indices greater than 2 were observed in 65.7% of patients, and GM indices between 0.5 and 1.5 were found in 25.7%. Variable GM indices were observed in the remaining 14.3% of patients [34]. Most patients were classified incorrectly according to the European Organisation for Research and Treatment of Cancer/Mycoses Study Group (EORTC/MSG) consensus definitions, usually in the probable category instead of the possible category, because the mycology criterion was met. The mean time needed to clear the antigen after discontinuation of the antibiotic therapy was 5.5 days, with a half-life of 2.4 days [34].

Although the PA-ELISA is standardized for detection of GM in serum, the antigen can be detected in other body fluids of patients who have invasive aspergillosis, including cerebrospinal fluid (CSF), urine, and bronchoalveolar lavage (BAL) fluid [35]. The published clinical experience with GM detection in these specimens, however, is limited to case reports, retrospective studies, and low numbers of cases with proven infection.

1,3-β-D-glucan

Glucans are glucose polymers joined by glucosidic linkages between C-1 on one residue and C-2, C-3, C-4, or C-6 on the next glucose residue with two possible configurations (ie, α- and β-linkages). α- and β- glucans are widely distributed in microorganisms and plants, but in contrast to α-glucans (eg, glycogens), the occurrence of β-glucans in animals is restricted to a few invertebrates. An overview of linkage composition, organization, and sources of α- and β-glucans is given by Stone and Clarke [36]. The 1,3-β-D-glucans with various molecular weights and degrees of branching may originate from a large variety of sources, including most fungi and yeasts, some bacteria, algae and plants, in which they have storage, structural, or protective roles [36]. They are water-insoluble structural cell wall components of these organisms, but may also be found in extracellular secretions of microbial origin. In fungi they are often present as an inner cell wall layer and are associated with other cell wall polymers, particularly polysaccharides, such as chitin. As major cell wall components, they are, together with 1,3-β-glucan hydrolases and synthases, involved in cell wall modifications during growth and morphogenesis [36].

1,3-β-D-glucan assay

A concentration as low as 1 pg/mL can be quantified spectrophotometrically by activation of factor G, a coagulation factor of the horseshoe crab [37]. BG specifically binds to the α subunit of factor G, activating its serine protease zymogen β subunit [38]. The activated factor G activates the proclotting enzyme of the horseshoe-crab (*Limulus polyphemus* or *Tachypleus tridentatus*) coagulation cascade, which in turn cleaves the chromogenic substrate Boc-Leu-Gly-Arg-p-nitroanilide, creating a chromophore that absorbs at 405 nm. The ability of linear BG to activate factor G has to exceed a critical value of 6800 Mw (DP 38) and increases with increasing Mw [39,40]. Low molecular-weight BGs are inactive even at concentrations as high as 100,000 pg/mL [39]. The single helical conformation is the dominant contributor to the activation of factor G [40], whereas for linkage type, Tanaka and colleagues [39] reported that linear 1,3-β-D-glucans, branched 1-3,1-6-β-D-glucans, and mixed linkage 1-3,1-4-β-D-glucans activated factor G. In addition, they also demonstrated that other polysaccharides, including endotoxin, did not exhibit such activity [39]. The BG assay was largely unreactive with 1,4-β-D-glucan, 1,6-β-D-glucan, and non-glucans containing 1,3-β-D-glucan linkages [39,41]. Furthermore, 1,2;1,3;1,6-α-mannan from *Saccharomyces cerevisiae* also showed low reactivity [41].

Because humans do not produce BG or BG-degrading enzymes, the presence of this component in the blood is presumed to indicate the presence of a fungal pathogen. The Fungi-Tec (Seikagaku Corporation) assay is widely used in Japan and uses the enzymes from *T tridentatus* for BG detection in plasma samples with a cutoff level of 20 pg/mL [37]. In contrast, a recently FDA-approved method has become available on the European and US markets (Fungitell, Associates of Cape Cod) using *L polyphemus* enzymes for BG detection in serum samples with a cutoff level of 60 pg/mL [41]. To measure BG levels in serum or plasma, the samples have to be treated with an alkaline reagent to convert triple-helix BGs into single-stranded BGs, which are more reactive in the assay [40,42]. The high pH also inactivates the serine proteases and serine-protease inhibitors in human blood that can give a false-positive and false-negative result, respectively [43]. These assays have been used to measure BG release in vitro by different fungal species and also to measure circulating BG levels in patients who have invasive fungal diseases.

BG is a pan-fungal marker, because the component is present in the cell wall of most medically important fungi, including *Aspergillus*, *Fusarium*, *Candida*, and *Trichosporon* [37,44]. Furthermore, also *S cerevisiae*, *Acremonium*, *Coccidioides immitis*, *Histoplasma capsulatum*, *Sporothrix schenckii*, *Blastomyces dermatitidis*, and *Pneumocystis jiroveci* can be detected by the assay [37,41]. Although various *Candida* spp, *S cerevisiae*, *Rhodotorula rubra*, *T beigelii*, and *A fumigatus* have been shown to release soluble BG into the culture fluid in parallel with in vitro fungal growth [45], *C neoformans* and *Cunninghamella bertholletiae* showed only a small reaction to the G test during their culture [45]. The reactivity of BG to factor G is known to be inhibited at high concentrations [46]; however, there was no evidence of overproduction of BG in culture supernatants of *C neoformans* [45]. Other studies showed that the BG assay is not useful for diagnosis of cryptococcosis and zygomycosis [47,48]. *P jiroveci* pneumonia (PCP) is also associated with circulating BG levels, because *P jiroveci* contain BG in their cyst wall [49].

Clinical studies

Until now only a limited amount of comparative studies have been done with the BG test (Table 2). The Fungi-Tec assay uses a cutoff level of 20 pg/mL and plasma samples for BG testing. This assay is widely used in Japan. Kami and colleagues [50] showed a sensitivity and specificity of 67% and 84%, respectively, in 33 patients who had invasive aspergillosis.

The Fungitell assay recommends a 60 pg/mL cut-off value with a definitive positive value above 80 pg/mL. These serum BG levels were chosen on the basis of a recent study of 30 candidemic subjects and 30 healthy adults [41]. Furthermore, this study showed that 60 pg/mL or more of this polysaccharide can be detected in serum of neutropenic patients who have a proven or probable invasive fungal infection [41]. Sensitivity and specificity ranged

Table 2
Performance of 1,3-β-D-glucan test in different clinical studies

Clinical study[a]	Cutoff used (pg/mL)	Sensitivity (%)	Specificity (%)	False positivity (%)	Ref.
Proven/probable IFI	60	100	90	4.3	[41]
Proven/probable IA	120	87.5	89.6	10.3	[6]
Proven/probable IFI	60	69.9	87.1	—	[48]
	80	64.4	92.4	—	[48]
Proven aspergillosis	60	80	—	—	[48]
	80	80	—	—	[48]
Proven candidiasis	60	81.3	—	—	[48]
	80	77.6	—	—	[48]
Proven cryptococcosis	60	25	—	—	[48]
	80	16.7	—	—	[48]
Candidemic/bacteremic patients	60	93.3	72.1	68	[51]
	80	86.7	77.2	56	[51]
Proven/probable IA	20	67	84	—	[50]

[a] Patients were considered to be positive if the level of BG was ≥20, 60, 80, or 120 pg/mL in at least one serum sample.

from 100% to 60% and 90% to 99%, respectively, depending on the number of positive sequential serum samples (1 to 3). Antifungal prophylaxis with caspofungin or itraconazole did not seem to affect the performance of the test [41], and the false-positive rate was 4.3%. A European study by Pazos and colleagues used a 120 pg/mL threshold to increase specificity of this test for diagnosis of invasive aspergillosis in 40 neutropenic patients and compared the test with the GM test using a threshold of 1.5 [6]. The sensitivity and specificity for GM and BG were identical, 87.5% and 89.6%, respectively. False-positive reactions occurred at a rate of 10.3% in both tests, but the patients showing false-positive results were different in each test [6]. Combination of the GM and BG test resulted in an increase of specificity to 100%. A recent multicenter clinical evaluation showed sensitivity for detection of invasive aspergillosis in 10 patients of 80% at 60-pg/mL and 80-pg/mL cutoff values [48]. For detection of invasive fungal disease (*Candida*, *Aspergillus*, *Fusarium*, *Cryptococcus*), sensitivity and specificity were 69.9% and 87.1%, respectively. The sensitivity was shown to be higher for subjects who had proven invasive fungal disease not receiving antifungal therapy compared with the subjects who were receiving antifungal therapy. Results from Pickering and colleagues [51] suggest that the Fungitell assay may be most useful for excluding invasive fungal disease because of the high number of false-positive results. Specificity was 77.2%, because 14 out of 25 bacteremic patients were BG-positive, 10 of these with gram-positive bacteremia. Also, other studies suggest that the assay may have value as a negative predictor of infections [52]. The actual value for diagnosis of invasive fungal disease has to be awaited.

Causes of false 1,3-β-D-glucan reactivity

As is clear from the aforementioned studies, one of the problems observed in the detection of BG is the occurrence of false-positive results, which decreases the specificity of the test [53]. As far as the specificity of the test is concerned, the only substance known to activate factor G is BG. Known causes of false-positive BG reactivity (ie, not related to invasive fungal disease) are hemodialysis with cellulose membranes [54–56], intravenous treatment with immunoglobulins [57,58], and specimens or patients exposed to gauzes and other BG-containing materials. A potential source of BG in drugs is the use of cellulose depth filters during the manufacturing process that might lead to variable levels of BG [59,60]. Albumin, coagulation factors, and plasma protein fractions manufactured using these filters have been shown to contain high levels of BG [59]. In addition, excess manipulation of a sample can result in contamination with BG [51]. Furthermore, dust samples contain high levels of BG [61]. The β-lactam antibiotic amoxicillin-clavulanic acid has recently been shown to contain BG and to cause BG reactivity in serum of patients following intravenous administration of the drug [62].

Although bacterial infections are suggested to be a possible cause of false BG reactivity [51,52], the only bacteria known to contain a β-1,3-glucan are *Alcaligenes faecalis* and *Streptococcus pneumoniae* [36,63]. Certain other streptococci are known to produce glucan [64], however, these are α-1,3-glucans [65]. Also certain gram-negative bacteria produce β-linked glucans, but these have β-1-2 and β-1-6 linkages [65,66]. In vitro testing of bacteria for BG reactivity should be done to determine if they contain cross-reactive molecules.

Two patients who were colonized with *Candida* showed "false" BG reactivity. Other patients who had intense colonization by *Candida* species, however, had negative BG levels [6]. Furthermore, fungal colonization (including oral, urinary, and bronchial colonization) did not increase the BG concentration to greater than 20 pg/mL [37]. Whether colonization might cause positive BG remains to be determined. The study of Yuasa and Goto [67] suggested that BG is released during the earliest stage of the invasive process of pulmonary aspergilloma, in which the fungus was considered not to have invaded the surrounding tissue or bloodstream.

In vivo kinetics, clearance, and immune response

Similar to GM, the kinetics of BG release in vitro and in vivo are poorly understood. A recent in vitro study with *A fumigatus* showed that BG and GM are released during logarithmic growth in the culture medium [68]. BG was detected somewhat later than GM and showed a decrease after 24 hours that was not caused by nutrient limitation (ie, glucose). Decrease of BG after 24 hours of in vitro growth has already been shown by Miyazaki and colleagues [45] for *C albicans* and was suggested to be caused by the enzyme β-1,3-glucanase. *A fumigatus* has been shown to produce cell wall-associated exo-1,3-β-glucanases and an endo-1,3-β-glucanase that might have a role in cell wall morphogenesis [69,70]. In other filamentous fungi exocellular β-glucanases also have been found and seem to have a role in hydrolyzing exocellular BGs for fungal catabolism. Whether this enzyme is clinically relevant remains to be established. Although elevation of the BG level in plasma paralleled the development and extent of *Aspergillus* infection in the animal model [71], the conditions at the infection site might influence the release of BG, especially during nutrient limitation [68]. Without a circulating fungal β-glucan catabolic enzyme, degradation of BG would not be accomplished in vivo, because humans lack these enzymes. That might explain the slow elimination of the antigen from plasma [57]. BG was detected in plasma and urine of patients after intravenous immunoglobulin therapy. A total amount of 150 pg/mL BG in the blood decreased to approximately 50 pg/mL in 5 hours after administration. During the first 2 hours, 23 ng was found in the urine, which was less than 5% of the total amount administered [57]. Another study showed that cells of *Candida* administered intravenously to mice were immediately deposited mainly in the liver as determined by ^{3}H-labeled cells. BGs were detected in these mice for at least 6 months by the BG assay. During this period the insoluble cell wall BG was gradually solubilized in these organs, by oxidative degradation by phagocytes, which use nonspecific oxidation reactions involving O_2, H_2O_2, and hypochlorous acid [72]. Intravenous administration of soluble forms of BG showed a 50% clearance rate of 5 hours from the blood and deposition in the same organs [72]. Because the cell wall BG is basically insoluble material in water, it is probably the soluble form that is present in blood of patients who have invasive fungal disease. The exact nature of the BGs that circulate in the blood remains unknown, however. The host lacks a BG catabolic enzyme and it is believed that BG is solubilized by the defense mechanism of the host or the metabolic process of the fungus [73].

BGs exhibit various biologic and immunopharmacologic activities, and the degree of these activities depends on the nature of the individual BGs (ie, molecular weight, degree of branching, conformation, and solubility in water) [73]. Many studies have shown that BG increases the function of macrophages, neutrophils, and other immunocytes [74,75]. Systemic intravenous administration to animals of BG microparticulates, however, has been shown to be associated with hypertrophy and hyperplasia of macrophage-rich organs, such as the liver, lung, and spleen. Specifically, granuloma formation has been observed [74,75]. When BG was converted to a water-soluble form, however, the undesirable side effects were eliminated while the immunologic activity was preserved [74]. Rice and colleagues studied the pharmacokinetics of different soluble BGs following intravenous and oral administration to animals [76,77]. Following oral administration, these BGs showed plasma peaks between 0.5 and 12 hours after translocation from the gastrointestinal tract into the systemic circulation. The BGs were bound and internalized by intestinal epithelial cells and gut-associated lymphoid tissue cells. Intravenous administration elimination half-lives ranged between 2.6 and 3.8 hours, whereas clearance varied between 42 and 117 mL/kg/h.

It has been suggested that a possible mechanism for establishing a fungal infection might be that fungi release soluble BG that blocks the BG receptors of phagocytes, permitting the fungus to escape host defense mechanisms [47].

Surveillance with diagnostic markers

A limited number of strategic studies that incorporate diagnostic markers have been performed. A decision analysis indicated that an approach based on surveillance with GM would lead to better identification of patients who require antifungal therapy without increasing the risk for incorrectly withholding antifungal therapy [78]. This preemptive approach was recently studied in hematology patients, showing that in patients undergoing GM surveillance, invasive aspergillosis was better identified than would be the case with an empiric management strategy [79]. The use of antifungals was also lower in the preemptive group as compared with the empiric group (17% versus 35%) [79]. Although the aforementioned study was a feasibility study, it supports an increasing role of diagnostic markers in the management of these patients.

With the number of available surrogate markers increasing, the role of each marker in the management of patients at risk for invasive fungal

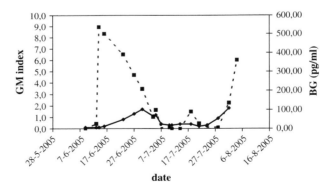

Fig. 1. Results of surveillance with BG of a neutropenic patient who had acute myeloid leukemia. A positive BG result (536.8 pg/mL) was obtained on June 16. GM and mannan were determined in the same sample but were negative (serum ratio, 0.1). A high-resolution CT scan of the chest showed no lesions consistent with invasive fungal disease. Mannan remained negative in consecutive samples, but the GM index started to increase in serum samples obtained 9 days (serum ratio, 0.8) after the first positive BG result. The patient was finally diagnosed with a proven invasive aspergillosis in the nasopharynx. Circulating BG levels are represented in the graph with a dotted line and the GM index with a solid line. Diagnosis of invasive aspergillosis was confirmed by nasopharyngeal biopsy on July 2.

disease needs to be studied. Although surveillance with multiple markers in high-risk patients seems to be a logical approach, cost issues certainly play a role. Also, the interpretation of results becomes more complex. The markers could be used to diagnose invasive fungal disease or to rule out the presence of invasive fungal disease, for instance, in persistently febrile high-risk patients. In addition, a marker could support true reactivity of another marker [80] or alternatively could confirm false reactivity. The time of first detection of circulating markers, however, might differ, and this may further complicate the interpretation. An example is shown in Fig. 1, in which several diagnostic markers were monitored in a neutropenic patient who had acute myeloid leukemia. BG was the first marker to become positive, which would indicate the presence of an invasive fungal infection. The diagnostic work-up in this situation is unclear given the broad range of fungi that may cause reactivity. GM and mannan (indicative of invasive candidiasis) were negative at that time. Only after 9 days was an increase of GM noted, and finally invasive aspergillosis of the nasopharynx was diagnosed.

Within the past decades much progress has been made in the development and clinical validation of diagnostic tools for opportunistic mycoses. The diagnostic markers are used in many centers that care for immunocompromised patients and help to identify those that require a diagnostic work-up or antifungal therapy. Nevertheless, to date no study has shown that approaches incorporating surveillance with non–culture-based diagnostic methods lead to a survival benefit.

References

[1] Marty FM, Cosimi LA, Baden LR. Breakthrough zygomycosis after voriconazole treatment in recipients of hematopoietic stem-cell transplants. N Engl J Med 2004;350(9):950–2.
[2] Morrell M, Fraser VJ, Kollef MH. Delaying the empiric treatment of *Candida* bloodstream infection until positive blood culture results are obtained: a potential risk factor for hospital mortality. Antimicrob Agents Chemother 2005;49(9):3640–5.
[3] Meyer M-H, Letscher-Bru V, Jaulhac B, et al. Comparison of mycosis IC/F and plus aerobic/F media for diagnosis of fungemia by the Bactec 9240 system. J Clin Microbiol 2004; 42(2):773–7.
[4] Hebart H, Loffler J, Meisner C, et al. Early detection of aspergillus infection after allogeneic stem cell transplantation by polymerase chain reaction screening. J Infect Dis 2000;181(5): 1713–9.
[5] Boutboul F, Alberti C, Leblanc T, et al. Invasive aspergillosis in allogeneic stem cell transplant recipients: increasing antigenemia is associated with progressive disease. Clin Infect Dis 2002;34(7):939–43.
[6] Pazos C, Ponton J, Del Palacio A. Contribution of (1- > 3)-beta-D-glucan chromogenic assay to diagnosis and therapeutic monitoring of invasive aspergillosis in neutropenic adult patients: a comparison with serial screening for circulating galactomannan. J Clin Microbiol 2005;43:299–305.
[7] Pfeiffer CD, Fine JP, Safdar N. Diagnosis of invasive aspergillosis using a galactomannan assay: a meta-analysis. Clin Infect Dis 2006;42(10):1417–27.
[8] Morelle W, Bernard M, Debeaupuis JP, et al. Galactomannoproteins of *Aspergillus fumigatus*. Eukaryot Cell 2005;4:1308–16.

[9] Herbrecht R, Letscher-Bru V, Oprea C, et al. *Aspergillus* galactomannan detection in the diagnosis of invasive aspergillosis in cancer patients. J Clin Oncol 2002;20:1898–906.

[10] Maertens J, Theunissen K, Verbeken E, et al. Prospective clinical evaluation of lower cut-offs for galactomannan detection in adult neutropenic cancer patients and haematological stem cell transplant recipients. Br J Haematol 2004;126(6):852–60.

[11] Stynen D, Goris A, Sarfati J, et al. A new sensitive sandwich enzyme-linked immunosorbent assay to detect galactofuran in patients with invasive aspergillosis. J Clin Microbiol 1995;33:497–500.

[12] Verweij PE, Masson C, Klont R, et al. Optimisation of the cut-off value of the Platelia Aspergillus ELISA. 16th European Conference on Clinical Microbiology and Infectious Diseases. 2006:S277.

[13] Mennink-Kersten MASH, Donnelly JP, Verweij PE. Detection of circulating galactomannan for the diagnosis and management of invasive aspergillosis. Lancet Infect Dis 2004;4:349–57.

[14] Marr KA, Balajee SA, McLaughlin L, et al. Detection of galactomannan antigenemia by enzyme immunoassay for the diagnosis of invasive aspergillosis: variables that affect performance. J Infect Dis 2004;190:641–9.

[15] Marr KA, Laverdiere M, Gugel A, et al. Antifungal therapy decreases sensitivity of the *Aspergillus* galactomannan enzyme immunoassay. Clin Infect Dis 2005;40:1762–9.

[16] Kwak E, Husain S, Obman A, et al. Efficacy of galactomannan antigen in the Platelia *Aspergillus* enzyme immunoassay for diagnosis of invasive aspergillosis in liver transplant recipients. J Clin Microbiol 2004;42:435–8.

[17] Husain S, Kwak EJ, Obman A, et al. Prospective assessment of Platelia Aspergillus galactomannan antigen for the diagnosis of invasive aspergillosis in lung transplant recipients. Am J Transplant 2004;4(5):796–802.

[18] Verweij PE, Weemaes CM, Curfs JH, et al. Failure to detect circulating *Aspergillus* markers in a patient with chronic granulomatous disease and invasive aspergillosis. J Clin Microbiol 2000;38(10):3900–1.

[19] Dalle F, Emmanuel Charles P, et al. *Cryptococcus neoformans* galactoxylomannan contains an epitope(s) that is cross-reactive with *Aspergillus* galactomannan. J Clin Microbiol 2005;43:2929–31.

[20] Rohrlich P, Sarfati J, Mariani P, et al. Prospective sandwich enzyme-linked immunosorbent assay for serum galactomannan: early predictive value and clinical use in invasive aspergillosis. Pediatr Infect Dis J 1996;15:232–7.

[21] Sulahian A, Boutboul F, Ribaud P, et al. Value of antigen detection using an enzyme immunoassay in the diagnosis and prediction of invasive aspergillosis in two adult and pediatric hematology units during a 4-year prospective study. Cancer 2001;91:311–8.

[22] Bretagne S, Costa JM, Bart-Delabesse E, et al. Comparison of serum galactomannan antigen detection and competitive polymerase chain reaction for diagnosing invasive aspergillosis. Clin Infect Dis 1998;26:1407–12.

[23] Maertens J, Verhaegen J, Demuynck H, et al. Autopsy-controlled prospective evaluation of serial screening for circulating galactomannan by a sandwich enzyme-linked immunosorbent assay for hematological patients at risk for invasive aspergillosis. J Clin Microbiol 1999;37:3223–8.

[24] Gangneux JP, Lavarde D, Bretagne S, et al. Transient aspergillus antigenaemia: think of milk. Lancet 2002;359:1251.

[25] Kami M, Kanda Y, Ogawa S, et al. Frequent false-positive results of *Aspergillus* latex agglutination test: transient *Aspergillus* antigenemia during neutropenia. Cancer 1999;86(2):274–81.

[26] Mennink-Kersten MA, Klont RR, Warris A, et al. Bifidobacterium lipoteichoic acid and false ELISA reactivity in aspergillus antigen detection. Lancet 2004;363:325–7.

[27] Mennink-Kersten MASH, Ruegebrink D, Klont RR, et al. Bifidobacterial lipoglycan as a new cause for false-positive Platelia *Aspergillus* enzyme-linked immunosorbent assay reactivity. J Clin Microbiol 2005;43:3925–31.

[28] Adam O, Aupérin A, Wilquin F, et al. Treatment with piperacillin-tazobactam and false-positive *Aspergillus* galactomannan antigen test results for patients with hematological malignancies. Clin Infect Dis 2004;38:917–20.

[29] Aubry A, Porcher R, Bottero J, et al. Occurrence and kinetics of false-positive *Aspergillus* galactomannan test results following treatment with beta-lactam antibiotics in patients with hematological disorders. J Clin Microbiol 2006;44:389–94.

[30] Mattei D, Rapezzi D, Mordini N, et al. False-positive *Aspergillus* galactomannan enzyme-linked immunosorbent assay results in vivo during amoxicillin-clavulanic acid treatment. J Clin Microbiol 2004;42:5362–3.

[31] Sulahian A, Touratier S, Ribaud P. False positive test for aspergillus antigenemia related to concomitant administration of piperacillin and tazobactam. N Engl J Med 2003;349: 2366–7.

[32] Walsh TJ, Shoham S, Petraitiene R, et al. Detection of galactomannan antigenemia in patients receiving piperacillin-tazobactam and correlations between in vitro, in vivo, and clinical properties of the drug-antigen interaction. J Clin Microbiol 2004;42:4744–8.

[33] Viscoli C, Machetti M, Cappellano P, et al. False-positive galactomannan Platelia *Aspergillus* test results for patients receiving piperacillin-tazobactam. Clin Infect Dis 2004;38:913–6.

[34] Bart-Delabesse E, Basile M, Al Jijakli A, et al. Detection of *Aspergillus* galactomannan antigenemia to determine biological and clinical implications of beta-lactam treatments. J Clin Microbiol 2005;43:5214–20.

[35] Klont RR, Mennink-Kersten MA, Verweij PE. Utility of *Aspergillus* antigen detection in specimens other than serum specimens. Clin Infect Dis 2004;39(10):1467–74.

[36] Stone BA, Clarke AE. Chemistry and biology of (1–3)-beta-d-Glucan. Melbourne, Australia: La Trobe University Press; 1992.

[37] Obayashi T, Yoshida M, Mori T, et al. Plasma $(1 \rightarrow 3)$-beta-D-glucan measurement in diagnosis of invasive deep mycosis and fungal febrile episodes. Lancet 1995;345(8941):17–20.

[38] Takaki Y, Seki N, Kawabata SS, et al. Duplicated binding sites for $(1 \rightarrow 3)$-beta-D-glucan in the horseshoe crab coagulation factor G: implications for a molecular basis of the pattern recognition in innate immunity. J Biol Chem 2002;277(16):14281–7.

[39] Tanaka S, Aketagawa J, Takahashi S, et al. Activation of a limulus coagulation factor G by (1, 3)-β-D-glucans. Carbohydr Res 1991;218:167–74.

[40] Aketagawa J, Tanaka S, Tamura H, et al. Activation of limulus coagulation factor G by several (1, 3)-β-D-glucans: comparison of the potency of glucans with identical degree of polymerization but different conformations. J Biochem (Tokyo) 1993;113:683–6.

[41] Odabasi Z, Mattiuzzi G, Estey E, et al. Beta-D-glucan as a diagnostic adjunct for invasive fungal infections: validation, cutoff development, and performance in patients with acute myelogenous leukemia and myelodysplastic syndrome. Clin Infect Dis 2004;39(2): 199–205.

[42] Saitô H, Yoshioka Y, Aketagawa NU, et al. Relationship between conformation and biological response for $(1 \rightarrow 3)$-β-[INSERT shppict]-glucans in the activation of coagulation factor G from limulus amebocyte lysate and host-mediated antitumor activity. Demonstration of single-helix conformation as a stimulant. Carbohydr Res 1991;217:181–90.

[43] Tamura H, Tanaka S, Obayashi T, et al. A new sensitive microplate assay of plasma endotoxin. J Clin Lab Anal 1992;6(4):232–8.

[44] Obayashi T, Yoshida M, Tamura H, et al. Determination of plasma $(1 \rightarrow 3)$-beta-D-glucan: a new diagnostic aid to deep mycosis. J Med Vet Mycol 1992;30:275–80.

[45] Miyazaki T, Kohno S, Mitsutake K, et al. $(1 \rightarrow 3)$-beta-D-glucan in culture fluid of fungi activates factor G, a limulus coagulation factor. J Clin Lab Anal 1995;9:334–9.

[46] Kakinuma A, Asano T, Torii H, et al. Gelation of Limulus amoebocyte lysate by an antitumor (1 leads to 3)-beta-D-glucan. Biochem Biophys Res Commun 1981;101(2):434–9.

[47] Miyazaki T, Kohno S, Mitsutake K, et al. Plasma $(1 \rightarrow 3)$-beta-D-glucan and fungal antigenemia in patients with candidemia, aspergillosis, and cryptococcosis. J Clin Microbiol 1995; 33(12):3115–8.

[48] Ostrosky-Zeichner L, Alexander BD, Kett DH, et al. Multicenter clinical evaluation of the $(1 \rightarrow 3)$ beta-D-glucan assay as an aid to diagnosis of fungal infections in humans. Clin Infect Dis 2005;41:654–9.

[49] Shimizu A, Oka H, Matsuda T, et al. $(1 \rightarrow 3)$-beta-D glucan is a diagnostic and negative prognostic marker for Pneumocystis carinii pneumonia in patients with connective tissue disease. Clin Exp Rheumatol 2005;23(5):678–80.

[50] Kami M, Fukui T, Ogawa S, et al. Use of real-time PCR on blood samples for diagnosis of invasive aspergillosis. Clin Infect Dis 2001;33(9):1504–12.

[51] Pickering JW, Sant HW, Bowles CA, et al. Evaluation of a (1- > 3)-beta-D-glucan assay for diagnosis of invasive fungal infections. J Clin Microbiol 2005;43(12):5957–62.

[52] Digby J, Kalbfleisch J, Glenn A, et al. Serum glucan levels are not specific for presence of fungal infections in intensive care unit patients. Clin Diagn Lab Immunol 2003;10(5): 882–5.

[53] Kawazu M, Kanda Y, Nannya Y, et al. Prospective comparison of the diagnostic potential of real-time PCR, double-sandwich enzyme-linked immunosorbent assay for galactomannan, and a $(1 \rightarrow 3)$-beta-D-glucan test in weekly screening for invasive aspergillosis in patients with hematological disorders. J Clin Microbiol 2004;42(6):2733–41.

[54] Obayashi T, Tamura H, Tanaka S, et al. Endotoxin-inactivating activity in normal and pathological human blood samples. Infect Immun 1986;53(2):294–7.

[55] Kato A, Takita T, Furuhashi M, et al. Elevation of blood $(1 \rightarrow 3)$-beta-D-glucan concentrations in hemodialysis patients. Nephron 2001;89(1):15–9.

[56] Kanda H, Kubo K, Hamasaki K, et al. Influence of various hemodialysis membranes on the plasma $(1 \rightarrow 3)$-beta-D-glucan level. Kidney Int 2001;60(1):319–23.

[57] Ikemura K, Ikegami K, Shimazu T, et al. False-positive result in Limulus test caused by Limulus amebocyte lysate-reactive material in immunoglobulin products. J Clin Microbiol 1989; 27(9):1965–8.

[58] Ogawa M, Hori H, Niiguchi S, et al. False-positive plasma $(1 \rightarrow 3)$-beta-D-glucan test following immunoglobulin product replacement in an adult bone marrow recipient. Int J Hematol 2004;80(1):97–8.

[59] Usami M, Ohata A, Horiuchi T, et al. Positive $(1 \rightarrow 3)$-beta-D-glucan in blood components and release of $(1 \rightarrow 3)$-beta-D-glucan from depth-type membrane filters for blood processing. Transfusion 2002;42(9):1189–95.

[60] Anderson J, Eller M, Finkelman M, et al. False positive endotoxin results in a DC product caused by $(1 \rightarrow 3)$-beta-D-glucans acquired from a sterilizing cellulose filter. Cytotherapy 2002;4(6):557–9.

[61] Douwes J, Doekes G, Montijn R, et al. Measurement of beta$(1 \rightarrow 3)$-glucans in occupational and home environments with an inhibition enzyme immunoassay. Appl Environ Microbiol 1996;62(9):3176–82.

[62] Mennink-Kersten MASH, Warris A, Verweij PE. Detection of circulating 1,3-beta-D-glucan in patients receiving intravenous amoxicillin-clavulanic acid. N Engl J Med 2006; 354:2834–5.

[63] Honda S, Sugino H, Asano T, et al. Activation of the alternative pathway of complement by an antitumor (1-3)-beta-D-glucan from *Alcaligenes faecalis* var. myxogenes IFO 13140, and its lower molecular weight and carboxymethylated derivatives. Immunopharmacology 1986; 11(1):29–37.

[64] Inai S, Nagaki K, Ebisu S, et al. Activation of the alternative complement pathway by water-insoluble glucans of *Streptococcus mutans*: the relation between their chemical structures and activating potencies. J Immunol 1976;117:1256–60.

[65] Banas JA, Vickerman MM. Glucan-binding proteins of the oral streptococci. Crit Rev Oral Biol Med 2003;14(2):89–99.

[66] Tang L, Weissborn AC, Kennedy EP. Domains of *Escherichia coli* acyl carrier protein important for membrane-derived-oligosaccharide biosynthesis. J Bacteriol 1997;179(11): 3697–705.

[67] Yuasa K, Goto H. 1, 3-β-D-glucan in patients with pulmonary aspergilloma. Mediators Inflam 1997;6:285–7.

[68] Mennink-Kersten MASH, Ruegebrink D, Wasei N, et al. In vitro release of galactofuranose (gal*f*)-antigens, 1, 3-β-D-glucan and DNA, surrogate markers used for diagnosis of invasive aspergillosis. J Clin Microbiol 2006;44:1711–8.

[69] Fontaine T, Hartland RP, Diaquin M, et al. Differential patterns of activity displayed by two exo-beta-1,3-glucanases associated with the *Aspergillus fumigatus* cell wall. J Bacteriol 1997; 179(10):3154–63.

[70] Fontaine T, Hartland RP, Beauvais A, et al. Purification and characterization of an endo-1,3-beta-glucanase from *Aspergillus fumigatus*. Eur J Biochem 1997;243(1–2):315–21.

[71] Mitsutake K, Kohno S, Miyazaki T, et al. Detection of (1–3)-beta-D-glucan in a rat model of aspergillosis. J Clin Lab Anal 1995;9(2):119–22.

[72] Miura NN, Miura T, Ohno N, et al. Gradual solubilization of *Candida* cell wall β-glucan by oxidative degradation in mice. FEMS Immunol Med Microbiol 1998;21:129.

[73] Ishibashi K, Miura NN, Adachi Y, et al. The solubilization and biological activities *of Aspergillus* β-(1, 3)-D-glucan. FEMS Immunol Med Microbiol 2004;42:155–66.

[74] Williams DL. Overview of (1, 3)-β-D-glucan immunobiology. Mediators Inflam 1997;6: 247–50.

[75] Zekovic DB, Kwiatkowski S, Vrvic MM, et al. Natural and modified (1,3)-β-D-glucans in health promotion and disease alleviation. Crit Rev Biotechnol 2005;25:205–30.

[76] Rice PJ, Lockhart BE, Barker LA, et al. Pharmacokinetics of fungal (1–3)-beta-D-glucans following intravenous administration in rats. Int Immunopharmacol 2004;4:1209–15.

[77] Rice PJ, Adams EL, Ozment-Skelton T, et al. Oral delivery and gastrointestinal absorption of soluble glucans stimulate increased resistance to infectious challenge. J Pharmacol Exp Ther 2005;314:1079–86.

[78] Severens JL, Donnelly JP, Meis JFGM, et al. Two strategies for managing invasive aspergillosis: a decision analysis. Clin Infect Dis 1997;25:1148–54.

[79] Maertens J, Theunissen K, Verhoef G, et al. Galactomannan and computed tomography-based preemptive antifungal therapy in neutropenic patients at high risk for invasive fungal infection: a prospective feasibility study. Clin Infect Dis 2005;41(9):1242–50.

[80] Millon L, Piarroux R, Deconinck E, et al. Use of real-time PCR to process the first galactomannan-positive serum sample in diagnosing invasive aspergillosis. J Clin Microbiol 2005; 43(10):5097–101.

ELSEVIER
SAUNDERS

Infect Dis Clin N Am
20 (2006) 729–734

INFECTIOUS
DISEASE CLINICS
OF NORTH AMERICA

Index

Note: Page numbers of article titles are in **boldface** type.

doi:10.1016/S0891-5520(06)00076-6
id.theclinics.com

Moving?

Make sure your subscription moves with you!

To notify us of your new address, find your **Clinics Account Number** (located on your mailing label above your name), and contact customer service at:

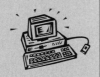

E-mail: elspcs@elsevier.com

800-654-2452 (subscribers in the U.S. & Canada)
407-345-4000 (subscribers outside of the U.S. & Canada)

Fax number: 407-363-9661

Elsevier Periodicals Customer Service
6277 Sea Harbor Drive
Orlando, FL 32887-4800

*To ensure uninterrupted delivery of your subscription, please notify us at least 4 weeks in advance of move.